A Nation in Pain

A NATION IN PAIN

Healing Our Biggest Health Problem

Judy Foreman

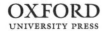

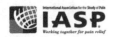

OXFORD
UNIVERSITY PRESS

Oxford University Press is a department of the University of Oxford.
It furthers the University's objective of excellence in research, scholarship,
and education by publishing worldwide.

Oxford   New York
Auckland   Cape Town   Dar es Salaam   Hong Kong   Karachi
Kuala Lumpur   Madrid   Melbourne   Mexico City   Nairobi
New Delhi   Shanghai   Taipei   Toronto

With offices in
Argentina   Austria   Brazil   Chile   Czech Republic   France   Greece
Guatemala   Hungary   Italy   Japan   Poland   Portugal   Singapore
South Korea   Switzerland   Thailand   Turkey   Ukraine   Vietnam

Oxford is a registered trademark of Oxford University Press in the UK and certain other countries.

Published in the United States of America by
Oxford University Press
198 Madison Avenue, New York, NY 10016

Library of Congress Cataloging-in-Publication Data
Foreman, Judy.
A nation in pain : healing our biggest health problem / Judy Foreman.
   pages cm
ISBN 978-0-19-983720-5 (hardcover); 978-0-19-023179-8 (paperback)
1. Chronic pain—United States.   2. Chronic pain—Treatment—United States.   3. Opioid abuse—
United States—History.   4. Pain—Alternative treatment.   I. Title.
RB127.F672 2013
616'.0472—dc23
2013015742

9 8 7 6 5 4 3 2

Printed in the United States of America
on acid-free paper

To Ken

CONTENTS

INTRODUCTION

In this book, I will argue that lack of adequate pain control is one of the most urgent health problems in America. In my research over the last five years, I have interviewed nearly 200 scientists and physicians, as well as countless patients, a few lawyers, and a handful of government officials. I have amassed a roomful of books on pain and hundreds upon hundreds of scientific papers.

I have found that there is an appalling mismatch between what people in pain need and what doctors know. Pain is the main reason that patients go to doctors, but most doctors know almost nothing about it, much less how to treat it. Doctors get only a few hours of pain education throughout four years of medical school. Even veterinarians get more.

The government, specifically the National Institutes of Health, the country's premier research establishment, isn't much better. It spends only about 1 percent of its vast budget on pain research, despite the fact that chronic pain is now considered a disease in its own right and is a bigger problem than heart disease, cancer, and diabetes *combined*. Indeed, federal spending on chronic pain is actually going *down*.

Culture wars over prescription pain relievers play into all this, too. I discovered that opioids (narcotics) are like airplane food—not great, but hard to get enough of when you're in need. But opioids are all too easy to get if you are a street abuser. Tragically, politics still means the government is focused more on punishing abusers than helping patients.

Nor does our healthcare reimbursement system get it right. It skimps on things that take a doctor's time—like talking to patients—and rewards interventions like surgery and injections that may or may not help.

I got into all this the hard way, with excruciating neck pain that came on, seemingly out of the blue, a few years ago. Like other pain patients, I trekked from doctor to doctor looking for help—and once, in desperation, to the emergency room, where I felt I was viewed more as a potential drug-seeker than as a person in severe pain.

I am better now. I tried much of what you'll read about in the second half of this book—opioids, NSAIDs, physical therapy, exercise (lots), meditation, acupuncture, massage, steroid injections, and Botox—pretty much everything except surgery and marijuana. I learned that nothing really cures pain, but that lots of things can help a little, and that adding them all together can decrease it a bit more.

Today, I count myself lucky. I am no longer living in pain. But I have come to believe that the failure to better manage pain borders on "torture by omission." Many people—some of whose stories you will read in the coming pages—are still living in pain, though, as you'll see, some manage to live extremely fulfilling lives.

Whatever your pain now—or the pain of someone you love—I hope this book will help you to better understand your pain and fight for the care you need.

Judy Foreman
Cambridge, Massachusetts
June 2013

HOW TO READ THIS BOOK

If you're a patient who's outraged at the way you've been treated—or not treated—for your pain, Chapter 1 is a must-read. Chronic pain is a problem of staggering proportions, yet many people with chronic pain feel utterly alone.

If you truly, deeply, absolutely hate science, just skim through Chapter 2 on how the body turns acute pain into chronic pain and Chapter 3 on the genes that rev pain up or damp it down. Even just skimming these chapters should convince you that, no matter what you've been told, your pain is not all in your head. If you're a physician, these chapters are a must-read—chances are that much of the research discussed was never taught in medical school.

If you're a woman and believe your pain has been dismissed in part because of your gender, Chapter 4 is for you. Especially if you believe the myth that women don't feel pain as much as men!

Even if you don't have kids, Chapter 5 is an eye-opener because of the appalling way we have undertreated—and still undertreat pain in children.

Researching Chapter 6, the mind–body section, was one of the highlights of this book for me. You'll read about the complex overlap between pain and depression, how the habit of "catastrophizing" (fearing the worst) can make pain worse, and how cognitive behavior therapy, distraction, meditation, hypnosis, and biofeedback can make it better. Significantly better.

Chapters 7 and 8 are about the "opioid wars," the clash between two epidemics—the epidemic of undertreated pain and the epidemic of prescription pain reliever abuse. You'll see that, while opioids can be abused, they are nowhere near as addictive as most people, including doctors, think. You'll learn the difference between *dependence* and *addiction*, about the mixed results of government efforts to monitor prescription pain relievers, and about the limits of opioids themselves. Sadly, opioids are not nearly as effective, especially in the long term, as one would hope. Clearly, something better is needed.

One such "something" is the focus of Chapter 9, which lays out an entirely new approach to treating pain not with opioids, but with drugs that act on specialized immune cells called glial cells. It's news to most people, but the immune system actually interacts with the nervous system to turn acute pain into chronic pain. This is good news because it gives scientists new drug targets, potentially reducing the need for opioids.

I decided to include an entire chapter (Chapter 10) on marijuana because it is so often overlooked in pain management. The science behind marijuana's efficacy for pain is fascinating. In fact, our bodies actually make our own marijuana-like substances. I explore in detail the risks and benefits of marijuana, as well as the political challenges to its wider use.

In Chapter 11—traditional Western treatments for pain—I assess the safety and effectiveness of a wide range of treatments including electrical stimulation, transcranial magnetic stimulation, injections, nerve-killing techniques, surgery, and new drugs in the pipeline. Hopefully, you will find some options that you may not have tried.

In Chapter 12—complementary and alternative treatments—I again take a strongly evidence-based look, this time at acupuncture, massage, energy healing, spinal manipulation (chiropractic), diet and vitamins, and even magnets and magnet field therapy. You may be surprised, as I was, at what I found.

Chapter 13 on exercise is a big upper. The evidence in favor of exercise for pain relief is very strong: In many, if not most, cases of chronic, non-cancer pain, exercise not only does not do damage—people's biggest fear—it can often make pain so much more manageable that life becomes livable, and fun, again.

Chapter 14 suggests a way forward to make better pain care a higher national priority. I argue that better pain management is a fundamental human right, and that failure to treat pain amounts to "torture by omission." I argue that the government should establish an institute or center for pain research within the National Institutes of Health. That medical schools should dramatically increase the hours dedicated to pain education. That licensing and accrediting organizations should be held accountable for making pain education a requirement for continued licensure of physicians.

Finally, I urge people with chronic pain to do as people with disabilities, breast cancer, and AIDS have done so successfully in recent years—to shed their isolation and shame and make their voices heard for the pain control they deserve.

A Nation in Pain

CHAPTER 1

The Enormity of the Problem

OVERVIEW

I never knew such pain existed. Several years ago, my neck suddenly went bonkers—a long-lurking arthritic problem probably exacerbated by too many hours spent hunching over a new laptop. On a subjective scale of 0 to 10 (there is no simple objective test for pain), even the slightest wrong move—turning my head too fast or picking up a pen from the floor—would send my pain zooming from a 0 to a gasping 10.

Sitting in a restaurant was agony if the table was too high, which forced my arms and shoulders up. So was sitting in the movies, looking up to see the screen. Shifting from sitting or kneeling on the bed to lying down was excruciating—there is simply no way to do it with a bad neck. Even silly little things like bending forward to try and paint my toenails became impossible.

During these episodes, which happened many times a day for months, I couldn't talk through the pain, though mere words couldn't have captured the pain's intensity anyway. So new, shocking, and incomprehensible was all this that I felt utterly alone, convinced that no one had ever felt like this before. But, of course, I was not alone. America, as I soon discovered, was then—and is still—in the midst of a chronic pain epidemic.

At first, I tried to cope by myself, with handfuls of ibuprofen, lots of stretching, and extra computer breaks. I kept on working as a nationally syndicated health columnist based at the *Boston Globe* and I kept hosting my weekly radio talk show. I also kept going to the gym and swimming three times a week. I kept singing and performing with my classical music group, too. And, of course, I kept hanging out with friends and family. Best of all, I continued to enjoy a new romance.

But as the months ticked by, the pain only got worse, so I sought help from the medical system, a system I thought I knew well, having covered it for decades. In fact, as the *Globe's* "Health Sense" columnist, I probably had the best address book in town, filled with the names of hundreds of eminent doctors. A funny thing happens, though, when you become a powerless patient, not an on-top-of-things journalist. The medical system I encountered as a person with pain was shockingly different from the one I thought I knew. And it was almost completely unprepared to help.

My first doctor, a young, female physiatrist (rehabilitation specialist) who came highly recommended, was initially nice. But over the course of our visits and escalating medications and injections, she seemed to grow angry when I didn't get better. At one point, she told me, rather coldly, that we had 10 minutes, during which we could either talk or I could get "trigger point" injections. Then, during what would end up being our last visit, she seemed to imply that my pain was caused by some emotional problem. I wanted to scream, "You bet I'm emotional—I'm in agony!"

Eventually, a magnetic resonance imaging scan (MRI) would show several almost-herniated disks in my cervical spine, as well as vertebrae sliding over each other (a condition called spondylolisthesis) and bone spurs stabbing my nerves. My facet joints (small joints that help stabilize the spine) showed arthritic damage. (I was actually lucky. Many people with back and neck pain have normal MRIs, while other people with no pain have disastrous-looking scans, a puzzle doctors can't figure out. At least mine showed something.)

More technically, what appeared to be happening was that my inflamed, irritated cervical nerves were firing almost nonstop, causing the trapezius muscle in my left shoulder and neck to spasm. The spasming in turn caused my head to twist bizarrely toward my shoulder (a condition called cervical dystonia), where it would stay "frozen" for long periods, forcing me to use both hands to turn my head back to a more or less normal position. The resulting pain was twofold: a searing, burning nerve pain that ran in a straight line from my neck to the top of my left shoulder, as if acid were dripping right onto the nerve, and severe muscle spasms.

After eight months of no progress—despite temporarily giving up work, swimming, the radio show, and singing—I finally began to get better when I saw a team of doctors at the New England Baptist Hospital in Boston. They *believed* me. They gave me time, cortisone shots, and very rigorous physical therapy called "boot camp."

I was grateful, of course, but sobered. Despite my familiarity with the medical system, it took eight doctors, multiple physical therapists, an acupuncturist, several massage therapists, an ergonomic consultant (who got me to buy all new office furniture), and more drugs, including opioids, than I had ever imagined I'd need before I began to get better. It's wonderful that I finally got the help I needed. Some people never do. This shouldn't happen in a country as medically sophisticated as ours. And yet it does.

* * *

One hundred million American adults live in chronic pain, according to a 2011 report from the prestigious Institute of Medicine, an arm of the National Academy of Sciences.[1] In 2010, that was more than 40 percent of the US adult population, 235 million.[2] That is a staggering figure, to be sure, and it's based on one massive study.[3] But it fits with other estimates.

A 2012 Gallup telephone survey of more than 353,000 American adults found that 47 percent were suffering from some type of chronic pain, a figure that translates to 111 million people.[4] Other estimates put the prevalence at about one-third of adults.[5, 6] A 2008 telephone survey of nearly 4,000 randomly selected Americans found that on any given day, 27 to 29 percent said they had been in pain during three randomly selected 15-minute periods that day.[7] A 2006 telephone survey of 46,394 Europeans in 15 countries showed that 19 percent had suffered pain for six months or longer, with pain in the moderate to severe range.[8]

To be sure, not everyone suffers chronic pain as badly as I did. But many have it much longer, and much worse. In fact, some people in chronic pain—a tenth to a third, depending on the estimate—hurt so badly they can't function.[9, 10, 11, 12]

Usually defined as pain lasting three to six months or more, chronic pain is vastly different from short-term, acute pain. It can transform life.

In some cases, it can literally shrink the brain. It can turn the nervous system into a runaway, self-sustaining nightmare in which the body may no longer even need stimulation from the outside world to produce pain—revved-up nerves keep doing it all by themselves.

In a way, chronic pain is a kind of perverse learning—connections among pain nerves actually get stronger and stronger. Eventually, even the slightest touch, like a feather on the skin, can feel like the scalding burn of a blowtorch, a condition technically called allodynia. This is not simply acute pain that lasts too long. It is the nervous system run amok—biologically, psychologically and socially, a whole new problem.

Not surprisingly, for some people with chronic pain, suicide can seem the only way to stop the agony. In the course of my conversations with physicians who treat chronic pain, I heard of a man with shingles (intense pain caused by the chickenpox virus) around the eye that didn't respond to any treatment; the man committed suicide. I heard of a surgeon who wound up in the emergency room of his own hospital, having in desperation used a scalpel on his back to try to cut out a nerve with shingles. I have heard of the opposite situation, too—people in severe pain who had signed Do Not Resuscitate (DNR) orders and then cancelled them once their pain was brought under control.

Overall, the risk of suicide for people in chronic pain is roughly twice as high as for other people, and the risk is highest for people with severe, chronic headaches.[13, 14] In Chapter 7, you'll meet a Salt Lake City truck driver with excruciating headaches, a man named Hyrum Neizer, who would be dead today if his wife hadn't walked in on him with a gun in his mouth. Even when people with severe, chronic pain don't contemplate actual suicide, 17 percent say they often just want to die.[15]

As we'll see repeatedly throughout this book, the medical system does a terrible job of educating doctors about pain. In fact, doctors themselves are often shocked, when they accidentally become pain patients, at how little their colleagues know about pain.

Howard Heit, a McLean, Virginia, gastroenterologist, was on his way to a meeting at the National Institutes of Health in Bethesda, Maryland, in 1986 when another car hit him head-on. The accident left him in a wheelchair for 20 years (until a new operation finally helped). For decades, he was in severe pain. "My life as a gastroenterologist was over," he told me. "I had muscle spasms 24/7."[16] "It became apparent to me that my fellow physicians had no idea about pain or how to treat it. If this was being thrown back at me, as a physician, as a male—and I went to school on a Division One football scholarship at the University of Pittsburgh—if this is happening to me, what is happening to the average person coming to a doctor?"

The fact is, said Paul Konowitz, an ear, nose, and throat specialist at the Massachusetts Eye and Ear Infirmary, doctors "don't do pain well."[17] Konowitz became a pain patient in the spring of 2004, when he came down with a rare autoimmune disease called pemphigus vulgaris. In this disease, the immune system attacks mucous membranes all over the body, creating excruciating blisters in the mouth, nose, tongue, eyes, and larynx: "It was horrifically painful," he said. Here he was, a physician married to another physician, with medical contacts all over Boston, arguably the world's medical mecca. Yet his chronic pain, and later his attempts to wean himself from opioid drugs, were so unbearable he became suicidal. "We had to figure it out for ourselves and we had an advantage—we had the background and people to talk to."

"What happens," explained New York dermatologist-turned-pain-patient David Biro, "is that we [doctors] are trained on this medical model. [But] when you have done everything you can on the medical model and there's no progress, we are not used to going to the next level. What do we do? We say, 'Go see somebody else. Go see a shrink.'"[18] Biro, now in his late 40s, was 30 when he developed a life-threatening condition called paroxysmal nocturnal hemoglobinuria, for which he needed a bone marrow transplant. The worst pain came after chemotherapy had caused ulcers up and down his gastrointestinal tract, and total body irradiation, which caused such a bad burn on his scrotum that the skin came off: "That was beyond excruciating."

Fortunately, his acute pain did not become chronic. But its severity prompted him to write three books. And his transition from doctor to pain patient left scars, partly because some of his doctors couldn't empathize: "It was very unnerving," he told me. "There's such an urgency about pain. You need to have the other person know in order to help you, but there's a divide between the sufferer and the outside observer. Pain brings these boundaries between people...into such acute focus."

Mark Cooper, a biophysicist who studies pain at the University of Washington in Seattle, was in graduate school when he had his first major attack of spasmodic torticollis, a painful condition in which muscles in the neck go into spasm, pulling the head to the side for weeks, months or years.

One day, Cooper had a whole body spasm that twisted his trunk sideways. "Every time I tried to pull, it pulled back," he told me.[19] Eventually, doctors decided it was a pinched nerve in his neck. But if Cooper had not been a pain scientist himself, he believes his doctors might never have made that diagnosis: "If I had been a woman or if I hadn't had a background in neurobiology, I believe that what happened to me might have been viewed as psychogenic pain."

Karen Binkley, an allergist and an associate professor of medicine at the University of Toronto, had to diagnose her own pain problem, too.[20] In 2007, she tripped over the elliptical exercise machine in her house and broke her little toe. No big deal. She got an X-ray, wore stiff shoes, and seemed to get better. Then the pain returned. Another X-ray. The bone hadn't healed. A cast. More pain. Weirdly, her foot started to turn pale. It swelled. Her toes turned blue. The skin looked too shiny. Slowly, the strange blue color crept up to her thigh. Her regular doctor was away, so she saw two other family doctors, then an orthopedic surgeon, and a podiatrist. All her friends are doctors, so she picked their brains, too. It was only when she finally began digging through her old medical school texts that she hit upon a likely diagnosis: reflex sympathetic dystrophy (now called complex regional pain syndrome, or CRPS), a neuroinflammatory problem. She bounced that idea off her regular doctor, who agreed with the diagnosis. But it still took visits to two pain clinics and help from a website for patients before she found doctors who understood CRPS. "It was only because I was a physician that I had the knowledge and resources to help research my care myself," she told me. "I would be institutionalized if I had not been a physician and been so persistent."

WHY DOCTORS KNOW SO LITTLE ABOUT PAIN

There is a good reason why doctors know so little about pain: Medical schools barely teach it. This is not just an American problem. In 80 percent of the world, pain biology and modern principles of pain relief and palliative care still aren't taught to medical students.[21]

To be sure, there are an estimated 3,000 to 4,000 US physicians who *do* understand pain and are certified as pain specialists. But they can't possibly attend to the millions of people in chronic pain.[22] That burden falls on primary care physicians, who are typically the first stop for people in chronic pain. And they get virtually no pain education at any point in their careers—medical school, subsequent residency programs, or later on in the continuing medical education (CME) courses that they must take to keep their licenses valid.

Over a lunch of diet Cokes and lobster salad one balmy fall day in Boston, Joseph Martin, the genial, white-haired, former dean of Harvard Medical School, told me how many hours of pain education Harvard Med students get during four years of medical school. Let's just say I was shocked. He and colleagues have tried to boost pain education, he added, but even so, he said, "We do not sufficiently educate students about pain and pain management."[23] University of North Carolina pain researcher Mark Zylka put it more succinctly: "I teach a one-hour lecture on pain to medical students. That's about all they get."[24]

Even veterinary students get more.

In 2009, a team of researchers from the University of Toronto surveyed 10 major Canadian universities that train doctors, nurses, dentists, pharmacists, and physical or occupational therapists. The team also surveyed four veterinary schools. The research design was hardly rocket science: They simply asked faculty members at the schools how much pain education their students were getting. The majority *didn't even know*. Sixty-seven percent "were unable to specify designated hours for pain," as the authors put it, adding understatedly that this "may suggest it [pain education] is not a priority."[25] As for the faculty members who could answer the question, the responses were still dismal. Across all the years of medical training, students got an average of 13 to 41 hours of pain education. Veterinary students got more than twice that—87 hours on average.

In 2011, British researchers from King's College in London found much the same thing.[26] They surveyed 19 professional schools of dentistry, medicine, midwifery, nursing, occupational therapy, pharmacy, physiotherapy, and veterinary science. On average, students got 12 hours of pain education, with physical therapists and veterinary students getting the most. But in many schools, pain education accounted for less than 1 percent of the curriculum, and only two programs fully utilized the curricula recommended by the International Association for the Study of Pain. And most pain education was taught the old-fashioned way—by lectures—which is not the best way to instill empathy for people in pain.

In a survey by the American Association of Medical Colleges, which represents 135 accredited medical schools, it was the same story. Among the schools that did attempt to teach about pain, on average, they offered 8 to 16 hours—over four years of medical school![27] Most recently, Johns Hopkins University researchers reported in 2011 on a study of 117 US and Canadian medical schools. They found that "pain education for North American medical students is limited, variable and often fragmentary."[28] Over the course of four years in US medical schools, they found, the median number of pain teaching hours was nine. Canadian medical students got twice that.

Not surprisingly, the Hopkins study found, many of the topics that the International Association for the Study of Pain (IASP) says should be part of a core curriculum on pain received "little or no coverage." Only four US medical schools had a required course on pain. And "a large number of US medical schools are not reporting any teaching of pain and an equally large number devote fewer than five hours to the topic," the Hopkins researchers found. "Given the recent advances in pain science, it is perplexing that pain education in medical schools remains so limited." The Institute of Medicine, in a major 2011 report on chronic pain, put it this way: "Most people in pain are cared for by primary care physicians who likely received little initial training or experience in best practices in pain management.... Too many physicians harbor outmoded or unscientific attitudes toward pain and people with pain."[29]

When pressed, doctors themselves admit this. A 2001 national survey by Harvard Medical School researchers revealed that half of doctors in primary care practice felt only "somewhat prepared" to counsel patients about pain management.[30] A 2006 survey of 111 primary care physicians, medical residents, nurse practitioners, and physician assistants found much the same thing—they felt inadequately prepared to treat pain.[31] A different 2006 survey, this one by the Association of American Medical Colleges, again showed the same pattern. One-quarter of graduates admitted their pain education was inadequate, a figure that had improved only slightly in a repeat survey in 2011.[32, 33, 34] Yet another survey, in 2007, queried 500 primary care physicians at 12 academic medical centers. Once again, only about one-third—34 percent—felt comfortable treating people with chronic, non-cancer pain.[35]

It's a vicious cycle. Because they learn so little about pain in medical school, few young doctors have any desire to become pain medicine specialists. In fact, a 2010 survey by the Association of American Medical Colleges found that from 2006 to 2010, not a single graduating student wanted to go into pain medicine. The prevailing attitude is perhaps best captured by what happened at the University of Washington in Seattle. When professors there asked graduating medical students what they would do when faced with a real pain patient, one student spoke for many: "Run!"

We are stuck, in other words, with a medical education system that is out of sync with the reality of chronic pain in America. "There is absolutely no feedback between the real world of the practitioners and what's taught in medical schools," says pain specialist John Loeser, a neurosurgeon at the University of Washington.[36] "The medical school curriculum is the last vestige of the feudal system in post-modern America. The curriculum is owned by the faculty of the school." There are some strategies, which we'll discuss in Chapter 14, that could change this. But it won't be easy.

"There's no way of putting new material into the curriculum without taking something out," Loeser told me. "That's why it's a feudal system. Each department owns a piece of the curriculum and nobody is willing to say, 'We will delete our material so you can have time for pain material.'"

Still, a few medical schools are trying. At Johns Hopkins, neurologist Beth Murinson developed a pioneering program.[37] It took six years of planning, but Murinson's team created a four-day course for first-year students that covers not just the neurobiological mechanisms of pain but delves deeply into the strong emotions that pain triggers in both patients and physicians. The idea was to have all 118 students undergo a brief experience with intense pain—in this case, a common experimental procedure called the cold pressor test. (I've undergone this test myself as part of the research for this book. You immerse your hand in icy water and see how long you can stand it. It really hurts. Like me, the students found this a powerful emotional lesson—they expressed surprise at how much distress this short experiment caused.)

The course was immensely successful. Not only did the students acquire basic knowledge about pain, they became more empathic. After the course, many students actually wanted to go into pain medicine.

ECONOMIC COSTS OF CHRONIC PAIN

Chronic pain, of course, is not just a biological, psychological, and social burden. It is an enormous economic burden as well, by some accounts, *the* leading reason that patients go to doctors.[38, 39] It costs the country more than cancer, heart disease, and diabetes *combined* and accounts for 42 percent of all visits to hospital emergency rooms.[40]

Figuring out the true economic costs of chronic pain, of course, is no simple task. To prepare its 2011 report on chronic pain, the Institute of Medicine hired a team of outside health economists from the Johns Hopkins Bloomberg School of Public Health and George Washington University. The economists concluded that chronic pain *conservatively* costs the country $560 to $635 billion a year in direct medical costs and lost productivity, way above the previous best guess of $100 billion a year developed in the late 1990s by the National Institutes of Health.[41] The bill for chronic pain lands mostly in the lap of the federal government. Medicare alone accounts for one-fourth of all US expenditures for pain. And the government has to absorb another loss as well—lost tax revenues because of lost productivity due to pain.[42]

But, as with anything economic, it wasn't easy getting to this bottom line, in part because the true costs of pain are tangled up with the costs of treating other diseases. How do you classify chronic pain, anyway? By body part affected? By severity? By the diseases it's associated with? And how many things do you include in the grand total? The economists decided to include the costs of direct health care for pain plus lost productivity attributable to pain. But even that is not simple. In terms of people in persistent pain, the economists decided to count only adults living in regular communities, not people in the military, nursing homes, or prisons, or children under 18. For the people they did count, the economists estimated that direct incremental healthcare costs due to pain every year ranged from $261 billion to $300 billion. This includes, but is not limited to, medical appointments, hospital stays when the primary diagnosis is pain, and medications.[43]

When it comes to lost productivity, the economists used three estimates: $11.6 billion to $12.7 billion for *days* of work missed, $95.2 billion to $96.5 billion for *hours* of work lost, and $190.6 billion to $226.3 billion for *lower wages* (because people in chronic pain may not be able to work as hard or compete for the same raises.) They did not count the impact of chronic pain on personal caregivers—like spouses or adult children who miss work to take care of family members in pain. Nor did they count the lost productivity of people traditionally not considered of working age—those younger than 24 and older than 65.

Partly because health care is so expensive in this country, Americans spend more per capita on chronic pain than in some other countries, the economists found. They compared healthcare costs for chronic pain in the United States with those in Australia and found that the per capita pain costs here were $1,842 to $2,072 (2008 figures), more than 43 percent higher than in Australia.

A different comparison is also striking, the economists found. A person with moderate chronic pain generates healthcare expenditures that are a whopping $4,516 higher than costs for someone without pain. And if the person has not moderate but severe pain? That person costs $3,210 more than a person with moderate pain! The most expensive pain conditions in America, by the way, are headache ($14 billion), arthritis ($189 billion), and back pain ($100–200 billion).

In theory, there could be better ways to pay for chronic pain care, starting with changes to the reimbursement system so that physicians would be paid for spending more time talking with patients, not just being "needle jockeys" focused on money-making procedures.

That kind of change is a pipe dream for most American doctors. But in Canada, it's a reality for some, including Yoram Shir, director of the pain center at McGill University in Montreal. He has the luxury of sufficient funding from both public and private sources. "There's a major difference between Quebec and the rest of the world," he told me.[44] "I have a huge advantage here. In the US, pain centers survive on procedures because they stick needles into bodies. That gives you more money.

Here, we are not driven by money. I can just give you recommendations to the best of my knowledge."

UNDERFUNDING OF PAIN RESEARCH

With chronic pain so prevalent and so expensive, you might assume that the federal government is spending wildly on pain research.

It isn't.

Shockingly, only about 1 percent of the $30.8 billion (2012) budget for the National Institutes of Health (NIH), the premier driver of bio-medical research in the country, is devoted primarily to pain research.[45, 46, 47] In fact, the money in the NIH budget allocated to research on chronic pain conditions has declined in recent years.

The NIH spent $386 million of its $30.9 billion budget in 2011 on "pain conditions—chronic," which, by my calculation, comes to 1.2 percent; in 2012, it spent $358 million of its $30.8 billion budget on this category, which by my calculation comes to 1.1 percent. (The NIH does not expressly budget by category and insists that it is misleading and incorrect to calculate percentages this way because actual spending figures can change and because research categories are not mutually exclusive.[48] The NIH would not specify how much of its budget does go to chronic pain.) To be sure, there are several different ways to estimate how much—or, more precisely, how little—NIH spends on chronic pain research. (The NIH gets about 90 percent of the federal spending on pain.[49])

David Bradshaw, a pain researcher at the University of Utah, regularly combs through the latest NIH budget figures on pain, both acute and chronic.[50] His method is straightforward: "I am looking at everything—all initiatives, intramural projects, extramural projects, etc." Working with a small team of fellow researchers, he starts by trying to come up with as many "search words" as possible to plug into his computer. Among the search terms he uses are "nociception" (perception of pain), "pain," "headache," "migraine," and the names of a number of specific pain conditions such as "fibromyalgia," "temporomandibular joint disorder," and so on. Then he laboriously goes through every project that the NIH funded in a particular year, checking the abstracts and titles of scientific papers using his search terms. The goal is to not overlook any project designed to investigate pain but, at the same time, to screen out studies that don't have pain as the main focus. Using this method, Bradshaw's team found that, as of 2009 data, NIH spending on pain research constituted about 0.45 percent of the total budget,[51] and things haven't changed much.

At the NIH itself, they count things somewhat differently, though the total support for chronic pain research is still tiny. Since 2008, NIH has had a feature on its website call RePORT so that Congress can figure out what the NIH was spending on what. It is designed so that a person can plug in search terms like "pain" or "chronic pain" and see which NIH-supported projects contain those terms and thus get an idea of how much and what kind of research the agency funds.

So I tried it. I typed in "pain," and the program helpfully changed that to "pain conditions—chronic." Sure enough, in 2011, NIH spent $386 million on chronic pain, out of a total budget of $30.9 billion. That's 1.2 percent, higher than Bradshaw's estimate, but not much.[52, 53, 54, 55] (And, as noted above, in 2012, NIH estimated it would spend less—$358 million—on chronic pain and less overall as well, $30.8 billion, which means the percentage spent on chronic pain actually went *down*, to 1.1 percent.[56, 57])

That's bad enough. But the more basic problem is that nobody is really in charge of pain research at NIH. Although there are "institutes" and "centers" within NIH for almost every disease one could think of, there is no such institute for pain.

To the extent that the federal government is involved with pain at all, pain research is spread out over many NIH institutes and programs. There is the Pain Consortium, set up in 2003, that tries to coordinate pain efforts. But it doesn't have much clout.[58] A recent report from the Senate Committee on Appropriations noted, that "eight years later, it is clear that the NIH must do more. Although every Institute and Center deals in some way with pain, none of them 'owns' this critical area of research."[59] There's another government group also trying to coordinate pain research, the Interagency Pain Research Coordinating Committee. But aside from having meetings, it's not clear how much of an impact these efforts have had so far.

This scattershot approach has big consequences. With no bureaucratic home, chronic pain—and the money to study it—gets lost in the shuffle. Diseases and conditions that have their own institutes at NIH get "line items" in the federal budget, which means that they can expect a certain amount of funding every year. Because there is no pain institute, there is no line item for pain. "Pain is an orphan within medicine. No one owns it," according to Scott Fishman, an anesthesiologist and pain researcher at the University of California, Davis.[60]

"Because there is no single institute funding pain at NIH, there is not a coordinated allocation," said Philip Pizzo, dean of the School of Medicine at Stanford University and chair of the Institute of Medicine (IOM) committee that wrote the 2011 pain report.[61] "When we tried to get the data, the Institutes sent us lots of abstracts related to funding different projects but it is really not possible to sort this out," he wrote me. "The bottom line is that whatever the actual funding, it is clearly less than might be allocated. For example, pain costs the nation more than cancer, heart disease and diabetes together. But the funding for pain research is only a fraction of that allocated to these disorders." The IOM committee did discuss setting up a pain institute, Pizzo said. But those discussions were doomed from the outset. The committee felt that setting up a new institute was simply "not a viable option" at the moment.

That's a shame.

"I think that what pain needs is a home and a budget and program staff like exists for other research areas at the NIH," in the words of Kathleen Foley, arguably the world's top pain and palliative care expert, and a neurologist at Memorial Sloan-Kettering Cancer Center in New York. "Until it has such an effort, pain research will not have much traction."[62]

There's one other important point here. Because there's so little federal funding available, scientists trying to study pain often feel they have no choice but to turn to drug companies for research money. Just because a drug company pays for research does not automatically mean the results of that research are invalid or distorted.

But it sure does raise red flags. At the very least, the sheer prevalence of so much industry-funded research creates the *appearance* of a conflict of interest. The appearance alone makes it difficult to know which research to trust.

HUMAN COSTS: THE DAY THE FILING CABINETS
FELL ON CINDY STEINBERG

Cindy Steinberg's life changed forever at 10 a.m. on March 3, 1995. She was in her 30s, a product development manager for a learning technology company just outside of Harvard Square in Cambridge, Massachusetts. She had a great husband and a two-year-old daughter. She had never missed a day of work, even working the day she went into labor. On that terrible day in 1995, her company was moving offices. "I was on the phone to a client and went outside my office to open a drawer to retrieve a file. Unbeknownst to me," she told me, "moving men had dismantled the cubicles and stacked them against the back of my file cabinet. I opened the drawer and the whole filing cabinet and 10 cubicle walls started coming at me. I turned to get away but I wasn't fast enough. The drawer struck me in the middle of my back and knocked me over. I was crushed underneath the filing cabinet and cubicle walls."[63] She has not had a minute—much less a day—ever since without pain, and often has several days a week with "horrible pain, a constant burning, gnawing ache." The crash tore ligaments and nerves in the middle of her back, between thoracic disc levels 7 and 10.

Incredibly, for the first five years, she kept working, running meetings for staff and contractors, as well as for her Fortune 500 corporate clients, lying flat on her back. At the end of many days, she would go home in tears. During those years, she traipsed from doctor to doctor—orthopedists, orthopedic surgeons, physiatrists, neurologists, anesthesiologists, a neurosurgeon, every specialist she could think of. She did physical therapy, various kinds of injections, acupuncture, and massage. "I was in total disbelief that I could be in this much pain and there wasn't anyone or anything that could really help me," she recalled. She was shocked that so many doctors treated her in a "demeaning, disbelieving, dismissive and distrustful" manner.

Finally, five years after her accident, she did find a doctor, an osteopath, who helped. "He was the first person who really listened to me, who understood," she said. He was appalled that she was still trying to work and convinced her that the only way to get a partial handle on her pain was to quit. "Walking away from a career I loved and had spent years developing was the hardest thing I had ever done," she said.

Her new life work became managing her own pain, currently with an antidepressant that helps with nerve pain, frequent exercise, and muscle relaxants. But her spine is still so unstable that she can't hold herself up long; when she tries, the muscle spasms can become unbearable. So she stays upright for an hour or so, then lies down for 25 minutes, back and forth, all day long. "It gets worse the longer I am upright sitting or standing," she said. She still goes to concerts at Boston's Symphony Hall, but lies down at intermission. When she flies, she buys two seats so she can lie across them.

She is shocked that there are so many other people suffering in chronic pain as she is. That could change, of course, and I hope it will. But it will take what the Institute of Medicine report called a "cultural transformation" in how we deal with chronic pain.[64]

In fact, unless we as a society begin to deal better with chronic pain, the problem will probably continue to get worse. Among other things, the worsening obesity epidemic means that growing numbers of people will get related diseases such as diabetes, which causes painful neuropathy. The heavier the nation becomes, the more people wind up with painful knee and hip problems, which often lead to surgery. If postoperative pain from these surgeries is not well managed, the result can be long-term pain.[65, 66] The healthcare system itself will likely keep driving the chronic pain epidemic, too.[67] Most surgical patients, for instance—an estimated 80 percent—have at least some postoperative pain, yet fewer than half report adequate pain relief. Inadequately treated acute pain often leads to chronic pain. Even for routine operations like hernia repair, breast and thoracic surgery, leg amputations, and coronary bypass operations, 10 to 50 percent of patients wind up with persistent pain that, in a substantial minority, becomes severe.[68, 69]

And then, paradoxically enough, there's cancer. All the wonderful progress we've made in recent years against cancer carries a dark side for chronic pain. Chemotherapy, life-saving as it can be, can induce its own kind of chronic nerve pain. Moreover, the better doctors do at treating people with cancer, the more cancer survivors—60 to 85 percent at last count—there are who live with pain.[70, 71] Cancer pain is so routinely undertreated that nearly one in every two cancer patients suffers needlessly.[72]

Even if the chronic pain epidemic were not destined to grow for these reasons, it's probably already worse than we think. The Institute of Medicine's estimate of 100 million Americans in chronic pain doesn't include people in the military, prisons, or nursing homes. Or children.[73]

And even if it did, we might *still* not get the full picture because of the erratic way data on chronic pain are currently tracked. Federal health agencies mostly track traditional *diagnoses* like arthritis or diabetes, not chronic pain, the problem that actually drives people into the health-care system. And almost nobody tracks pain on a longitudinal basis, a serious problem given that chronic pain by definition lasts three to six months and, more often, years. Nor do many measures of chronic pain reflect how severely it interferes with daily functioning.

"We used to think of pain as only a sensory experience," says Clifford Woolf, a neurologist and pain genetics researcher at Children's Hospital in Boston. But "there has been a shift in our thinking, chronic pain is not just a symptom. It is a disease of the nervous system. This insight really changes the way we understand pain."[74] Other researchers, too, now believe chronic pain is far more than just a symptom of something else; it is a neurological disease in its own right.[75]

We are, in other words, just beginning to understand how large the problem of chronic pain is in America. And unfortunately, it's probably much worse than we think.

CHAPTER 2

What Is Pain, Anyway?

OVERVIEW

"What in heaven's name is going on?" It was a question that nagged at me every night. (For reasons I never did understand, my neck pain always got worse around midnight, just when I wanted to go to sleep.) The pain made no sense. I had had no injury. No car wreck. Yeah, I worked all day on a laptop in ergonomically disastrous postures, but so does everybody else. Physically, I had never been stronger. I had taken up competitive US Masters swimming in my late 50s and turned out to be pretty good at it, qualifying regularly for Nationals—and even the World Championships—in several events.

I was also happier than I had been in years. After suffering through my late husband's 11-year battle with two kinds of cancer, I did a lot of heavy grieving after he died, then pulled myself together and signed up for Match.com. There, to my astonishment and delight, I met a wonderful new man. That relationship was going well (we are married now). Work was going well, too. So I could not imagine what was wrong with my neck. Why did it always hurt on the left, never the right? Why did I get a burning, shooting pain in a straight line from C-7, the lowest cervical (neck) joint, down to my shoulder? Why did my muscles spasm so much my head would get locked into a crooked position (cervical dystonia) for long periods of time?

When this sudden immersion into the world of chronic pain began five years ago, I set out on a journey to understand my own pain and to unravel the secrets of pain in general. It has been a fascinating trip—with a happy ending, at least so far—that has taken me to the outer frontiers of molecular biology and the inner reaches of the brain and mind. In this chapter, I will share the highlights of what I have learned so you can better understand your own pain, while sparing you, hopefully, excessive details and impenetrable jargon. I'll describe briefly the different kinds of chronic pain and how the nervous system works, particularly the ways that pain signals travel in the body up to the brain—where we actually "feel" pain—and the ways nerves running back down to the body help damp pain down.

Most important, we'll talk about crucial new insights into chronic pain. That it physically changes the nervous system, literally causing the loss of brain tissue. That chronic pain (pain lasting three months or more) is not just a symptom of something else, but is often a *disease* of the nervous system in its own right. That it's not just the nervous system that gets revved up in chronic pain, but some parts of the immune system, too—specifically, microglial cells. That, with luck, brain scanning technology may soon allow doctors to "prove" that a person is in pain, a vast improvement over just listening to (and often, not believing) his or her story.

For the record, throughout this book I will use the official definition of pain: "an unpleasant sensory and emotional experience associated with actual or potential tissue damage, or described in terms of such damage."[1] This comes from the International Association for the Study of Pain (IASP), the world's top pain research group. The IASP adds—and this is crucial—that "the inability to communicate verbally does not negate the possibility that an individual is experiencing pain and is in need of appropriate pain-relieving treatment."

To my surprise, I learned that in many pain syndromes, an obvious, physical injury or cause of chronic pain can never be found, a puzzle that is a source of enormous frustration to people with pain and doctors alike. Doctors call these real, but mysterious, conditions *functional pain syndromes*. In other words, although pain often *is* triggered by an initial, sensory experience, that isn't always the case. The acute pain of labor, for instance, has an obvious cause; the chronic pain of fibromyalgia, which is associated with changes in the central nervous system, often does not.[2]

Legendary Canadian pain researcher Ronald Melzack was one of the first to realize how wickedly complex chronic pain is. He developed the *neuromatrix theory*, the idea that pain is the result of output from a widely distributed network of nerves—not a straightforward stimulus-response to sensory input.[3] Nowadays, researchers know it's even more complicated than that. Chronic pain is now seen as a *biopsychosocial* phenomenon, not just a linear response to an unpleasant stimulus, but an ever-changing, almost living thing, an intricately interwoven tapestry that includes not just physical sensations but also our emotional responses to pain and our emotional responses to other people's emotional responses to our pain. No wonder it's so hard to understand someone else's pain. Given this complexity, it's not surprising that different regions of the brain.—the prefrontal cortex, amygdala, hypothalamus, hippocampus, primary and secondary somatosensory cortex, to name just a few—all contribute to the overall experience of pain.[4] Indeed, precisely how active each given region is at any moment can change dramatically, as high-tech, moment-by-moment images of the brain show.

Things can be so malleable, in fact, that some people with chronic pain are able to look at real-time brain scan images of their own brains in pain and learn, via biofeedback, to change their perception of pain. For the better.[5] But usually, it's not that easy. Author Melanie Thernstrom captured this beautifully in her 2010 book, *The Pain Chronicles*.[6]

"To be in physical pain," she wrote, "is to find yourself in a different realm—a state of being unlike any other, a magic mountain as far removed from the familiar world as a dreamscape." And the longer the pain persists, she continued, "the more excruciating the exile becomes. *Will you ever go home?* you begin to wonder, home to your normal body, thoughts, life?"

Harvard professor Elaine Scarry put it eloquently in her 1985 book, too. "To have great pain," she wrote, "is to have certainty; to hear that another person has pain is to have doubt. (The doubt of other persons, here as elsewhere, amplifies the suffering of those already in pain)."[7]

One of my hopes for this book is that, with the growing understanding of pain, some of those doubts—and some of that suffering—can be dispelled.

Chronic pain comes in four basic "flavors"—nociceptive, inflammatory, dysfunctional, and neuropathic, which describe different ways of understanding how pain signals travel in the nervous system. Sometimes, chronic pain can be a combination of these types. Cancer pain, for instance, is often a combination of nociceptive, inflammatory, and neuropathic, depending on how big the tumor is and where it lodges. Historically, scientists thought about pain in terms of its etiology—that is, what caused it: an injury, a tumor, an infection, and so on. Increasingly, they are turning to a different method, says Clifford Woolf, a pain researcher at Boston Children's Hospital.[8] It's the pain *phenotype* that counts, he says, particularly when it comes to classifying the various subtypes of neuropathic pain. The pain phenotype refers to the unique collection of symptoms of each person with pain; the idea then is to link each phenotype to specific, underlying neural mechanisms.[9, 10]

So here we go.

Nociceptive pain is that instant, intense reaction you get when you hit your thumb hard with a hammer or cut your finger with a knife. The word *nociception* simply means the perception of a noxious, or unpleasant, stimulus. Compared to other types of pain, nociceptive pain is relatively simple—essentially an on–off switch. To trigger nociceptive pain, it takes a pretty big (that is, a high-intensity) wallop. If you just touch your hand lightly with a hammer, you won't feel pain. The usual stimuli for nociceptive pain are mechanical forces, like that hammer, too much heat or cold, and chemicals, including acids.[11, 12] Less obviously, nociceptive pain also happens when some part of the body is subject to unusual mechanical force, like the grinding of bone-on-bone in osteoarthritis of the knee, or injury to an organ like the heart, when it is deprived of oxygen. The way neurologists see it, the bone grinding in osteoarthritis and the oxygen deprivation in the heart are pretty similar to the external stimulus of hitting yourself with a hammer in the sense that they don't come from any problem intrinsic to the nervous system itself.

Nociceptive pain is basically "good," or adaptive, because it serves an important, biological purpose: It alerts you to danger and lets you know about your now-damaged tissue, which motivates you to be gentle with the damaged area until it heals. It's comparatively straightforward, too.

You thwack your thumb with the hammer, pain signals travel along a nerve, or, more often, a number of nerves, from your thumb to the spinal cord, get handed off to another set of nerves that run up through the brainstem to the cortex, or thinking part of the brain. End of story. When your thumb heals, it's all over—pain nerves quiet down and you forget all about it.

Inflammatory pain is a bit different. While it takes a big wallop to trigger nociceptive pain, both big wallops and smaller ones can trigger inflammatory pain; then, once that sore thumb swells up and gets all red, even the slightest touch can hurt. Inflammatory pain persists as long as the tissue remains damaged and swollen. In a sense, inflammatory pain, like nociceptive pain, is somewhat "good," or adaptive, in the sense that inflammation does good things, including the secretion of natural chemicals called cytokines that act to promote healing. But inflammatory pain can also be "bad," or nonadaptive, because pro-inflammatory cytokines amplify, or rev up, the transmission of pain signals along nerves.[13] Indeed, with inflammatory pain, nerves rev up in both the central nervous system (the brain and spinal cord) and in the periphery—our arms, legs, and everything else—becoming overactive and hypersensitive, to the point that you can end up with more pain than you started with.

The third type of pain, dysfunctional pain, is really nasty, and, as its name implies, it serves no purpose at all—it's totally useless, maladaptive, and devoid of any redeeming virtues. In dysfunctional pain conditions like fibromyalgia, irritable bowel syndrome, and some types of headache, pain can be triggered without any external pain stimulus at all, at least as far as scientists can tell. With dysfunctional pain, there's no damage to the nervous system itself and no inflammation. As with inflammatory pain, there *is* sensory amplification, or revving up, of pain signals in both the periphery and central nervous systems.[14]

Worst of all, in many ways, is the fourth type of pain, neuropathic pain, the most complicated of the pain problems.[15, 16] Neuropathic pain is caused by damage to the nervous system itself. In a sense, neuropathic pain is to the nervous system what AIDS is to the immune system. The AIDS virus attacks the immune system, the very system that is supposed to deal with viruses. Neuropathic pain attacks the nervous system itself by altering the way nerves function—an insult to the very system that is supposed to deal with pain. This, of courses, makes treatment extraordinarily tricky. While nociceptive pain, that simple kind, is all over when it's over, neuropathic pain goes on and on, long after the initial trigger, if there was an obvious one, is history.

Like dysfunctional pain, neuropathic pain can occur without any obvious external pain stimulus, and it, too, gets amplified and revved up in both the peripheral and the central nervous systems. Neuropathic pain occurs in conjunction with many diseases and different types of damage to the nervous system, including trauma to nerves (as in surgery), pressure on nerves (as from a herniated disc in the neck or back), injury from toxic chemicals landing on nerves (as in chemotherapy), infection from neurotropic viruses like herpes zoster, and so on. A truly dramatic demonstration of the differences between neuropathic and inflammatory pain was reported in late spring 2012 by University of California, San Francisco pain researchers Allan Basbaum and Joao Braz.[17] Their team transplanted fetal cells that make gamma-aminobutyric acid (GABA), a chemical pain inhibitor, into mice with neuropathic pain. The cells dampened neuropathic pain but did not affect inflammatory pain.

HOW THE NERVOUS SYSTEM TRANSMITS PAIN

Researchers and physicians use a lot of jargon when they talk about the nervous system, but the concepts are fairly simple. The central nervous system consists of the brain and spinal cord and is chock full of nerve cells. Interestingly, scientists have recently discovered that other cells called microglial cells—which are part of the immune system—also live amidst the nerve cells and contribute mightily to the processing of pain signals. (In fact, the overlap between the nervous and immune systems in pain processing is so important I've given it a whole separate chapter—Chapter 9.) Here's the snapshot version of how the nervous system works: Electrical signals travel along sensory nerves from the periphery—our limbs—to a specific structure in the spinal cord called the dorsal horn. There, the nerves release chemicals that communicate with a second nerve cell that runs all the way to the brain, where a third nerve cell takes the stimulatory message to various regions of the brain where we feel what we interpret as pain.

Perhaps the most impressive thing about nerve cells is their sheer number. In the adult human brain alone, Harvard Medical School neuroscientist Gary Brenner told me, there are an estimated 100 billion neurons with perhaps 100 trillion connections.[18] Put differently, there are more brain cells at a dinner for 10 people than all the stars in the Milky Way galaxy.[19] And then there's the peripheral nervous system— all the nerves *outside* the brain and spinal cord.

The peripheral nervous system is divided into the *somatic* nervous system, which means the nerves just under the skin, and the *autonomic* nervous system, nerves everywhere else. The autonomic nervous system is further divided into two branches: *sympathetic* and *parasympathetic*. (Scientists sometimes also refer to a third division, the enteric nervous system, which controls the gastrointestinal tract and is often called "the second brain" because it can operate on its own and has direct connections to the central nervous system.) The sympathetic system is in charge of the famous fight-or-flight response, the body's instantaneous reaction to stress via the hormone adrenaline. Well-known signs of the sympathetic response are increased heart rate and blood pressure, constricted blood vessels, and sweating. The parasympathetic system is the quieter partner, dominating things while the body is at rest. Normally, the two systems act in concert to produce homeostasis.

The raison d'être of the entire nervous system, of course, is to convey information from the outside world to the brain or from one part of the body to the brain, all of which is accomplished by translating a huge variety of incoming information into bite-sized electrical and chemical signals. Nerve cells, also called neurons, are electrically excitable and come in three basic types: sensory neurons, which respond to light, touch, sound, chemicals, and other stimuli and are the most important nerve cells for pain; motor neurons, which act on signals from the brain and spinal cord to make muscles contract; and interneurons, neurons in the central nervous system that "talk" only to other nearby neurons. Scientists also use the word *nociceptor*—this just means a subcategory of sensory nerves that responds to the noxious, tissue-damaging stimuli that cause pain. Each nerve cell consists of a cell body, where the nucleus of the cell resides, one axon, and a bunch of filaments called dendrites that look like the messy split ends of a strand of hair and function as receiving centers for incoming information.

Axons are incredibly long filaments that can extend a meter or more. When bundled together into fibers and further bundled into cables, they're called *nerves*. The sciatic nerve, the longest nerve in the body (and famous for the leg pain it causes), has one long axon that runs from the base of the spine down to the foot. Interestingly, nerve fibers carry information at different speeds. The so-called A-delta fibers, which are relatively large in diameter and are covered with myelin, convey information very fast and are major players in pain transmission. C fibers, which are skinnier, conduct pain information 15 times more slowly because they are not coated with myelin. A-beta fibers, which carry information from the skin about touch and pressure but not pain, are the biggest and fastest fibers. But the most amazing thing about these nerves is how specialized they are for receiving different types of information—from mechanical, chemical, thermal, or other stimuli.[20, 21] In fact, the specialization of these nerves is so fine-tuned that there are different thermal receptors for responding to fairly small differences in temperature.

For instance, a receptor called TRPV1, located on the tip of certain nerves, is programmed to detect heat above 109 degrees Fahrenheit. It also responds to "hot" substances like capsaicin, the ingredient in chili peppers, and to acid, as well as to an endogenous fatty substance called anandamide, which is somewhat like marijuana. TRPV2, a closely related receptor, detects hotter temperatures—above 126 degrees Fahrenheit. Still another receptor, TRPA1, detects cold temperatures—less than 63 degrees Fahrenheit—and responds to mustard oil and wasabi as well. (Not surprisingly, targeting drugs to these receptors, and fiddling with the genes that make the receptors, is a hot area of research.[22]) Acid-sensing receptors are also exquisitely sensitive. By studying the highly painful and toxic venom of the Texas coral snake, researchers have shown that acid-sensing channels in sensory nerves play a much larger role in pain than previously thought.[23, 24]

Once all this this incoming sensory information is collected by the receptors, the next task of the nervous system is to transport it to the brain, a problem for which evolution has come up with a remarkably elegant solution: pass information *along* a nerve cell electrically and *between* one nerve and the next, chemically.

Incoming information enters the system through dendrites (those "split ends") and exits at the other end of the nerve cell through an axon. When information reaches this far end of the axon, the axon releases chemical messengers that float into a narrow gap called a synapse. In the synapse, waiting dendrites from the *next* nerve cell in the chain pick up the chemical signal, convert it to an electrical message that travels through the second nerve to *its* axon, which in turn pumps out *its* chemical messengers into the synapse for the dendrites from the third nerve in the chain to pick up, and so on. Electrically, the passage of information works through impulses called *action potentials* that act like on–off switches, giving a nerve a simple message: to fire or not. It is an all-or-nothing, yes–no, binary system.

Like any other cell, nerve cells are encased in a two-layer, insulating membrane. It is in this fatty membrane that the receptors, also known as ion channels, lie. Some ion channels are *voltage-gated*, which means they are activated by electrically charged ions that flow back and forth across the membrane in and out of the cell. Others are *chemically gated*, which means they are activated by chemicals—neurotransmitters—floating around outside the cell. In its normal, resting state, the interior of the nerve cell has a negative charge compared to the outside. It's a big difference. There are 10 times more sodium ions outside the cell than inside. (With other charged particles, such as potassium, it's the other way around—the concentration of potassium ions is 20 times higher inside the cell than outside.)

When the nerve receives a signal—say, mechanical pressure on your thumb or an acid on an acid-sensitive dendrite—sodium from the outside rushes into the cell through sodium channels. The sudden influx of sodium *depolarizes*, or reverses, the electrical charge. Now the outside of the cell has the negative charge and the inside, the positive. The cell "thinks" of this as an unnatural state and immediately seeks to correct it by having potassium ions rush outside. Once this happens, the electrical balance returns to normal.

Sodium channels, in other words, act as molecular amplifiers, turning small electrical signals into action potentials that can conduct for long distances along an axon.[25] The short-lived change in the electrical charge—just milliseconds long—is passed step by step from one little section of the axon to the next. In many axons, these sections are covered with myelin, but there are tiny gaps (called nodes) between the sections, and it's actually in these gaps that the sodium channels lie. So when sodium rushes in through these channels, the change in electrical charge "jumps" across the gap with enough electrical energy to depolarize the next section of the axon, then the next and the next, all along the axon. In technical jargon, this is called a *wave of depolarization*. (In nerve cells that don't have a myelin sheath, there's no gap for energy to jump across, so transmission of the signal is slower.) With potassium channels, researchers have recently shown that two channels in particular (called K2P) may be especially important in pain sensation and chronic pain.[26, 27] And a new family of ion channels that respond to mechanical force also appears to play a role in pain—and touch—sensation.[28, 29, 30] Specific proteins convert mechanical stimuli into electrical signals.

When the wave of depolarization reaches the end of the axon, that's when the mode of information transfer changes from electrical to chemical, with the release of a chemical—a neurotransmitter—that lands on receptors in the dendrites on the other side of the synapse to keep the signal going, nerve after nerve. But the chemical—neurotransmitter—signals can carry different messages. If the neurotransmitter is *excitatory*, as happens with the chemical glutamate, the result is an increase in nerve activity and, ultimately, continued transmission of the pain signal. (Obviously, one way to stop transmission of a pain signal would be to block the glutamate receptor; there are drugs, such as the anesthetic ketamine, that can do this. But these drugs have too many side effects for chronic, widespread use.) On the other hand, if the neurotransmitter is *inhibitory*, or calming, like the neurotransmitter GABA, the result is a dampening of pain.

Granted, this is pretty esoteric stuff, but it matters. Think of this—with gratitude—the next time you go to the dentist. It's only because scientists have unraveled these basic mechanisms that they were able to come up with excellent local anesthetics such as lidocaine that work by blocking sodium channels. With sodium channels blocked, the wave of depolarization never happens and pain signals—from a dentist's drill—never get going.

But the story, of course, doesn't end here. It ends in the brain. In order to actually "feel" pain, signals must travel upward from the dorsal horn in the spinal cord to the brain, specifically, to the brainstem and also to the thalamus (the spinothalamic tract) and finally to the rest of the brain, where perception of the pain finally occurs.

As pain signals pass through the spinal cord, cells in the dorsal horn act like a gate, either sending the signal straight on up or modifying it. Some designated nerve cells (the thick, myelinated ones that detect touch as opposed to pain) also kick in at this point. This is a good thing because it means that if you thwack your thumb with a hammer and then rub your thumb hard, the touch nerves can overpower the pain nerves, somewhat decreasing pain. Once pain signals get to the brainstem, the brainstem begins sending electrochemical signals downward (called *descending modulation*) to try to block incoming pain signals.[31] In fact, some of the drugs that help control pain—anticonvulsants, opioids, and antidepressants—work in part by enhancing this descending modulation. In the dorsal horn, that all-important relay station in the spinal cord, the downward-moving, pain-blocking signals do help somewhat, and they act in several ways. One is by slowing the release of pain signals coming in from the periphery. Another is by blocking the receptors into which the chemical pain signals land in nerve cells across the synapse.

But even as the brainstem "tries" its best to dampen pain, some pain signals manage to keep going upward, eventually reaching the thalamus. Here, they get passed on to three main areas of the brain: the somatosensory cortex in the parietal lobe, which tries to figure out where in the body the pain is coming from; the limbic system, which adds emotional importance to the pain; and the frontal cortex, the part of the brain behind the forehead that governs thinking and gives meaning to the pain. (And meaning really counts. For instance, severely injured soldiers, brimming with feelings of heroism and nobility, have long been known to report significantly less pain than similarly injured civilians, whose pain has no lofty meaning.[32] Similarly, childbirth hurts like hell—but we see it as beautiful, at least afterward, because we get a lovely, new baby for our efforts.)

The somatosensory cortex—and a fascinating little site inside it called the *homunculus* (Latin for "little man")—have been the site of some of the most profound discoveries in science.[33] In the 1940s, pioneering neurosurgeon Wilder Penfield operated on epileptic patients who were awake and could talk. (The brain itself does not have receptors to detect noxious stimuli, so an acute injury to the brain, such as surgery, is not painful.[34]) He applied mild electrical currents to different areas on the surface of the brain and asked patients where in their bodies they felt a tingling or movement. From this information, he was able to create a map that showed where sensations from different parts of the body are processed in the somatosensory cortex.[35, 36] The homunculus is a grotesque-looking but kind of adorable little thing, essentially a very distorted map of the body.

The first thing you notice about this map is that a hugely disproportionate amount of brain tissue is devoted to sensations coming from the mouth, tongue, lips, face, and hand. Obviously, this suggests that information coming from these areas is extremely important for survival. Like other parts of the nervous system, the homunculus is also quite plastic, or changeable. For instance, the homunculus hand of a concert pianist would look quite different from that of a newborn baby. Rats have a *ratunculus*, and the rat's little body map exaggerates information coming from the whiskers. The homunculus also plays a role in the mysterious problem of phantom limb pain. Many, though not all, people who by accident or surgery, wind up with an amputated arm, leg, breast, or other body part often feel pain in the missing body part, and sometimes it's excruciating. Someone with a missing arm, for instance, may feel as though the fist on that limb is tightly clenched, with the fingernails digging painfully into the palm. For years, as often happens with things doctors can't readily explain, it was assumed that phantom pain was psychological.

But it's not psychological, as some ingenious experiments have shown. For instance, in the homunculus, the area that maps sensations coming in from the face is located very close to the area for incoming information from the hands, as University of California, San Diego neurologist V. S. Ramachandran has dramatically demonstrated with a person whose left arm was lost in a car crash. As an experiment, Ramachandran touched the patient's cheek with a Q-tip, then asked him what he felt. The man said he felt his cheek being touched—but his phantom thumb as well. Perhaps, speculated Ramachandran, the somatosensory cortex noticed that it was not getting any more information from the left arm, because it was missing, and somehow the space in the homunculus that *was* allocated to the arm got taken over by nerves from the face.[37]

Ramachandran figured out a way to help some people with phantom limb pain. Using a box with two armholes cut in the side and a mirror placed inside, he would have the person place his good arm and his stump through the holes, then look inside. What the person "saw," because of the mirror, was the illusion that he had both arms. He then asked the person to clench and unclench his good fist. Because of the mirror, the person actually "saw" both fists clenching and unclenching. By unclenching the "good" fist, it felt to him as if both fists opened, which, over time, relieved the pain in the phantom.

HOW THE BODY TURNS ACUTE PAIN INTO CHRONIC PAIN

In a sizable percentage of (unfortunate) people, a series of unhappy events conspires to turn acute pain into chronic pain. In fact, one of the puzzles in pain research today is to figure out why this happens in some people and not others, a question that falls to scientists who study pain genes. (See Chapter 3 on pain genetics.)

Chronic pain—usually defined as pain lasting three months or longer—is not just acute pain that doesn't go away. It is the result of fundamental changes in the nervous system itself. When pain becomes chronic, it is no longer just a symptom of something else, but can become a disease in its own right. It quite literally changes the brain, in some cases causing a loss of gray matter equivalent to 20 years of aging, as Northwestern University neuroscientist Vania Apkarian showed dramatically with brain scans in 2004.[38]

So, how does this change occur? The transformation of pain involves *neural plasticity*, or the changeability of the nervous system, and *sensitization*, which means nerve cells become more and more responsive to weaker and weaker pain signals, as if, like good students, they "learned" to get better and better at transmitting pain. This results in a kind of runaway hyperarousal of the nervous system that some call "wind-up." In fact, the properties of nerve cells can be altered so much that the pain is no longer coupled to the presence, intensity, or duration of noxious stimuli.[39] It is now physically transformed from short-term, acute pain into a long-term, *self-perpetuating* phenomenon.[40, 41, 42, 43, 44] This "learned" hypersensitivity occurs in both peripheral and central nerves.

In the periphery, several important things happen, and two in particular. Nerves that used to be responsive only to nasty—noxious—stimuli "learn" to react to benign substances as if they were noxious, too. And nerves become hyperresponsive—extra sensitive—to the original noxious stimuli, too. It's almost as if the system gets addicted to all the excitement, craving more and more stimulation. Scientists call this ugly, new state of affairs allodynia. The system is so overrevved that the brain now responds to the most benign of stimuli—like a feather stroking the skin—as if it were a burning blowtorch. Mere touch now triggers excruciating pain.

Consider what happens in inflammatory pain. In inflammation, immune cells—with the best of protective "intentions"—begin secreting chemicals called cytokines, among them TNF-a, interleukin 1B, specific pain messengers like bradykinin and prostaglandin E2, and even the normally benign nerve growth factor (NGF). (In embryos, NGF guides the development of new nerves in embryos, but it can also rev up the pain response.) Together, these chemical messengers and others act on the tips of nerve cells in the periphery, making them increasingly sensitive to pain signals. Inflammatory diseases such as rheumatoid arthritis are prime examples of the cycle of misery caused by this revved-up process.

But sensitization doesn't just occur in the periphery: It happens in the central nervous system, too, starting in the first signal relay station in the spinal cord, the dorsal horn. That's the place where axons from peripheral nerves spurt out their chemical signals to waiting dendrites of nerve cells across the synapse, spurring the transmission of pain signals up to the brain. A key player in this process is the excitatory neurotransmitter glutamate. When glutamate is released by the axon of a C fiber, it floats across the synapse and lands on several different types of receptors: most important, receptors called NMDA. When triggered by glutamate, ion channels—in this case, for calcium—open up in the receiving cell. This triggers a cascade of chemical steps inside the cell, the net result of which is that the cell puts even more NMDA receptors on its surface. This, of course, makes the cell extra sensitive to pain, allowing even more pain signals to get through.

While glutamate and other chemical messengers like substance P and BDNF (brain-derived neurotrophic factor) rev up short-term pain fast through calcium channels, other transmitters land on different receptors in the receiving cell and start a slower revving up process that keeps the pain signals going longer term by actually acting on genes. Once this hypersensitivity process gets started in the central nervous system, it takes less and less stimulation from peripheral nerves to keep it going.

This has huge potential implications. To keep central sensitization to a minimum, it helps, as nurses often put it, to "keep ahead of the pain." In one study, when doctors gave prostate surgery patients spinal injections of pain relievers *before* surgery, the patients had less pain afterward than those treated conventionally.[45] If further research confirms this, one of the most straightforward ways to reduce the amount of chronic pain in this country would be to provide better control of acute pain after surgery.

But it's not just that the nervous system learns to react to a benign stimulus like the stroke of a feather as if it were a blast from a blow torch, or that the nervous system becomes hyper-responsive to genuinely noxious stimuli. In some kinds of pain, particularly neuropathic pain (damage to the nervous system itself), what happens is that once a nerve is injured and gets revved up, the firing of electrical impulses can keep going *without any trigger* at all from the periphery.

It's as if the nerves get on a roll, turned on by having been turned on before, eventually becoming free of the need for a triggering event. The nerves learn to fire spontaneous, or *ectopic*, signals all by themselves. Worse yet, it's not just the nerves that once *were* triggered that gallop away with all these spontaneous, ectopic signals. Nearby nerve cells get caught up in the process as well, just like the flu spreading from person to person. At the most basic, neurological level, pain, too, becomes contagious, spreading from one nerve to the next. (I remember it well. That killer-burning feeling in my left shoulder and those fiery jolts of electricity shooting from my neck to my shoulder took on a life of their own. Now I understand why.) Adding significantly to the changeover from acute to chronic pain is the fact that nerves that are injured can actually change the activity of their genes, in many cases, *increasing* the activity of genes that pump out substance P, BDNF, and another pain molecule called neuropeptide Y.

And the body plays yet another nasty trick. The "good" neurotrans-mitters, like GABA, and another called glycine, chemicals that nor-mally quiet the nervous system down, now get deranged themselves. During the process of sensitization, the beneficial inhibitory function of GABA and glycine gets turned on its head—these neurotransmit-ters literally change sides in the battle, revving up pain signals instead of quieting them down. In other words, with sensitization, not only do nerves *increase* transmission of pain signals, they also *decrease* their normal methods of damping down pain. After a while, some of the GABA-producing nerves in the spinal cord even die off altogether, per-haps from sheer overwork and exhaustion: They just can't cope any-more with the onslaught of incoming pain signals.

And even all this is, unfortunately, only half the story. Making mat-ters even worse is that immune cells also get into the act. Years ago, early neuroanatomists dubbed these cells *glia*, Greek and Latin for "glue," though there are other, less lofty, translations as well, including "slime," or "snot," says University of Colorado neuroscientist and glial cell researcher Linda Watkins.[46] Shocking as it may seem, glial cells—there are three types: astrocytes, oligodendrocytes, and microglia—outnumber nerve cells in the central nervous system by 10 to 1. In the developing brain, they do good work, guiding wandering neurons to the right destinations and helping them form synapses.

But, like Jekyll and Hyde, glial cells also have a dark side. If they become activated by chemical pain signals from nerves, they send out their own chemical signals that increase chronic pain. As if adding insult to injury, if a person is taking morphine to control pain, glial cells actu-ally steal some of it to further rev up pain signals. Glial cells spring into action whenever the body senses that it is in some kind of physiological distress—from pain, but also from things as diverse as physical trauma, chemotherapy, diabetes, direct nerve damage, inflammation, and even bits of blood leaking out from blood vessels. Linda Watkins calls these chemical distress signals "alarmins."

The minute an alarmin lands on a receptor called TLR-4 (toll-like receptor number 4) on the surface of a glial cell, the glial cell begins pumping out huge numbers of cytokines called IL-1 (interleukin 1), IL-6 (interleukin 6), and TNF (tumor necrosis factor). These cyto-kines, like most molecules in biology, are both "good" and "bad."

IL-6, for instance, is great at its "day job" as an immune stimulant. If you get an infection, it's IL-6 that signals the brain to produce fever, thus raising body temperature, which in turn helps kill bacteria. IL-1 is a "good" cytokine, too, in its normal, immune-boosting role: It helps white blood cells flock to the site of an infection to fight bacteria. But these pro-inflammatory cytokines, particularly Il-1, are devils as well as angels. They are *neuroexcitatory*, meaning they rev up nerve cells to carry pain signals faster and faster.

Specifically, the cytokines pumped out by glial cells land on sensory nerves that carry pain signals up to the brain. This amplifies the original pain signal, making nerve cells fire faster and faster, generating ever more pain signals headed for the brain. The relatively recent discovery that glial cells play a major role in turning acute into chronic pain has revolutionary implications. If drugs can be developed to stop glial cells from amplifying pain signals—and scientists are working on this now—that would be a breakthrough in pain treatment because it would provide an alternative, nonnarcotic approach to pain control. Granted, once again, this is pretty intense biochemistry. But understanding what's going on chemically validates the fact that chronic pain is not "all in one's head."

IMAGING: INSIDE THE BRAIN IN PAIN

For the first time, scientists using modern brain scanning techniques, particularly functional magnetic resonance imaging (fMRI), can now look noninvasively inside the brains of people in chronic pain—in real time. This is a major step forward, not just because it adds significantly to understanding how chronic pain affects different parts of the brain, but because it makes real, explicit, and *visible* a phenomenon that, until now, has been totally subjective. As researchers Irene Tracey and Catherine Bushnell put it, fMRIs are at long last providing objective proof that the physical, emotional, and cognitive suffering of people with chronic pain is real.[47]

In 2011, Stanford University researchers led by neuroscientist Sean Mackey showed that they could use fMRI scans along with fancy computer algorithms to detect specific patterns of brain activity and, in essence, to tentatively diagnose pain—in the research lab.[48] If this technology pans out, doctors may no longer need to rely solely on a person's self-report of pain because they would be able to "see" it on a scan. (Of course, because no test is perfect, it's possible that people in real pain might be dismissed as faking if they "flunked" such a test.) In the study, the researchers put volunteers in the brain scanner and then applied heat to their forearms, producing moderate pain.[49] The scanner recorded brain patterns with and without pain and then analyzed the patterns to create a computerized model of what experimental, thermal pain looks like. Researchers then had the computer analyze the brain scans of other volunteers to see whether it could detect brain activity suggestive of thermal pain. The computer got it right 81 percent of the time.

We're still a long, long way away from using fMRI as a diagnostic test for pain, Mackey told me.[50] But it is a major first step—with enormous legal, as well as clinical, implications.[51]

Hundreds of thousands of legal cases every year depend on "proving" the existence of pain, though the technology could cut both ways.[52] Some people may be able to use fMRIs to prove to skeptical insurers and employers that their pain is real, that they are not malingering and they merit compensation. But no scientific test, including fMRI, is perfect. Some insurers and employers may be able to argue that fMRIs are not yet sophisticated enough—or that the tests may indicate some kind of general brain arousal, like anxiety or distress, but not pain specifically, which could cast doubt on patients' claims.

The most dramatic finding from MRI scans that measure brain structures (as opposed to function) in people in chronic pain is how much that pain causes loss of brain tissue, though no one really knows the exact cause of this loss—an important unresolved question. The first evidence of this came in 2004 with studies by A. Vania Apkarian of Northwestern University Feinberg School of Medicine. Using brain scans, he showed that people with chronic back pain have 5 to 11 percent less gray matter in their brains than healthy people.[53] (Gray matter consists primarily of the cell bodies of neurons in the brain; white matter consists of the axons of these cells, which look white because of the fatty, myelin sheath that surrounds them.)

Normally, it would take 20 years of aging to lose this many brain cells, Apkarian found. Significantly, his team also showed that the decrease in the prefrontal cortex and thalamus was linked to the length of time a person had chronic pain. Since then, other researchers have found similar losses of brain tissue in people with fibromyalgia, irritable bowel syndrome, tension headaches, the facial pain of trigeminal neuralgia, and other chronic pain problems.[54, 55, 56, 57] Even phantom pain and spinal cord injury can trigger losses of gray matter.[58, 59] (Interestingly, when given to people with pain, opioids—formerly called narcotics—can also produce changes in the volume of 13 specific regions of the brain's "reward" circuitry, though whether these changes are beneficial or harmful is not clear.[60])

Changes in the brain due to pain constitute one of nature's cruelest tricks. Catherine Bushnell and Irene Tracey have shown that chronic pain damages the thinking centers of the brain,[61] as Greg Scherr, a 50-year-old California stockbroker now disabled by chronic back pain, discovered to his dismay.[62] Scherr somehow fractured 11 vertebrae in his back, and no one can figure out why. "My vertebrae are fracturing like tempered glass," he says. A seemingly endless series of surgeries and medications has helped only minimally. Typically, when he wakes up in the morning, his pain is a 5 on a 0-to-10 scale. By the end of the day, it's often 8 or 9, depending on how much sitting or standing he has done. And that is despite three opioid medications. Often, he spends an entire day lying down in the fetal position. Recently, he's been getting relief with thrice-weekly deep-tissue massage to relieve his cramped muscles and learning to live "in the sandbox that I now have to play in and NOT doing things outside that box to cause me more pain and additional fractures."[63]

But the worst part of his long ordeal, for both Sherr and his wife of more than 25 years, is his memory loss. On the days when he is able to drive the short distance to the store, he announces that he's going for coffee and the paper, to which his wife usually adds, "Get milk." He often forgets the milk and has no recollection of her asking him. It wasn't until he was filling out a pain questionnaire from his insurance company that asked about memory problems that he put it together. "Son of a bitch," he said to himself. "That's what it's from. You'd never think a bad back would affect memory."

Nobody knows exactly how chronic pain wipes out gray matter. One unproved idea is that the cells simply poop out and die from metabolic exhaustion; in other words, they burn out from overwork. A provocative study from McGill University researchers might support this idea. Women who have had the painful genital condition called vulvodynia for only a few years have *increased* gray matter, as if their brains were scrambling to cope with all the incoming pain signals. But women who have had vulvodynia for more than a few years have *decreased* gray matter.[64]

But there's a conundrum here. If brain cells really are dying because of chronic pain, it's hard to explain the emerging good news that some brain damage caused by chronic pain may be reversible! Germany's Arne May, from the University Medical Center in Hamburg, studied 32 people with osteoarthritis in one hip who were scheduled for total hip replacement surgery. (Osteoarthritis of the hip, which can cause debilitating pain, is an appealing problem for pain researchers to study because, unlike most other types of pain, surgery can truly fix the problem, eliminating pain 88 percent of the time.[65]) Before the surgery, the researchers documented decreases in gray matter in several parts of the brain including the anterior cingulate cortex, the right insular cortex, the operculum, the dorsolateral prefrontal cortex, the amygdala, and the brainstem. They then looked at 10 of the patients after surgery. In all 10, hip pain had disappeared and there was an *increase* in gray matter in several of the previously affected areas.[66] Seven months later, Irene Tracey of Oxford University published similar conclusions on 16 patients undergoing hip surgery.[67] And in 2011, McGill University researchers similarly showed that effective treatment of patients' low back pain restored normal brain function.[68]

Brain scanning has revealed some other remarkably specific changes accompanying chronic pain. One study in people with fibromyalgia, for instance, showed that "catastrophizing" about pain (imagining the worst) is a mental phenomenon separate from depression and linked to very specific brain regions—those associated with attention and anticipation.[69] In a different study, researchers showed that a very specific area of the medial prefrontal cortex—right behind the forehead—was extremely active and tightly linked to the intensity of chronic back pain.[70]

A number of specific brain regions now appear to be changed by chronic pain, including the insular cortex, thalamus, cingulate cortex, somatosensory cortex I and II, and the prefrontal cortex.[71, 72] It's good news that scientists have been able to document such changes in the emotional and cognitive parts of the brain.[73] These discoveries make clear and visible the subjective experience of many people with pain—that when pain is chronic and intense, emotions are intensified and it's difficult to think straight.

Lastly, fMRIs are beginning to document precisely where in the brain opioid drugs like morphine—and drugs that block morphine—work. You can take a human brain, give it a drug, and see patterns of activation, David Borsook, a Harvard Medical School neurologist, told me.[74] Just as one would expect, when he maps the actions of morphine and the opioid blocker naloxone, they show opposite activation patterns. This suggests that brain scanning will increasingly be useful not just to document chronic pain but to test which drugs might be most effective in which people with pain.[75, 76, 77]

ASSESSING PAIN: MEASURING HOW MUCH YOU HURT

My mother died in my arms a number of years ago—my mother, her two poodles, and me all snuggled up together in her bed at home. She had been in a semi-coma for several days—quite peaceful, actually. During those long days, I sat nearby and watched, amazingly peaceful myself. I became a student of her face, a face that was almost as familiar to me as my own. I learned to watch for the telltale signs that, despite her apparent unconsciousness, the pain from her terminal leukemia might be breaking through the drugs she was taking.

When that happened, her eyebrows would draw together, and the muscles around her eyes would contract, creating crow's feet where, despite her 79 years, she had barely had them otherwise. The muscles in the middle of her face would contract, too, wrinkling her nose a bit and slightly raising her upper lip. (Interestingly, mice in pain do much the same thing, as researchers from McGill University and elsewhere have shown: Their eyes squeeze shut, their noses and cheeks bulge, and their whiskers stand on end.[78] Rabbits express their pain similarly with facial changes: Their whiskers move, their noses bulge, and their eyes narrow.[79])

Sometimes, it wasn't her face that I noticed so much as a general rest-lessness—she would move her legs and wiggle around on the bed as if trying to get rid of something, or trying to get comfortable. Whenever I noticed what seemed to be signs of increasing pain, I asked the hospice worker and nurse, both of whom were there with us, whether it was time to increase her pain medications. Often, we did. I was utterly sure that I was accurately assessing her pain by these cues.

But was I? It turns out that assessing someone else's pain is trickier than you might think. Functional MRIs, as we've just seen, may be one way. But even if they were infallible, objective tests for pain, very few people in pain have an fMRI machine in their bedrooms.

So, as a practical matter, that leaves other methods: looking at the faces of people in chronic pain, for example. Asking people to rate their pain on numerical, linear, or pictorial scales. Asking them to keep track of pain using electronic scales on iPads or other personal digital devices. Or, as doctors have done for generations, asking people to describe their pain verbally. And combining a few well-chosen questions with a very focused physical exam—in under 15 minutes. All of these methods—even simply rating pain on a scale of 0 to 10—can be helpful. But they all have serious drawbacks, too, partly because chronic pain is intrinsi-cally such a subjective phenomenon.

For instance, looking at a person's face as he or she grimaces in pain turns out to be pretty accurate—if the observer is a layman. (*Accurate* meaning that the observer's rating of the pain correlates fairly well with the patient's, and, to some extent, with fMRIs as well.) But if the observer is a healthcare professional, watch out. Research shows that the professionals—the very people you would hope would be most attuned to facial pain cues—routinely *underestimate* their patients' pain. And if the doctor in question has reason to suspect—as doctors are often trained to do—that the person is not really in pain but is just seeking drugs, the tendency to misread and underestimate facial cues becomes even worse.[80, 81, 82]

The attempt to capture pain in some sort of orderly fashion really began in 1975 when Canadian psychologist Ronald Melzack developed what has become known as the McGill Pain Questionnaire.[83] The ques-tionnaire divides pain into different types by the words people in pain use to describe it. For instance, to specify the temporal qualities of pain, the questionnaire asks people to pick one of the following words: "flickering," "quivering," "pulsing," "throbbing," "beating," or "pounding." To capture the spatial aspects of pain, the questionnaire asks people whether their pain is "jumping," "flashing," or "shooting." The questionnaire also asks about so-called punctate pressure—that is, whether the pain feels "pricking" or more severe, like "stabbing." It asks about thermal features of the pain, from "hot" to "searing"; about the "dullness" of pain, from "dull" to "heavy"; and about the overall pain, from "annoying" to "unbearable."

Although some pain clinics still use the McGill Questionnaire, many now use other methods. For young children, many doctors use the "faces" scale, in which the child picks the one picture of a face out of six that most closely matches his or her pain. These scales show a range of faces: from a happy face showing no pain to a scrunched-up face grimacing in agony. Partly because the faces scales have so few gradations, they're pretty awful from a scientific point of view, Donald Price, a University of Florida neuroscientist, explained to me.[84] A bit better is the simple 0 (no pain) to 10 (the worst pain imaginable) numerical scale, and even better is a numerical scale with finer gradations, from 0 to 100. Personally, I found the 0–10 scale helpful because it allowed me to take heart from even tiny decrements in pain. There were many days—and nights—when I ranked my pain at 10++++ on the scale. Deep breathing, lying still, meditating as best I could, even just trying to focus on a TV show, could sometimes drop the pain a tiny notch or two. This simple scale also helped me keep track of what activities or physical positions made my pain better or worse, and which treatments knocked it down a number or two.

But numerical scales have a flaw, at least for researchers trying to assess the efficacy of pain medications.[85] The problem is that the scales are linear and can't easily reveal ratios, such as the amount of improvement a certain drug or treatment provides. For that, a ratio scale such as the visual analog scale (VAS) is better. In general, the VAS scales correlate quite well with fMRI assessments of pain. What's really important, however, for both patients and doctors, is to know how pain is affecting a person's ability to function and participate in the activities of daily life. Even better, says Harvard Medical School professor of anaesthesia Robert N. Jamison, are electronic versions of this kind of scale.[86]

A number of commercial pain tracking programs and e-diaries are available online.

And even better than simple e-diaries are pain-tracking systems that use what psychologists call *ecological momentary assessment.* A hand-held device beeps at random times during the day, prompting a person to enter data on his or her current pain rating and mood. This is more reliable than asking people to remember—at the end of the day, or in a doctor's office a month later—what their pain has been like. The take-home message for people with chronic pain is that there's growing evidence that if they present these factual e-diaries to their doctors, doctors are more likely to change medications to improve pain control.[87, 88]

But there's an even more promising pain assessment method in the works—combining better-designed questions with highly focused physical exams in the doctor's office. The idea, says pain researcher Clifford Woolf of Boston Children's Hospital, is to get the *phenotype* of a person's pain. This means using the person's own verbal description of pain to figure out precisely what kind of pain the person has in order to get at the underlying neurological mechanisms. Pain described as "burning," for instance, may be different from pain that makes a benign experience like taking a shower excruciating. The verbal descriptions often point to different mechanisms.

Woolf's team has now developed a program called the Standardized Evaluation of Pain (StEP) that involves just six questions and 10 physical tests. It's cheap, low-tech, takes only 15 minutes, and is helpful for figuring out, for instance, whether a person's back pain is neuropathic—that is, caused by damage to the nervous system itself, or not. In fact, the StEP system seems able to predict with 90 percent accuracy (even better than a brain scan) what kind of pain a person has.[89] In one study of 137 people in pain, STeP was able to distinguish *axial back pain,* that is, nonspecific pain that does not travel to the buttocks, legs, or feet and is not associated with a specific anatomical problem, from *radicular back pain* (also known as sciatica), which is neuropathic pain caused by inflammation of the nerve root and bulging discs or bone spurs in the lower region of the spine.

This difference matters. If the pain is axial, the best treatment may simply be nonsteroidal anti-inflammatory drugs (NSAIDs). But if it's radicular, the best choices may be gabapentin (Neurontin) or dulox-etine (Cymbalta).

And, finally, what about the old-fashioned technique that I used with my mother, simply looking at a person's face and trying to gauge the degree of pain? Since my mother couldn't talk and I knew her very well and had no trouble believing that her terminal cancer was causing pain, I suspect that my assessment of her face and body language probably was pretty accurate. It did give me a sense of how much pain she was in. Besides, as a practical matter, my family and I had already agreed that if there was any doubt, we would err on the side of overmedicating her, since it was clear to all of us that she was dying.

But in less extreme situations, important questions remain: How accurate are facial cues in conveying pain? How well do observers read these signals? Why do doctors do worse at this than other people? Can a person fake pain expression? How much does an observer's own history of pain, or lack thereof, influence how he or she rates someone else's facial cues? And what happens, as it often does with health profession-als, if the observer's training is geared more toward spotting potential drug abuse than toward treating pain?[90]

Facial cues, it turns out, are a reasonably accurate way for the per-son to communicate pain, says psychologist Kenneth Prkachin of the University of Northern British Columbia. But from the observer's side, things can get muddied, with a big confounder being how much pain the observer has encountered in his or her own life. Prkachin has found that observers who have had chronic pain in their own or their families' lives rate patients' facial expressions of pain much higher than observers who haven't.[91] This is important. If an older person experiencing pain is seen by a young doctor who has never yet had significant chronic pain, that doctor might underestimate that person's pain.

But doctors, and some other healthcare professionals, routinely underestimate patients' pain, regardless of their own personal experi-ences with pain. Study after study going back to the late 1990s shows that healthcare professionals minimize patients' pain far more than nonhealthcare professionals do.[92] If an ordinary person downgrades a patient's facial expression of pain by 10 percent, healthcare profession-als downgrade it by 15 to 20 percent, Prkachin told me. All of which, of course, contributes to dismissing a person's pain as "all in his head."

In a clever experiment, Prkachin and European colleagues video-taped people with shoulder pain being asked to move their shoulders in a painful way. The videotapes were then shown to 120 healthcare professionals, who were divided into three different groups and told to rate the patients' pain.[93] One group saw only the videotaped faces. The second group saw the videotaped faces and was also given the patients' numerical pain ratings. The third group was given the same information as the second group, but was also told that the patients were probably cheating and were faking their expressions of pain to seek narcotics.

The healthcare professionals all routinely underestimated the patients' pain. But those who got the patients' own pain ratings as well gave estimates closer to the patients' own rating. And the healthcare professionals who were told the patients might be cheating underestimated pain just as badly as the group that saw only the faces. (Interestingly, a 2011 study from McGill University suggested that observers are more likely to think men are faking pain than women.[94])

If doctors really want to make more accurate assessments of facial pain cues, psychologist Kenneth Craig has a suggestion: Pay attention to the timing of facial cues. Facial cues, after all, are subject to both voluntary and involuntary muscle movements. When a person is faking, he or she often gets the timing of winces and grimaces wrong. The timing of facial cues during faked pain are out of sync and typically exaggerated, Craig explained, almost like a caricature of pain expression.[95]

But I have a suggestion, too. Obviously, healthcare professionals see so much pain every day that they may become numb to it and fail to read facial cues right. But when in doubt, they could err on the side of believing the patient.

CHAPTER 3

The Genetics of Pain

OVERVIEW: ONE GENE, TWO REMARKABLE FAMILIES

You might be tempted to think—as many scientists themselves thought until fairly recently—that it's pretty much of a crapshoot which people in pain, after similar diseases or surgeries, would wind up in intense, even chronic pain, and which would sail through. All anybody really knew was that people were different. As Norwegian researchers put it in a 2009 paper, "Among people with the same condition, pain ratings typically cover the entire scale from 'no pain' to 'the worst pain imaginable.'"[1]

But why? Why, for instance, do only one in 10 people over 50 who get shingles—that painful problem caused by the same virus that causes chickenpox—go on to develop an even longer lasting pain syndrome called postherpetic neuralgia?[2, 3, 4] Why doesn't everybody get it?

Millions of people have diabetes, too. But only 60 to 70 percent develop a kind of nerve damage called neuropathy, usually tingling or numbness. And only 13 percent of these go on to develop persistent painful neuropathy.[5] Why don't they all wind up with this debilitating pain?

It's possible, of course, to explain some individual differences in the experience of chronic pain as psychological. After all, emotions, especially the tendency to "catastrophize," can make pain worse (see Chapter 6). Gender plays a huge role, too (see Chapter 4). So do other factors, including stress. In fact, pain researchers have recently shown that there is an extremely complex interrelationship among genes, gender, and stress.

That said, scientists now know that genes—those 25,000 regions in our DNA that we all inherit from our parents—are especially crucial. In fact, unraveling the role that genes play in how susceptible a person is to pain is, in some ways, the most exciting scientific frontier in pain research. Indeed, the central question of chronic pain research has moved from "What causes chronic pain?" to "Of all the things that cause chronic pain, how come they usually don't?" as McGill University pain geneticist Jeffrey Mogil puts it.[6]

Scientists now think that genes control perhaps 50 percent of susceptibility to chronic pain. (*Genetic susceptibility*, by the way, means the likelihood that you'll get a chronic pain condition like, say, osteoarthritis; *genetic sensitivity* means how much it hurts if you do have a chronic pain condition.) "Across a number of different kinds of pain, genes seem to be at least half the driver of how much pain you experience," says pain geneticist Clifford Woolf of Children's Hospital in Boston. "Genes give us an amazing and powerful tool to begin to understand how pain is generated."[7]

For one thing, the more that scientists can figure out which genes contribute to chronic pain susceptibility, the more new drug targets there are. That's important because the standard drugs now used for chronic pain—opioids—are only partially effective and carry significant side effects. For another, the more scientists understand the genes that underlie individual differences in chronic pain susceptibility, the more researchers can "personalize" medications—that is, they can look at an individual's genome (all the DNA in a person's body) and figure out which drugs are most likely to help. For instance, an estimated 7 to 10 percent of Caucasians are born with a nonfunctioning gene that normally makes an enzyme that converts codeine (inactive) to morphine (active).[8] If I were one of those people and a doctor gave me codeine, I would *not* get the pain relief that a person with the gene would get and, sadly, I *would* get some of the side effects.

There's yet another reason why it's important to find pain genes. Given how often people are told that the pain is all in their heads, the more scientists can prove—by tracing pain susceptibility and sensitivity to the genes we are born with—that pain has a biological basis, the more respect people in chronic pain will get, and the better doctors will treat them.

* * *

As a child, Pam Costa, now a 48-year-old wife, mother, and psychologist in Tacoma, Washington, thought it was normal to walk to her elementary school in the gutter. After all, the gutter usually had nice, cool water in it, which soothed the burning pain in her feet. Sometimes, if no other option were available, she'd stick her feet in the toilet to cool them off. "I couldn't understand why the other kids didn't have to do the same thing," she told me. "It was very perplexing. I thought that everybody's feet burned all the time and other people were just stronger than I was."[9]

Burning pain was certainly normal in her family—30 other people in her extended family had it. Three of her cousins committed suicide because of unrelenting pain, and one died from an apparently accidental overdose of pain relievers. "My mother grew up coming home from school and soaking her feet in ice along with her five cousins," she recalled. "All the kids would sit around the bathtub with their feet in it." Pam Costa herself has needed daily opiate drugs for nearly 30 years, and even so, her pain is barely controlled.

A different kind of normal prevails for Ashlyn Blocker, now a teenager in Patterson, Georgia. Since birth, she has been unable to feel any pain at all, which might seem like a blessing, though it's not. Among other things, it means she and her parents have to monitor her body daily for injuries and infections that might otherwise go undetected.[10]

Strange as it may seem, both Ashlyn Blocker and Pam Costa have mutations in the same gene, a gene called SCN9A. Both mutations are exceedingly rare, but of high interest to researchers because of what they can teach us about the mechanics of pain. (A gene mutation is a permanent change in the DNA sequence of a gene; mutations can involve whole stretches of DNA or just a single building block. Gene mutations can be acquired from a parent or acquired during a person's lifetime, although the latter kind of acquisition is very rare.)

By chance, Ashlyn inherited a recessive mutation in the SCN9A gene from each of her parents, John, a telephone technician, and Tara, who has a degree in physical education. John and Tara each have one normal, dominant copy of the gene, as well as an aberrant copy. That one "good" gene is enough to allow them to process pain normally. Their other two children are also normal. But with two copies of the "bad" gene, Ashlyn can't process pain signals.

In its normal, healthy form, the SCN9A gene helps the body make "voltage-gated sodium channels" called Nav1.7 channels, little openings in nerve cells through which charged particles called ions flow in and out. So far, scientists have discovered 10 sodium channels. Sodium channels exist in large numbers only on excitable cells—nerve cells, muscle cells, and specialized muscle cells in the heart.

The job of sodium channels is to transmit messages along a nerve. When a nerve cell receives a signal such as contact with a nasty acid, that signal is converted into an *action potential*, which, like an electric current flowing through a copper wire, travels along the long axons of nerve cells. This is triggered when sodium from outside the cell rushes in through the sodium channels and briefly changes the electrical charge of the cell—a process called depolarization. The end result is the firing of the nerve, which causes the pain signal to be passed up from the periphery through the spinal cord to the brain, where pain is finally felt, kind of like the body making a telephone call to the brain.

Because of her mutation, Ashlyn's sodium channels do not conduct sodium ions properly and so do not pass on pain signals. In technical jargon, this is called a *loss-of-function mutation*. (Mutations in the gene for this sodium channel also can cause loss of smell.[11]) But this wasn't obvious at first. Nobody noticed that, even as a baby, Ashlyn could feel no pain, remembers her mother.[12] All they could see was that she seemed happy, cheery, and easygoing. But when she was six months old, her left eye became inflamed. Antibiotics didn't help, so the family pediatrician suggested a visit to an ophthalmologist. That visit revealed a massive corneal abrasion.

I can personally attest that a corneal abrasion hurts like crazy—but not for Ashlyn. She "was happily interacting and giggling," her mother Tara recalls. Suspicious, the ophthalmologist referred the family to a geneticist. As they waited for that appointment, Tara and John began noticing other strange things. While Ashlyn was teething, she bit all the skin off the tip of her finger and would bite her lips and tongue bloody. "We think she could feel *something*," Tara says. But whatever the sensation was, it wasn't pain.

The geneticist didn't know what specific gene might be at fault, but it was clear that Ashlyn's insensitivity to pain was genetic, permanent, and dangerous. When she was three, Ashlyn burned her hand seriously, but didn't even cry. Tara found her in the backyard simply staring at her red, blistered hand. Another time, during a family camping trip, Ashlyn broke her ankle. "She came back with dirt and grass on one side of her body," Tara says. "But when we asked her what happened, she said, 'I don't know.'" It took two days for the ankle to swell enough for her parents to realize it might be broken. Impressively, even though she can't feel pain herself, Ashlyn has learned to be sympathetic when she knows someone else is in pain. "She understands the concept," Tara says.

Finally, in 2006, when Ashlyn was seven, the Blockers found out which gene was defective. British researchers at the University of Cambridge discovered that a particular mutation in the SCN9A gene keeps people from feeling pain.[13] Once the results from that study were published, Ashlyn's doctor, rheumatologist Roland Staud at the University of Florida, checked her stored DNA and found that she had that very mutation.[14] That fit with earlier stories of people with congenital pain insensitivity, including a 1932 report of a carnival performer dubbed "The Human Pincushion." In their 2006 report, the British researchers also noted a similar story—a 10-year-old Pakistani street performer who, feeling no pain, would jab knives through his arms and walk on burning coals. (He died at age 13 from injuries he suffered jumping off a roof.) The research team subsequently tracked down six people with the same genetic mutation from three related families in Pakistan.

As for Ashlyn, as long as she marries a man with two normal SCN9A genes, she won't pass on pain insensitivity to her children. Which made me remark to Tara, half-joking, "At least when she is in labor, Ashlyn won't feel pain." To which Tara replied, "But how will she know when to go to the hospital?"

Instead of a loss-of-function mutation in the SCN9A gene, like Ashlyn has, Pamela Costa has the opposite—a *gain-of-function mutation*, which means that instead of not working at all, her sodium channels work overtime, ramping up pain signals day and night, every day of her life. (There are other gain-of-function mutations in SCN9A that cause more subtle changes in sodium channels.[15, 16, 17]) Pam's mutation causes erythromelalgia, also known as "burning man syndrome" or "burning feet syndrome," which affects several hundred people worldwide. Coping with erythromelalgia is almost impossible to describe in words, though Pam tries: "Imagine being born with this and never having an escape from it. That's what's so disheartening."[18]

As with Ashlyn Blocker, it was not obvious right away when Pam was born that she carried the terrible gain-of-function mutation. To Pam's mother, who has a milder form of the problem, red, painful feet were simply a fact of life. Pam's maternal grandfather had had the same thing, as did his siblings and many of her cousins. When Pam was a baby, she did scream all the time, but her parents and grandparents attributed it to colic. They didn't know what to make of the fact that she refused to keep booties or covers on her feet, either. By fourth grade, when her gym teachers made all the kids run around a track, Pam would collapse in agony after 50 feet. The teachers thought she was a behavioral problem, even though she was trembling and crying in pain. "It felt like my feet were on fire," she says.

It was not until she was 11 that doctors at the Mayo Clinic in Minnesota and other doctors in Birmingham, Alabama, where most members of her extended family live, were able to put together a pedigree, tracking this dominant gene throughout the extended family tree. Knowing that she would pass the gene on to her children, Pam and her husband adopted a child.

Remarkably, Pam has, despite severe pain, managed to work at two university teaching positions. She can't walk far or exercise aerobically because becoming hot makes the pain worse. But she does yoga and lifts weights three times a week at her physical therapist's office, after which the therapist wraps her in cool gel packs to ease the pain enough so she can drive the eight blocks home. "I push through it because I want my heart and bones to be healthy," she says. She hates taking opioid drugs—she takes a type that lasts for 12 hours and does not produce a "high." The drugs have wreaked havoc on her colon, as opioids often do. To control constant constipation, she has to do, in essence, a partial colonoscopy prep to clean herself out every day. The few times she has tried to get off opiates, she developed such excruciating pain that her blood pressure soared to a dangerous 250 over 140 mm Hg. (Normal is 120 over 80.)

The only time in her life that she had no pain was when she emerged from surgery to remove her appendix. When she woke up in the recovery room, the anesthesia drugs were still working. "Oh, my God," she remembers saying. "My feet don't hurt. It's incredible not to be in pain."

Scientists began zeroing in on the kind of mutation Pam has in 2004, when a Chinese dermatologist discovered two families with an inherited form of erythromelalgia. He tracked the problem to a mutation in the *SCN9A* gene and wrote it up in a genetics journal.

A world away, Stephen Waxman, a neurologist at Yale University who had been studying the *SCN9A* gene for other reasons, read the Chinese paper and had one of those rare *eureka!* moments. "You had to pull us off the ceiling," he remembers.[19] "We had done all the work on the normal *SCN9A* gene. We had the gene literally sitting in our refrigerator!" The Chinese team had described exactly where in the DNA the troublesome mutation lay, so it was almost child's play for Waxman's team of 20-odd scientists to create the same mutation in their gene, put it into cells, and see what happened.

What happened blew their minds. The mutation caused pain nerves in the dorsal root ganglia to fire abnormally, becoming hyperactive. In other words, the mutation allowed sodium channels to become activated much more easily than normal and to stay turned on longer—a classic case of gain-of-function. It was as if the nervous system's sensory nerves, like "telephone wires," could now pick up static and amplify it in such a way that the brain felt that these painful signals were constantly present. Waxman's team and others, including a Dutch group, have since discovered more than a dozen families around the world with this gain-of-function mutation.[20] "These people feel like hot lava is being poured onto their bodies," says Waxman. And, unlike Ashlyn's situation, in which it takes two recessive genes to cause the problem, it takes only one copy of the gain-of-function mutation—because it's a dominant gene—to wreak lifelong misery.

Which raises an obvious question: Can overactive sodium channels be tinkered with to relieve pain? One way would be to use the anesthetic drug lidocaine, which does indeed reduce pain by blocking sodium channels. Lidocaine—plus its oral form, mexiletine—does help a few people with sodium channel mutations.[21] Another sodium channel blocker, carbamazepine, has also been shown to help a few people in a family with a gain-of-function mutation.[22]

But so far, most existing sodium-channel blocking drugs are nonspecific—that is, they block multiple sodium channels, not just the ones that cause pain, but "good" ones in our muscles, heart, and brain as well.[23, 24, 25, 26] "I suspect that I might be able to cure pain with lidocaine," Waxman of Yale told me. But at least with traditional formulations, "the dose would be so high" that it would block lots of nerves. That could "cause heart arrhythmias and would affect the brain, too, making people confused or sleepy." In fact, it could be lethal. Currently, a number of pharmaceutical companies are working on better versions. "There is a lot of work going on with Nav1.7 specific blockers. We hope that, in the not-too-distant future, there will be a new class of highly effective pain medications with few, if any, CNS [central nervous system] side effects," says Waxman.[27]

HOW HERITABLE IS SUSCEPTIBILITY TO CHRONIC PAIN?

Back in 1999, McGill's Jeffrey Mogil picked 11 common laboratory mouse strains and ran all the mice through 12 common pain tests. He found that susceptibility to pain is quite heritable—it often runs in families—and ranges from 30 to 76 percent.[28, 29]

Obviously, that means that other factors—including psychological and environmental—also play significant roles in pain sensitivity. But the mouse results encouraged human pain geneticists to delve more deeply into the heritability question with that time-honored research technique: studying identical twins. Identical twins have the same genes but often manifest disease differently because of different environmental exposures and experiences.

In 2004, British researchers looked at 1,064 women, including 181 identical twin pairs and 351 fraternal twin pairs, and concluded that low back and neck pain were significantly heritable. For low back pain, there was a 52 to 68 percent chance that if one identical twin had the problem, the other did, too. For neck pain, the figure was 35 to 58 percent.[30]

Three years later, another British team looked at twins to study experimental, as opposed to clinical, pain.[31] They recruited 51 pairs of identical twins, as well as 47 pairs of fraternal twins, all of them women. They brought the women into the lab and put them through many of the same tests that Mogil had used in mice: heat pain thresholds, responses to dilute hydrochloric acid, and the like. Just as in the mouse studies, the researchers found sensitivity to pain was 22 to 55 percent heritable.

That same year, Norwegian researchers also did a twin study of pain sensitivity, looking at 53 pairs of identical twins and 39 pairs of fraternal twins, both male and female. In their research, they added an extra test—sensitivity to an extreme cold stimulus.[32] Intriguingly, the cold and heat pain stimuli produced different effects. With cold, there was a 60 percent chance that one twin would have the same response as the other; with heat, there was only a 26 percent chance. Puzzling, isn't it? Among other things, the different results from hot and cold stimuli show how careful researchers—and drug makers—need to be in the pain tests they choose to study.

The Danes and Finns have also found significant heritability in pain susceptibility. A huge Danish study of 15,328 male and female twins found that inherited susceptibility explained 38 percent of lumbar (lower back) pain, 32 percent of thoracic (mid-back) pain, and 39 percent of neck pain.[33] A Finnish twin study of 10,608 twins found that susceptibility to fibromyalgia was 51 percent inherited.[34] Other studies have documented a strong hereditary link for migraines, menstrual cramps, back pain in general and sciatica specifically, as well as osteoarthritis.[35] With osteoarthritis (OA), twin studies have shown that heredity probably accounts for 39 to 65 percent of the knee problems and 60 percent of hip problems—at least in women.[36]

To be sure, there are some caveats in all this, as with twin studies in general. If a disease were totally heritable in a simple way, you would expect that if one identical twin had it, the other would, too. But, as we've seen, it's rarely that straightforward. With twin studies in general, notes Mogil, "heritability is like a glass of water. Is it half full or half empty?"[37]

Part of this variability is beginning to be explained by the emerging field of epigenetics, which refers to changes in proteins (histones) that are associated with DNA and help determine what genes are actually expressed. (Histones are the main components of a structure called chromatin, around which DNA wraps itself.) These epigenetic changes—such as the attachment of a chemical called a methyl group to DNA—can actually be passed down from one generation to another even though there is no change in the DNA itself. With pain, University of Texas researchers have shown that epigenetic changes that occur near a certain gene in response to inflammation or nerve injury can "lead to persistent pain by altering pain-modulating pathways."[38] The net result increases pain.[39]

This is all very sophisticated science, to be sure, but the basic idea is that a person's "genotype"—his or her genes—is not the same as that person's "phenotype." The manifestation of something as complex as chronic pain can involve *both* susceptibility genes and epigenetic changes that—in response to a person's environment and experience—can change whether those genes are expressed or not. In other words, a person's environment can enhance or repress the genes he or she is born with. That's part of the reason why identical twins with the same genes don't always get sick with the same disease, including chronic pain.

THE HOTTEST GENES TO WATCH

While the *SCN9A* gene is obviously important, researchers are now busy deciphering dozens more pain susceptibility genes. Ultimately, the idea is to put together a "panel" of pain genes that could provide a genetic risk profile for each person. This way, for instance, doctors could identify *before surgery* which patients would be likely have intense pain afterward or to have acute postsurgical pain turn into chronic pain. Those people could have their pain treated more aggressively.

There are various ways to figure out which genes contribute to pain susceptibility.

One way is to "think backward." Once it's known which particular neurological mechanism transmits pain—such as a nerve receptor for heat or acid—scientists can look for the gene that makes that receptor. Another way to hunt for pain susceptibility and sensitivity genes is through "linkage analysis." Scientists take two or more strains of mice, and run them through various tests of experimental pain. Some strains of mice turn out to be more sensitive to certain types of pain than others, while some strains are strikingly pain resistant. Scientists then look at the DNA—the whole genome—of the different strains and see where the genes differ. The implication is that the differences in genes may account for the differences in pain sensitivity.

In humans, scientists often do something similar, genome-wide association studies (GWAS). They start with two groups of people, one with a certain disease, like chronic pain, and the other without. They then compare the genomes of both groups in hopes of finding genes that have different forms (alleles) in the sick versus the healthy people. Again, at least in theory, the different genes might be responsible for the different "phenotypes," that is, having chronic pain or not.

Yet another major approach to finding pain genes is to use a *microarray* (also called the *gene chip method*), which involves RNA, not DNA. (DNA is a long, double-stranded chain of molecules called nucleotide bases that is the master blueprint for our genes; DNA makes RNA, which is a single strand of nucleotides that carries the code for all the proteins in our cells.)

In the gene chip technique, scientists compare mice that are in pain with mice that are not. (There are multiple ways—including a mouse "grimace scale"—to tell whether a mouse is in pain.[40]) The scientists then sacrifice the mice and take samples from specific tissues such as the dorsal root ganglia, the first relay station for pain signals in the spinal cord, looking for RNA. Since different genes are active, or "turned on," in animals with pain as opposed to those not in pain, finding the RNA produced by pain nerves is a step toward identifying the pain genes themselves.

Still another way to understand pain genes is to create special strains of mice in which a possible pain gene is "knocked out" (deleted altogether; these mice are then *knockout mice*) or "knocked down" (made somewhat less active; the mice are then *knockdown mice*). Then these mice are tested for their sensitivity to pain.

One of the world's busiest pain genetics labs belongs to McGill's Jeffrey Mogil. Mogil is a friendly, energetic, curly-haired man better known as "the mouse guy." As we talk, he gestures toward his inner sanctum, the home, at any one time, to dozens of strains of mice. On the wall hangs a poster of a mouse genome, a colorful diagram showing every one of the 22,000 genes that a mouse is born with. (That's roughly the same number of genes as a human.) As he guides me through the door, I am assaulted by that unmistakable odor—eau de mouse—common to many biological labs. Here, in their pristine little cages, live black mice, white mice, black-and-white mice, brown mice, and even "redheaded" mice, though these actually look sort of yellow. The mice are all carefully bred to create colonies of mice that are all genetically identical to one another, a process that takes 20 generations. The mice are labeled and studied for their susceptibility to pain and their responsiveness to pain-relieving medications.

Mogil keeps meticulous track of his own and other scientists' searches for mouse pain genes, updating findings every week on his Pain Genes Database, where he lists the results of all published knockout mouse studies. At last count, researchers had found roughly 370 potential pain genes, with new ones being discovered almost daily. "I've got six or seven in my pocket right now," Mogil told me. Still, it's a daunting task. "We're putting together a 1,000-piece puzzle. We are nowhere near putting it all together."[41]

In addition to the sodium channel genes that play such a huge role in the lives of Ashlyn Blocker and Pamela Costa, scientists are exploring genes that control other ion channels, particularly channels for calcium and potassium. For instance, if just one tiny speck of DNA is changed in a potassium channel gene, people who inherit this mutation are at significantly higher risk for pain, as demonstrated by genetic studies of 1,359 patients.[42] Indeed, an estimated 18 to 22 percent of the population inherits two copies of this mutation—one from each parent—and thus is at significantly higher pain risk. An additional 50 percent of people inherit one copy of the mutation and are at somewhat higher risk. People who inherit no copies of the mutation are the lucky ones—they are at lowest risk.

On the flip side, geneticists have found a mutation in a calcium channel gene that seems to *protect* against pain rather than raise the risk.[43] This mutation appears to make people *less* sensitive to pain, at least to pain triggered by intense heat. People who inherit this gene mutation also appear to be less susceptible to chronic back pain. If scientists can find a way to mimic the proteins that this gene makes and use them as drugs, this could provide a novel approach to treatment, particularly for chronic back pain.

Migraine headaches, too, have a clear genetic susceptibility. Indeed, migraines, which afflict an estimated 20 percent of adults, have long been known to run in families. Numerous genes are involved in triggering migraines, says neurologist Michael Moskowitz of Massachusetts

General Hospital in Boston.[44] One type of migraine called familial hemiplegic migraine has been linked to problems in ion channels for both calcium and potassium.[45] (A different gene variant on chromosome 8 has been linked to an even more common form of migraine.[46])

But it's not just genes for ion channels that pain geneticists are chasing. One of the most important of these is a gene called *GCH1*, which was found in 2006 by Clifford Woolf and others.[47] This gene makes an enzyme that controls production of a molecule called BH4, which scientists joke could stand for "Big Hurt."[48, 49] People who have high levels of BH4 experience more pain, while people with less BH4 experience less. Encouragingly, it's now possible to predict which people are likely to be more or less sensitive to pain by screening for only three single nucleotide polymorphisms (SNPs), which are tiny bits of DNA.[50]

Another "favorite" gene of pain geneticists is *COMT*.

"We all have the *COMT* gene," medical geneticist Luda Diatchenko of the University of North Carolina told me.[51] "But some people have a form of the gene with high activity, and some, the form with low activity. High activity is better. High *COMT* means low pain and low *COMT* means high pain." The luckiest 40 percent of Caucasians, says Diatchenko, have the high-activity form and are relatively *unsusceptible* to pain. In fact, these folks are only half as likely as normal to develop the painful jaw condition called temporomandibular joint disease (TMD).

COMT works in part by making enzymes that get rid of stress hormones like norepinephrine, William Maixner, director of the Center for Neurosensory Disorders at the University of North Carolina, explained to me.[52, 53] Since norepinephrine acts directly on nerves—thus boosting pain—*getting rid* of norepinephrine can reduce pain.

There's already good news emerging from this research. A common blood pressure drug, propranolol, which blocks norepinephrine, blocks pain, too. Genetic testing for *COMT* can help identify which people are most likely to benefit from the drug.[54, 55] There's another key finding emerging from the *COMT* research. The hormone estrogen decreases *COMT* activity. Because lower *COMT* means more pain, this may partly explain why women, who have more estrogen, experience more pain than men, as we'll see in the next chapter.

Other genes generating excitement are the *PAP* gene, which boosts the body's production of a pain-relieving substance called adenosine, and another gene that, when deleted in mice, reduced chronic pain.[56, 57]

Less exciting, unfortunately, is the research on genes that control receptors for opioids (narcotics). There are three main opioid receptors—mu, delta, and kappa—each of which is produced by separate genes. The hope, still unfulfilled, is that studying mutations in opioid receptor genes might lead to better opioid drugs, including forms of the drugs that are less likely to lead to addiction.[58] So far, the best studied is the gene that makes the mu-opioid receptor. At least three subtypes of mu receptors, and perhaps as many as 10, can be made as the gene gets chopped up and spliced in different ways by the body.[59] But, so far at least, the effort to link specific variants of opioid receptor genes to differences in susceptibility to pain and responsiveness to opioid drugs has been disappointing. A recent meta-analysis,[60] in which data from eight other studies were pooled, found no significant association between changes in an opioid receptor gene and the amount of opioid drugs needed to control pain.

HOPE FOR THE FUTURE

Nonetheless, pain geneticists are optimistic. One of the most ambitious efforts to decipher pain genes is the $25 million Orofacial Pain: Prospective Evaluation and Risk Assessment (OPPERA) project, funded by the federal government, and based at the University of North Carolina.[61, 62] The first part of the project is a prospective study in which 3,200 men and women, all healthy volunteers, have been tested in the lab for sensitivity to various kinds of experimental pain. They've also been put through psychological tests for anxiety and depression to see how those factors may influence development of pain. And they've had their blood drawn and saved for genetic testing. The idea is to follow them for five years and see who gets the notorious TMD.

The second part of the project involves people who already have the disease. It began with 200 TMD patients, with 1,000 more patients to be added over time. The idea is to compare the people with TMD with the 3,200 from the first part of the study who don't yet have the disease in hopes of finding genes that confer risk for TMD. If the OPPERA project can live up to the dreams of its creators, it could become a model for unraveling the many ways in which genes influence susceptibility to pain.

CHAPTER 4
Gender and Pain

THE LIONESS'S SHARE—IN THE REAL WORLD

I couldn't help but notice, as I took my screeching neck and smoldering frustration to doctor after doctor, that most of the fellow sufferers in the waiting rooms were female. This was something of a surprise since I, like many people, male and female, had subscribed to the notion that women are less sensitive than men when it comes to pain. If men had to give birth, so the mythology goes, the human race would disappear because no man could stand the pain.

But this prevalent belief is wrong. The disparity in men's and women's pain—especially in clinical situations but also, albeit more controversially, in experimental pain labs—is one of the more puzzling observations in medicine. Scientists are just beginning to realize, for instance, how significant an effect sex has at even the most basic biological level, the expression—activation—of genes, including the genes that control responses to intense, potentially pain-inducing stimulation.

In fruit flies, for instance, researchers from North Carolina State University have shown that males and females are different in the expression of a whopping 90 percent of all their genes.

In other words, for almost all genes in the fly's genome, sex plays a significant role in how active a particular gene is, how much it is "turned on" and how much of a role it plays in the animal's physiology and behavior.[1] Finding such sex differences in gene expression is exciting because it may point to important sex-related differences in pain processing biology, according to geneticist Inna Belfer of the University of Pittsburgh.[2]

In humans, the big picture is clear. Women are both more likely to *get* painful conditions that can afflict both sexes and to report *greater pain* than men with the same condition, according to studies over the last 15 years.[3] (Although we're focused on chronic pain here, women also have more *acute* pain than men even after the same surgeries, such as wisdom tooth extraction, gall bladder removal, hernia repair, and hip and knee surgery.[4, 5])

The fact that chronic pain is higher in women has been consistently observed, but it is not well understood.[6] In 2008, when researchers looked at the prevalence in 10 developed and seven developing countries, a sample that included 42,249 people, they discovered that the prevalence of any chronic pain condition was 45 percent among women, versus 31 percent among men.[7]

In a 2009 review, a different team of researchers similarly found that worldwide, women experience more irritable bowel syndrome, fibromyalgia, headaches (especially migraines), neuropathic pain (from damage to the nervous system itself), osteoarthritis, jaw problems like temporomandibular joint disorder (TMD), and musculoskeletal and back pain.[8]

A type of neuropathic pain called complex regional pain syndrome (CRPS) that can start with a minor injury to a limb also seems to stalk women.[9, 10] Women are 3.4 times more likely to get CRPS than men, according to a 2007 study by Dutch researchers who examined patient records from 600,000 patients.[11] A United Kingdom study on neuropathic pain came to fairly similar conclusions.[12]

Fibromyalgia, too, seems mainly to affect women. A few studies have failed to find significant sex differences in the prevalence of fibromyalgia (also called widespread pain), but many others have found such differences, including studies from Sweden, the Netherlands, the United Kingdom, Israel, and the United States.[13]

With osteoarthritis, the wear-and-tear joint disease of later life, both the prevalence and the severity are greater in women.[14, 15, 16] TMD is also far more common in women,[17] as are other types of facial pain, according to studies in Finland, Germany, Sweden, Turkey, the United States, Nigeria, and Brazil.[18] The same is true for irritable bowel syndrome

(IBS), a condition that causes abdominal pain and abnormal bowel movements. IBS is 3.2 times more common in women than men.[19] (Except, curiously enough, in India and a few other places around the world where the ratio is inverted.[20])

And, of course, headaches. With headaches in general and migraines in particular, women are much more likely to be afflicted. Over the course of a given year, the prevalence of migraine ranges from 3 to 33 percent in women, but from 1 to 16 percent in men. This pattern holds true in studies around the world.[21]

Overall, in other words, chronic pain tends to be a more severe and more complex problem for women.[22] In a massive 2012 study—the biggest of its kind—Stanford University researchers studying 11,000 patients confirmed this. They found that women reported more pain with disorders in the musculoskeletal, circulatory, respiratory, and digestive systems. For the first time, the Stanford researchers also found significant sex differences with acute sinusitis and neck pain.[23]

So, we know there are sex differences in pain. But why? And are there evolutionary reasons behind it? One theory, explained to me by University of North Carolina pain researcher William Maixner, is that females may have evolved sensory mechanisms that allow for greater acuity across sense organs in general.[24] Females are more sensitive to changes in smell, temperature, visual cues, and other stimuli that may signal danger. The fact that they are more attuned to pain makes some sense. Harold J. Bursztajn, a psychiatrist at Harvard Medical School, also suggested that a woman's ability to feel and be more sensitive to a child's pain may come with the price tag of higher sensitivity when feeling her own.[25]

But only recently have pain researchers begun to study the exact genetic, physiological, hormonal, and psychosocial factors that underlie sex differences. And that's largely because pain researchers have been hampered by one—rather shocking—fact: Most—in fact, 79 percent—of basic pain research in mice and rats is still done using males.[26]

Many pain researchers, McGill's Mogil among them, contend that this has been a catastrophe, and that the old rationale alleging that menstrual cycles make females too complicated to study is utterly bogus. This bias toward studying male rodents, he argues, is simply a product of inertia.

"Sex matters," concluded the prestigious Institute of Medicine in a 2001 report. "Sex, that is, being male or female, is an important basic human variable that should be considered when designing and analyzing studies in all areas and at all levels of biomedical and health-related research."[27]

But many researchers still don't take that to heart. While the National Institutes of Health now requires routine inclusion of both sexes in *human* studies, much animal research "continues to eschew females," says University of Florida pain researcher Roger Fillingim. Given that pain is mainly a female problem, this means research that excludes females is incomplete at best and invalid at worst.[28, 29]

To me, the implication is obvious: If researchers want to insist on studying just one sex, why not study only females?

THE LIONESS'S SHARE—IN PAIN LABS, TOO

It's not just clinical pain conditions that reveal the unequal burden of suffering. Sex differences have also shown up in lab experiments in which people voluntarily let scientists test their responses to potentially painful stimulation—with informed consent—though recent research suggests these differences may not be as significant as once thought.

I volunteered for some pain experiments at McGill University in Montreal, spurred partly by sheer curiosity and partly, I must confess, by the hope of proving objectively how tough I was (and therefore, despite my first doctor's lack of empathy, how tough I had been during my most intense bouts with neck pain).

So I asked neuroscientist Catherine Bushnell, then at McGill, to assess me using some of the pain testing routinely done in her lab. She agreed. Her assistant sat me down, explained what would happen, then cheerfully applied varying amounts of thermal stimulation to my inner arm. I was supposed to say when the sensation went from just plain heat to pain, as she kept track of the rising temperatures and how long it took me to cry "uncle."

In a separate test, she had me immerse my right hand in icy water for as long as I could stand it. I winced and grimaced—cold water really hurts!—but was delighted to learn from both tests that I had a higher than average pain threshold.

I felt like taking these results to that young physiatrist in a hospital outside of Boston who seemed not to believe me and had implied that my pain was all in my head. I wanted to say, "See? I really do have pain and I really am tough. Now do you believe me?"

* * *

Pain researchers are discovering fascinating things from lab experiments, but before we begin our discussion of them, a word of caution. It turns out that the gender of the experimenter—not just the gender of the subject—has an interesting effect on how men and women volunteers report their pain sensitivity—a reflection, no doubt, of the powerful role cultural expectations have on pain expression. In an interview, Karen Berkley, a Florida State University neuroscientist, explained to me that women are brought up to have permission to—and, in fact, are expected to—recognize problems more quickly and efficiently than men. Women are more sensitive to danger, and they will more quickly recognize a threat.[30]

In the pain lab, when the experimenter is a woman, men tend to report *less* pain (machismo in action!). Curiously, women's reports of pain do not seem to be influenced as much by the gender of the experimenter, at least according to research conducted more than 20 years ago by scientists at the State University of New York.[31]

More recently, British researchers confirmed the same thing.[32] They took two groups of male college students and two groups of females. A female experimenter tested one group of males and a male experimenter tested the other; the female students were tested similarly, one group by a man, the other by a woman. In all cases, the experimenters were dressed to emphasize their gender roles.

The men tested by a woman showed higher thresholds for pain—in other words, they seemed to be tougher—than those tested by a man. For the female students, ratings of pain were the same whether the experimenter was a man or woman. And lest you still doubt how much men care about how tough they appear, catch this. After University of Florida researchers told men in one experiment that women had tolerated the procedure better, the men then scored the highest pain tolerance of all.[33]

But the most intriguing—and controversial—findings from pain labs focus on the question of whether women in experimental pain situations truly have lower pain thresholds and lower pain tolerance than men. Observed differences have often been small, and are group *averages*, much like a height distribution. Just as, on average, most men are taller than most women, some women are taller than some men. It's the same at the extremes of pain sensitivity—some females are less sensitive to potentially painful stimulation than some men.

Historically, women have often been shown to be *more* sensitive to experimental pain stimuli than men—with lower pain *thresholds* (they report pain at lower levels of stimulus intensity) and lower *tolerance* (they can't bear intense painful stimulation as long).

It turns out in more recent studies, though, that the type of pain stimulus—heat, cold, mechanical pressure, electrical stimulation, ischemic pain (from tourniquets cutting off blood supply), and other methods—matters greatly. In a 2012 systematic review of 10 years' worth of pain lab data (122 scientific papers) on sex differences in healthy people (not people with pain), Canadian researchers found that men and women have comparable *thresholds* for cold and ischemic pain, but that women have lower pain thresholds for pressure than men.[34] As for *tolerance*, there is strong evidence, the Canadian team found, that women tolerate less heat and cold pain than men, but that tolerance for ischemic pain is comparable in men and women.

Previous research had shown that pain induced by mechanical pressure produces big sex differences in sensitivity,[35] and that electrical stimulation is more painful for women, too.[36] With thermal pain, women had also been found to be more sensitive to heat pain than men in 23 studies. The same holds true for pain induced by cold—in 22 studies reviewed, women proved more sensitive to pain.[37]

But overall, the experimental pain picture is muddy. Even 10 years' worth of lab data, the Canadian team concluded, have not produced a clear and consistent picture of sex differences in human studies, which prompts the question of how useful *experimental* pain studies are in understanding the clear, significant sex differences in *clinical* pain.

There is an important twist to this—it's what scientists call *temporal summation* of pain, adding up one's cumulative experience of pain. In the lab, this is measured by the gradual increase in a person's pain ratings as brief, potentially painful stimuli are delivered to the skin every three seconds or so.[38, 39] Women show higher pain summation scores, though, again, studies are mixed and some of the higher levels of temporal summation in women may be explainable by anxiety.[40]

This is a crucial idea, notes neuroscientist Joel Greenspan of the University of Maryland. The fact that women's brains tend to accumulate pain sensations more than men's is likely to be one reason why women are more susceptible to *chronic* pain—pain that adds up over time.[41]

And it's not just what men and women *say* about their pain when they're being tested in pain labs that highlights sex differences, but what their brain scans show, too. With heat pain as the painful stimulus, positron emission tomography (PET) scans show that women exhibit more pain sensitivity than men at the same level of thermal stimulation of the inner arm (122 degrees Fahrenheit).[42]

In a different PET scan study that used rectal distention as the potentially painful stimulus, UCLA researchers looked at 23 women and 19 men with irritable bowel syndrome (abdominal pain and abnormal bowel movements).[43] To be sure, some pain processing regions "lit up" similarly in men and women. But women's brains showed more activation in the limbic system, which processes emotions, while men's showed more activation in cognitive, or analytic, regions.

Harvard Medical School researchers have documented similar findings. With migraines, they found, women's brains react differently than men's, especially in the emotional reaction to the pain.[44] This difference fits with the idea that women often express pain in more emotional terms—and may indeed have stronger emotional responses to pain.

Of course, it's not just *increased* activity in certain brain regions that show responsiveness to pain, but *decreased* responsiveness—deactivation—in other areas that document what's going on in pain. In another study that used rectal distention as a pain stimulus, women showed evidence of deactivation in some brain areas, suggesting that they may actually get used to a certain amount of pelvic pain, perhaps because they are exposed so often to pain from menstrual cramps, endometriosis, pelvic inflammatory disease, and childbirth.[45]

While women are more likely to seek treatment for pain, they may be less likely to receive adequate treatment for it, though again, this is somewhat controversial. There is a "fairly extensive literature suggesting that physicians treat women and minorities less aggressively for their pain," noted researchers from the Albany Medical Center in a 2003 paper.[46] But the authors themselves did not find such a pattern. In fact, they found that, overall, comparable doses of opioids were selected for men and women, as well as for blacks and whites. And a 1995 study from Stanford University found that women sometimes get even more aggressive pain treatment than men. Women in the emergency room who came in with headache, neck pain, or back pain were perceived by providers as having more pain and got more powerful pain-relieving drugs.[47]

But, those studies aside, there is a lot of evidence pointing the other way—toward undertreatment of women.[48] One reason women may be undertreated is that when women talk about their pain, they use more emotional language and thus are often perceived by healthcare providers as exaggerating. Indeed, psychiatrists have developed standardized criteria to assess the way men and women portray their pain. According to these criteria, women are often deemed histrionic—that is, dramatic and emotional.[49] But a bigger reason is probably that doctors learn so little about pain in medical school that they may be just plain ignorant, or even shy, about some types of pain in women.

For example, consider Tarlov cysts. These are little sacs in the lower back that become filled with cerebrospinal fluid. The sacs then press painfully on nerve roots, causing pain in the genital and buttocks area. The cysts are overwhelmingly a female problem. Roughly 90 percent of cases occur in women, estimates Massachusetts General Hospital neuroscientist Anne Louise Oaklander. "Many women just do not reveal, even to their physicians, symptoms affecting their genitalia or anus, and this is the last thing that most spine surgeons want to discuss, either," she says. It all adds up to barriers for women seeking treatment.[50]

Undertreatment of pain in women should not be such a surprise, given the undertreatment of a number of medical conditions in women. With heart attacks, for instance, Canadian researchers reviewed the charts of 142 men and 81 women with comparable symptoms and risk factors and found that men were more likely to be given lipid-lowering drugs, get angiograms (to detect potentially clogged blood vessels), and to have coronary artery bypass surgery.[51] Women are also much less likely than men to be admitted to intensive care units, to get certain procedures (such as being put on respirators) once they get there, and to die after a critical illness, according to a large study involving nearly 25,000 critically ill patients in Canada.[52] And after heart surgery? A controversial 2007 Rhode Island study tracked the medications given to 30 men and 30 women who had just had coronary artery bypass surgery. The researchers were astonished to find that men got pain medications, while women got sedatives.[53]

Indeed, women's pain symptoms are often minimized. In one clever study, researchers from Georgetown University videotaped professional actors portraying people with chest pain. The researchers showed the videos to more than 700 primary care physicians and gave them data about each hypothetical patient. The doctors were much less likely to believe that the women had heart disease.[54] Similarly, when European researchers looked at the records of 3,779 heart patients, 42 percent of them women, they found that women were not worked up as thoroughly.[55] It was the same story in a Mayo Clinic study of 2,271 men and women who went to the emergency room with chest pain.[56]

Granted, chest pain is a tricky type of pain to evaluate, in part because women having heart attacks often exhibit different symptoms from men. But less complicated medical problems, like the knee pain of osteoarthritis, exhibit the same pattern. Women are three times less likely to get the hip or knee replacement that they need, and often don't get the surgery in a timely manner, says Mary I. O'Connor, a former Olympic rower who now heads the orthopedic surgery department at the Mayo Clinic in Jacksonville, Florida. "And when they do have the surgery, they often do not do quite as well as men. We call it the 'never catch up' syndrome."[57]

"A woman usually waits longer" to have surgery, says O'Connor, in contrast to a man, who usually seeks surgery before his pain becomes extreme. The surgery itself is equally beneficial for both sexes, but because a woman has typically had more advanced disease by the time she undergoes surgery, the result often "is not quite as good."[58] Even though women wait too long before having surgery, there may also be an "unconscious bias" at work that may make doctors less likely to *recommend* surgery to a woman with moderate knee arthritis, O'Connor thinks.

Canadian researchers looked into this very question, asking 38 family physicians and 33 orthopedic surgeons to evaluate one "standardized," or typical, male patient and one "standardized" female patient with moderate knee arthritis. That's the degree of arthritis in which it's a judgment call whether surgery is necessary or not.[59] (Two orthopedic surgeons confirmed that the male and female patients had the same severity of disease.) The odds of a surgeon recommending knee replacement, the Canadian team found, were 22 times higher for the male patient than the female.

Women are undertreated for abdominal pain, too. In Philadelphia, emergency room doctors kept track of 981 men and women who arrived with acute abdominal pain. The men and women had similar pain scores, but women were significantly less likely to get any kind of pain medication and were 15 to 23 percent less likely than men to get opiates specifically. Women also had to wait longer before they got any kind of pain medicine—65 minutes, on average, compared to 49 for men.[60]

Women with cancer and AIDS have also historically been more likely than men to get inadequate pain treatment.[61, 62]

A fascinating Swedish study also revealed gender biases. Using a modified version of a national exam for young doctors, the Swedish researchers described hypothetical neck pain in patients. Some of the hypothetical patients were male and some female; all were described as bus drivers who were living in tense family situations. The interns were more likely to ask female patients psychosocial questions, and more likely to request lab tests in the males.[63] Female interns were just as biased as males.

I hate to say it, but I believe it, based on my own experience.

HORMONES AND PAIN

If, as we've seen, women have more chronic pain conditions than men, the question then becomes, why? Why *do* women have more pain than men? There are several possible reasons.

One theory is that the chemical pathways that get activated inside nerve cells may be different in males and females. In studies with male rats, says neuroscientist Jon Levine of the University of California, San Francisco, the "secondary messengers" (chemicals that relay pain signals) are different in females and males. Male rats use three different secondary messengers; females use one.[64] Women also have more nerve endings in their skin than men, which could partially explain why women may be more sensitive to potentially painful stimulation, according to research from Massachusetts General Hospital in Boston.[65] Moreover, the nerve cells that convey information about intense stimulation are studded with receptors for sex hormones: testosterone and estrogen, in particular.

In fact, perhaps the most intriguing reason for sex differences in pain responsiveness may lie with these two hormones. But understanding this potential hormonal contribution has been nightmarishly tricky, as researchers have reported in a number of review papers since 1999.[66]

As young children, boys and girls show comparable patterns of pain until puberty. But once puberty hits, certain types of pain are strikingly more common in girls. Even when the prevalence of a pain problem is the same in both sexes, pain *severity* is often more intense in girls than boys.

Take migraines. Before puberty, boys and girls get roughly the same number. After puberty, the prevalence becomes 18 percent for women, and 6 or 7 percent for men.[67, 68] A similar pattern holds for TMJ, now called temporomandibular joint disease (TMD): no sex differences before puberty, significant differences afterward—women get it twice as often as men.[69] Indeed, as girls progress through puberty, chronic pain of various sorts—back pain, headaches, TMD, and stomach pain—worsens.[70, 71]

Overall, many researchers think that testosterone generally protects against pain, an idea illustrated dramatically in some rat studies. Newborn male rats that are castrated are unable to produce testosterone later, during puberty. The result? The animals become less sensitive to the pain-reducing effects of the opioid morphine.[72] If newborn female rats are *given* testosterone, they get *better* pain relief from morphine. (A word of caution, though: It's not clear how well pain findings in rats translate to people.)

As adolescence progresses, boys actually develop more pain *tolerance*, perhaps partly because of the flood of testosterone, says Lonnie Zeltzer, a pediatric pain specialist at the University of California, Los Angeles.[73]

But if the role of testosterone in pain is relatively straightforward (more testosterone, less pain), the role of estrogen is anything but. Genetics research suggests that estrogen down-regulates—or reduces—the activity of one of the leading "pain genes," called *COMT*. The job of the *COMT* gene is to chew up stress hormones like epinephrine. That means that if *COMT* activity is too low, the body can't get rid of stress hormones as well. Since stress hormones act directly on nerves to rev up pain, the net result of estrogen acting on *COMT* is more pain, says William Maixner, director of the Center for Neurosensory Disorders at the University of North Carolina.[74]

And other research, too, supports the "estrogen is bad" theory. At the University of Maryland, neuroscientist Richard Traub studies hormones and pain in rats. He starts by testing female rodents' sensitivity to pain, then takes out their ovaries (which make estrogen), and then tests them again. Without their ovaries, these females act more like males—that is, they're less sensitive to pain.[75] He then gives back estrogen to these animals. They soon go back to feeling pain, just as in the bad old days before their ovary surgery, says Traub.

You could think of menopause as the human version of this experiment. At menopause, women's ovaries stop pumping out estrogen, almost as if the ovaries had been surgically removed. To combat the symptoms caused by this precipitous drop in estrogen, many menopausal women begin taking exogenous estrogen—that is, estrogen not made naturally in the body but taken as a drug.

If the general theory—that estrogen increases pain—is true, you would expect that taking exogenous estrogen (hormone replacement therapy) would make pain worse. But it turns out that the "estrogen is bad" theory is too simplistic. Sometimes exogenous estrogen makes pain worse, but sometimes it doesn't. And sometimes it makes it better.

Several studies have shown that menopausal women who take hormone replacement therapy do have more back pain, and more pain from TMD as well, as the theory would predict. Linda LeResche, a pain researcher at the University of Washington, looked at the histories of more than 6,000 women over 40. She found that those who took hormone replacement therapy were 30 percent more likely to be referred for treatment of TMD.[76] She found much the same pattern in a different study of more than 6,000 younger women—those taking birth control pills were 20 percent more likely to be referred for TMD treatment.[77]

Back pain, too, clearly seems to be associated with hormone replacement therapy.[78,79] The same goes for thermal pain. University of Alabama researchers found that women taking hormone replacement therapy were more sensitive to heat stimulation than women not taking the therapy and than men.[80]

But other studies show no link between hormone replacement therapy and pain in older women. And still others show that when post-menopausal women *stop* taking hormone replacement therapy, their pain goes up: just the opposite of what the theory would predict.[81]

Similarly, some women with a history of migraines begin getting the headaches anew within a couple of weeks of *stopping* estrogen therapy.[82] And some pain conditions like trigeminal neuralgia that are more common in women typically don't start until after menopause.[83]

And have you ever wondered what happens when transsexuals take hormones to enhance the sexual characteristics of their "new" sex? Anna Maria Aloisi, a physiologist at the University of Siena, wondered exactly that. In a preliminary study, she tracked male-to-female human transsexuals who take estrogen to enhance female sex characteristics, and found that approximately one-third develop chronic pain, especially headaches. She also looked at female-to-male transsexuals who take testosterone to enhance male characteristics, and found that their chronic pain goes down.[84] All of which fits with the overall theory.

But no one is quite sure why these hormones have such effects. One theory is that testosterone dulls the excitatory pain pathways in the brain that would crank up pain, while estrogen may block the nervous system's pathways for *inhibiting* responses to potentially painful stimuli.

What makes unraveling the estrogen–pain link even more complicated, of course, is that in premenopausal women, estrogen levels rise and fall dramatically over the course of each menstrual cycle, with many women experiencing striking fluctuations in pain responsiveness at different points in the cycle. Pain in a number of conditions—including irritable bowel syndrome, TMD, headache, and fibromyalgia—changes significantly over the cycle.

But not always in the direction one might expect. Some women feel *more* sensitive to pain during times in their cycles when estrogen is low.[85] During pregnancy, when estrogen levels are high, some women experience *fewer* migraines and TMD pain, whereas after childbirth, when estrogen falls abruptly, the number of migraine attacks increase.

Given such complexity, a growing number of researchers now suspect that it's not the absolute level of estrogen that is key for pain, but rapid *changes* in hormone levels. "It's the *change* that produces the change," according to pain researcher Fernando Cervero at McGill University."[86]

PINK PILLS FOR WOMEN, BLUE PILLS FOR MEN?

One of the hottest questions tormenting pain scientists these days is why some opioid drugs—narcotics—work better in one sex than the other. No one doubts that the problem exists. It is clear that "there are sex differences in opioid analgesia," say Roger Fillingim of the University of Florida and Robert Gear of the University of California, San Francisco. What's unclear, they note, is "the direction and magnitude" of these differences.[87, 88, 89]

Part of the reason this is so hard to figure out is that answers vary depending on which pain assays, or tests, researchers use, whether they study rats or humans, whether they look at experimental pain in the lab or clinical pain in real patients, and whether the pain is acute or chronic. And, of course, which opioid drugs they are studying.[90]

What *is* clear, however, in both the rodent and human nervous systems, is that there are three major classes of opioid receptors: mu, delta, and kappa. These receptors are like magnets into which pain-relieving opioids fit. This lock-and-key setup is the same whether the opioids come from inside the body (endorphins) or are taken as drugs. Wherever the opioid comes from, a filled opioid receptor is a happy receptor—it acts quickly to reduce pain.

Morphine, the most commonly used opioid, binds to mu receptors, the largest of the three classes of receptors. Fentanyl, a drug that is 100 times more powerful than morphine, also binds to mu receptors.

Codeine does not bind strongly to mu receptors, but after the body turns codeine into morphine, it binds just fine.

Other, less frequently used drugs, such as Talwin, Nubain, and Stadol, are different. They bind primarily to kappa receptors. This is important because response to kappa opioids varies depending on sex and may even be specific to certain pain situations, such as tooth extraction.[91] (So far, there are no drugs designed to fit into delta receptors.)

All three receptors—mu, kappa, and delta—work roughly the same way. When the receptors are filled, they trigger a cascade of chemical events inside the nerve cell that ultimately block production of pain-boosting chemicals like substance P. The result? Decreased pain.[92]

At Georgia State University, neuroscientist Anne Z. Murphy is trying to unravel the mechanics of sex differences in response to opioids, especially with respect to chronic inflammatory pain. She focuses on an area of the brain called the periaqueductal gray (PAG), a processing center for morphine-type drugs.[93] To produce that inflammatory pain in a rat, Murphy injects a rat's paw with a solution called complete Freund's adjuvant (FRA), an oil, with a smidgen of tuberculosis bacterium thrown in. This injection stimulates an immune (inflammatory) response. The animal's paw quickly swells, and the rat starts "guarding" its now-hypersensitive paw. Murphy then gives the rats, male and female, morphine to stop the pain—with dramatic results.

Females require twice as much morphine as males to produce the same level of anesthesia.[94, 95] So, if morphine works better in male rats than in females, why might that be? Perhaps, Murphy reasoned, the answer might lie in the mu receptors onto which morphine binds.

Knowing that morphine binds to mu receptors and that the PAG brain region is loaded with mu receptors, Murphy decided to look more closely at PAG regions in males and females. Using a sophisticated radioactive staining technique called autoradiography, Murphy counted the number of mu receptors in the PAG area of male and female rat brains. Lo and behold, there turned out to be twice as many mu receptors in male rats as in females. (So far, nobody has done a similar experiment in people.) Murphy thinks this might explain why morphine is twice as effective in male rats. It conceivably might explain the difference in people, too.

In 2003, anesthesiologist Daniel Carr at Tufts University Medical School in Boston found that, following surgery, women report more intense pain than men and need at least 30 percent more morphine.[96]

But other researchers have doubts about all this. It's unlikely, says Robert Gear, a pain researcher at the University of California, San Francisco, that the sheer number of mu receptors is even close to the whole story. "Even if there is such a difference," he says, "I don't think it explains any sex differences in opioid analgesia."[97]

And a 2010 systematic review and meta-analysis of 50 studies on sex and opioid efficacy threw cold water on the whole idea, suggesting that there is actually *greater* morphine efficacy in women.[98] "Interestingly," wrote the authors, a team from Leiden University in the Netherlands, "while animal studies show a tendency for opioids to act more efficaciously in males, human studies are less clear.... Our observations that women display greater opioid analgesia than men are completely opposite to what has been found in the rodent literature."[99]

But it's actually even more complicated than that. In pain experiments in the lab, for instance, mu opioids may indeed be more effective in women, the Dutch researchers found. But clinical studies—with real pain patients—are more ambiguous, with some studies showing more mu opioid efficacy in men, and others, more efficacy in women. Curiously, when patients themselves control their analgesia—by pushing a button to release a dose of drug intravenously—men consumed more opioids.[100]

Again, the interesting question is why. If women consume fewer opioids, is it because they are feeling less pain? Or because they experience more or worse side effects from opioids, including negative mood, nausea, and vomiting.[101] In other words, women who control their own analgesia may deliberately underdose themselves to avoid the side effects.

That has been a leading theory since 1999, when a team of California researchers reviewed 18 studies to see how much pain-relieving medication men and women used after surgical operations. They found that there were no sex differences in some studies, and that in others, women indeed used less medication.[102] But most of the 18 studies did not actually assess pain—they looked only at medication use. So, again, women may have been underdosing themselves.

Morphine also seems to have a slower onset of action in women compared to men, which, in the short run, would make it appear to be less effective in women. Women also typically have more body fat than men, and since mu opioids become concentrated in body fat, this could mean lower blood levels, and hence less efficacy, in women. It's a complex picture, to be sure.

Luckily, things are a bit clearer with opioids other than morphine, particularly with drugs such as Talwin, Nubain, and Stadol that work on kappa receptors. In general, these drugs work better in women. More than 20 years ago, Robert Gear and Jon Levine of the University of California, San Francisco demonstrated this in people having their wisdom teeth extracted.[103, 104, 105] Since then, other studies from the same group have confirmed the greater effectiveness of kappa drugs in women.

There is, however, a strange twist to this: Kappa opioids seem to work especially well in women with red hair. In 2003, Jeffrey Mogil, the rodent geneticist at McGill University, and Roger Fillingim, a psychologist and human pain researcher at the University of Florida, joined forces to test a prediction of Mogil's theory based on mouse studies: that red-headed women would respond especially well to Talwin (pentazocine). They used fancy genetic mapping and found that one particular gene called Mc1R (for melanocortin-1 receptor) was key.

Women (and mice) with red hair (actually, yellowish hair in mice) or very fair skin have two mutant copies of the Mc1R gene, essentially rendering it useless. (This is analogous to animal experiments in which researchers deliberately "knock out" certain genes to see what happens). The Mc1R gene is in the pain circuit that contains kappa opioid receptors. Somehow, Mogil thought, knocking out this gene seems to allow activation of the kappa opioid system, producing analgesia.[106]

As Mogil and Fillingim discovered, this is exactly what happens in red-headed women, who have two mutant Mc1R genes. They get "significantly greater analgesia" from pentazocine than all other groups.[107] Indeed, pentazocine produces more analgesia in red-headed women than in non-red-headed women or men of any hair color. While many doctors don't know about this, the good news is that at least some obstetricians do.

An even more important wrinkle is the observation that the efficacy of opioids in women can vary depending on where she is in her menstrual cycle. In her studies, Murphy has found that the degree to which female rats respond to morphine varies according to the menstrual (estrus) cycle. When estrogen is highest, she says, morphine is the least effective, perhaps because estrogen *down-regulates*, or reduces the number or availability of, mu receptors. When estrogen is low, morphine works better, possibly because of more mu receptors.

But, once again, the picture gets complicated. Researchers from the University of Michigan have found just the opposite: that when women are in the high-estrogen phases of their cycles, there is an *increase* in mu activity.[108] And when the female rats were in low-estrogen periods of their cycles, there were reductions in mu receptor activity and more sensitivity to pain. This piece does fit with some—but not all—human data showing that women may be most sensitive to noxious stimulation when their estrogen is lowest, as just before their periods.

Basically, a straightforward theory to explain the data on sex and opioid efficacy remains "elusive," as the Leiden researchers put it.[109] Murphy, the Georgia neuroscientist, assesses the ridiculously complex interplay between sex and opioid response more bluntly: "It stinks, doesn't it?"

CHAPTER 5
Children in Pain

THE HORROR

Little Jeffrey Lawson weighed only 1 pound, 11½ ounces. But his tragic death in 1985 after heart surgery without anesthesia triggered a long-overdue uproar over the way doctors viewed pain in babies and children.

In those not-so-old days when Jeffrey was born, as a preemie, many doctors mistakenly believed that babies' nervous systems were too immature to process pain and that, therefore, babies didn't feel pain at all.[1,2] Or, doctors rationalized, if babies did somehow feel pain, it was no big deal because they probably wouldn't remember it. Besides, since nobody knew for sure how dangerous anesthesia drugs might be in tiny babies, doctors figured that if surgery was necessary to save a child's life, they'd better operate anyway—and comfort themselves with the hope that the child wouldn't feel pain. As one scientific paper from those days intoned, "Pediatric patients seldom need medication for relief of pain. They tolerate discomfort well."[3]

That's preposterous, obviously. But doctors had to have these self-protective beliefs for their own emotional survival, says Neil Schechter, a pediatric pain physician at Children's Hospital in Boston. "Doctors were not sure how to do anesthesia in babies. In response, they had to believe that the babies couldn't feel pain. They were too scared of the anesthetics."[4]

"It was a kind of natural denial," explains his Children's Hospital colleague, anesthesiologist Charles Berde. "It reduces your own cognitive dissonance to make up a story that there's no pain. People make up stories to comfort themselves."[5]

Comfort was something tiny Jeffrey clearly didn't get. As soon as Jeffrey was born, according to his mother, Jill Lawson, he was placed in the neonatal intensive care unit. He was put on a respirator but developed lung problems, a moderate brain bleed, as well as kidney and liver problems.[6,7] It soon became clear that something was wrong with his circulation, too.

In the developing fetal heart, there is a duct that connects the pulmonary artery and the aortic arch to allow most of the blood from the right ventricle to bypass the fetus's compressed lungs. Evolution presumably came up with this solution to protect the right ventricle from having to pump too hard against the high resistance in the lungs. The minute a newborn takes his or her first breath, the lungs open up, resistance drops, and the duct closes up, allowing normal circulation. But in Jeffrey, the duct did not close properly, a not-uncommon occurrence called patent ductus arteriosus. The remedy was surgery.

Jill, a Maryland housewife who had graduated from Penn State at 20 as an anthropology major, remembers being promised that the surgery would be done under anesthesia. It was not—as she and her husband, James, who worked in the bookbinding department of a Smithsonian library, would soon discover to their horror. During the 1½-hour procedure, Jeffrey was given only a paralyzing agent, Pavulon (pancuronium bromide), but no pain relievers, according to his mother. Although he could feel pain, he could not move, cry, or in any way indicate what he was feeling, except, of course, for the stress chemicals pouring into his bloodstream. Doctors cut holes on his neck, and a hole on the right side of his chest, put a catheter in a vein in his neck, and then cut open his chest along his breastbone. His flesh was then lifted up and his ribs pried apart to expose the heart for repair.

When Jeffrey died five weeks after the surgery, Jill, who was facing major surgery herself for a severe kidney infection, obtained his medical records. She remembers standing in the medical records office at the hospital, flipping through Jeffrey's records. She saw that he had been given the muscle relaxant, but no pain relievers. Stunned, she read on. When Jeffrey's chest was cut open, his blood pressure, pulse rate, and oxygen requirements all skyrocketed. Unmistakable signs of stress. And pain. Today, more than a quarter century later, she still feels guilt that she allowed this to happen to her son: "Parents are supposed to watch out for their children," she told me. "This is a very tender subject."

At the time, while still in shock, she got the anesthesiologist's name from Jeffrey's records and called her. "She tried to tell me that they had him on pancuronium. I said, 'But that has nothing to do with pain.' There was this silence." If the rationale for the lack of anesthesia was that Jeffrey was too sick to tolerate anesthesia, she wondered, wasn't he also too sick to have the surgery? When she finally managed to get a meeting with hospital staff, as she remembers it, one doctor commented that her upset was proof that parents shouldn't be allowed into the neonatal intensive care unit.

"They disowned it. They placed as much of it as they could on me for making problems. At one point, I was referred to as a 'poorly managed second-level patient.' They made the assumption that I was some kind of idiot. I was a housewife, and I didn't dress all that well. They treated me like I was some kind of low-functioning person."

Jill, whose writings eventually spurred necessary, though still-insufficient, changes in pediatric pain control, was shocked to discover that, far from being anomalous, undertreatment of pain in babies and children was common practice. It shouldn't have been. Even back in 1985, scientists, doctors, and nurses could—and should—have known that babies feel pain.

THE GROWING EVIDENCE

In 1974, Joann Eland became one of the first practitioners to document the undertreatment of children's pain. Then a nurse at the University of Iowa working on her master's thesis, she walked around the wards at her Iowa hospital and looked at the medical charts of 25 children aged four to eight who had had all sorts of surgeries—cleft palate repair, repair to the urethral opening at the tip of the penis, and so on.

Over their entire hospital stays, the 25 kids—collectively—got only 24 doses of pain medicine. Of these, only half were opioids (narcotics). Thirteen children received no pain medication at all, despite having had a traumatic amputation of a foot, removal of a neck mass, partial kidney removal, or other serious procedures.

Eland, who now has a PhD and is an associate professor, contrasted that poor pain management for children with what happened with 25 adults who had also had surgeries in the same hospital at the same time. Over *their* hospital stays, the adults—collectively—got 372 doses of narcotics (opioids) and 299 doses of non-narcotic pain relievers.[8]

Tragically, Eland's work didn't have nearly the impact it should have had across the country. But in her own hospital, her study did change the way kids were treated. Almost 20 years later, researchers again looked at the records of 25 children who had had surgery and found that 23 of 25 had had prescriptions for narcotics, with an average pain treatment of 3.3 doses per day.[9]

Even back in the early days, Eland wasn't the only one troubled by undertreatment of children's pain. In 1982, other researchers documented that children undergoing debridement of burns often got no anesthesia at all.[10] (Debridement is a notoriously painful procedure in which dead tissue is peeled off burn sites over and over again to let underlying skin grow and heal.) In 1983, pain researcher Judith E. Beyer of the University of Virginia tracked the use of postoperative anesthesia in 50 children and 50 adults who had had cardiac surgery. Nobody, not even the adults, got very good pain management. But at least the adults actually received 70 percent of the opioids that had been prescribed for them. The kids got only 30 percent.[11]

That same year, Australian researchers studied 170 children who had just had surgery. They found that 75 percent had inadequate anesthesia.[12] In 1986, Schechter compared 90 children and 90 adults undergoing identical surgical procedures—hernias, appendectomies, burns, and fractured femurs—at a variety of hospitals. He, too, found an "enormous disparity" in pain control: Adults got twice as many doses of opioids as children.[13]

But it took research into the basic neurobiology of brain development to begin to convince the medical world that babies and children did indeed feel pain and should be treated for it. Fortunately, this was a mission that British pain researcher Maria Fitzgerald plunged into with vigor. Fitzgerald began examining how the nervous system in newborn rats—and humans—changes under the assault of severe pain. In 1985, she published the first of a series of pivotal papers in which she tracked the postnatal growth of pain pathways. She showed not only that local analgesics can reduce the risk of subsequent chronic pain, but that untreated pain in infancy can have long-term adverse effects.[14, 15, 16, 17, 18, 19, 20, 21, 22] This was a huge revelation. It made unavoidably clear that if pain is inflicted on a preemie or newborn, it changes the developing sensory-neural system in ways that can be long-lasting.

But what really hammered that point home was a blockbuster paper in 1987 in the *New England Journal of Medicine*. The authors of that paper, pediatric pain specialists K. J. S. Anand, now at the University of Tennessee, and Paul R. Hickey of Children's Hospital in Boston, laid out irrefutable evidence that babies, and older children as well, do feel pain. Human newborns, they said, "do have the anatomical and functional components required for the perception of painful stimuli."[23] Citing study after study, they made the case that babies' nervous systems are indeed mature enough to process pain signals, that they react to pain with massive stress hormone release, and that anesthetics can— and should—be given to newborns undergoing surgery.[24, 25, 26, 27, 28, 29, 30]

In meticulous detail, with more than 200 citations in their *New England Journal* article, Anand and Hickey showed that newborns have at least as many nociceptive (pain) nerve endings in their skin as adults. Indeed, pain nerves are already developed in some areas of the skin as early as seven weeks' gestation, fairly early in a woman's pregnancy. By 20 weeks' gestation, the fetal brain has the full complement of nerve cells. (A more recent study has shown that by 35–37 weeks of gestation, fetuses can discriminate between mere touch and pain.[31])

Anand and Hickey also attacked head-on the argument that newborn babies couldn't feel pain because some of their nerve fibers are not yet myelinated—that is, not yet covered with a protective, fatty sheath. It is true that without this protective myelin coating, nerves do transmit pain signals slightly more slowly. But in babies, this slower transmission is more than offset by the fact that nerve impulses have much shorter distances to travel from the periphery to the brain, as Anand and Hickey pointed out. Babies, therefore, may be even quicker to feel pain than adults. They also have higher levels than adults of some pain neurotransmitters, such as substance P.

In fact, very young babies may actually be extra sensitive to pain because the descending, top-down pain control signals from the brain to the spinal cord haven't kicked in yet, observes Celeste Johnston, a nurse-turned-McGill-University-professor.[32] At least in rats, it takes 10–12 days after birth for the animals to be neurologically mature enough to activate these descending pathways.[33] Even during the birth process itself, it's clear that babies are actively trying to cope with pain. If the birth is comparatively easy for the baby—a vaginal or Cesarean delivery—newborns pump out three to five times higher levels of endorphins than adults do at rest. But if the newborns have more stressful deliveries—with breech presentation or a vacuum extraction—they show even higher levels of endorphins.[34, 35, 36] The babies, in essence, are trying to take care of their own pain.

Not surprisingly, the idea that babies feel pain fed into the debate over circumcision. Even as far back as the early 1970s, it was clear that if a newborn was circumcised without anesthesia, his sleep was disturbed.[37] And levels of the stress hormone cortisol rose sharply.[38] By contrast, if a newborn is given local anesthetic before circumcision, he does not show behavioral signs of pain and stress.[39] But it took decades before it became clear that uncontrolled pain during circumcision can sometimes have lasting effects. That was demonstrated in 1997, when Canadian pharmacologist Anna Taddio studied three groups of baby boys. One group was not circumcised. One group was circumcised after getting a local anesthetic called EMLA. The third group was circumcised after a placebo medication. Four to six months later, the infants were videotaped while they got standard vaccinations. The results were straight-line clear: uncircumcised babies cried the least during vaccinations, those circumcised but with EMLA cried a bit more, and those circumcised with placebo cried the most, strong evidence that EMLA can attenuate circumcision pain.[40, 41] (Today, many circumcisions are done with a different kind of anesthesia, a dorsal penile nerve block.)

And it's not just babies, but older children, too, who may suffer lasting effects from untreated pain. Research suggests that school-age kids with cancer who undergo painful procedures such as bone marrow aspiration or lumbar puncture experience more pain during subsequent procedures if they don't get good pain control the first time around.[42]

WE *CAN* TREAT CHILDREN'S PAIN, BUT *DO* WE?

In recent years, doctors and nurses have learned a lot about treating pain in babies and children, including how to use powerful opioid (narcotic) drugs safely.

Historically, infants and young children have been underdosed with opioids for fear of significant respiratory side effects, California pediatric pain specialists Lonnie Zelter and Elliot Krane noted in a 2011 pediatric textbook.[43] But with proper understanding of the way opioids work in young bodies, they say that children can receive effective relief of pain and suffering "with a good margin of safety."

For instance, it's been clear for decades that young children who receive good pain management during surgery fare better than those who don't.[44, 45, 46] To be sure, treating babies with opioids can get tricky. Adverse events, both major and minor, following anesthesia are about twice as common in young children as in adults. And the risk is highest, not surprisingly, in the newest, tiniest babies.[47] In newborns, the liver is so immature that it takes longer to detoxify drugs. That means that weaning babies off opioids can take longer and must be done with exquisite care so as not to trigger a new bout of pain.[48]

On the other hand, older children (aged two to six) actually clear drugs faster than adults. But this gets tricky, too, because faster clearance may mean that the child needs a new dose sooner. For example, a sustained-released oral morphine drug that an adult needs to take only twice a day requires three-times-a-day dosing in kids.[49] The point, though, is that doctors now know how to manage kids' pain—and gradual withdrawal from opioids—quite successfully.[50, 51]

Perhaps surprisingly, kids themselves can be pretty good at it, too. When given the chance, children as young as six can learn how to do patient-controlled analgesia, in which the patient pushes a button to administer a preset infusion of morphine.[52] Importantly, letting kids administer their own opioids does *not* increase drug complications. And many kids prefer this approach to getting repeated intramuscular injections of pain relievers.[53] (It's anxious parents who actually mess things up. They tend to either over- or underdose their children unless they receive a vigorous education program first.)

As for that ever-present concern about opioids—the fear of addiction—there's no need to go there. Many parents—and doctors—still harbor what California researchers Zeltzer and Krane call an "unrealistic fear of addiction."[54] In reality, research shows that "the rational acute or chronic use of opioids in children does not lead to a predilection or risk of addiction," unless that child is already at risk by virtue of genetic background and social milieu.[55] Even with kids, including teenagers, who do have substance abuse problems, Zeltzer and Krane note, it's important to emphasize that these young people, too, "are entitled to effective analgesic management, and that often includes the use of opioids."

For milder pain, non-opioid approaches can often help, including things that taste sweet, breastfeeding, pacifiers, cuddling, skin-to-skin contact, swaddling, and, for older children, self-hypnosis and cognitive-behavior therapy. Take, for instance, the common hospital practice of lancing a newborn's heel to draw blood for testing. It may look like nothing to an adult, but, as McGill's Celeste Johnston notes, "size-wise, it's like a knife in the foot of an adult."[56]

And it turns out that Mary Poppins was right: A spoonful of sugar really does help during heel lances and other minor procedures. A number of studies, including a major review of 44 other studies by the Cochrane Collaboration, an international group that analyzes medical research, have found that sucrose significantly reduces the length of time a newborn cries during a heel stick, though it doesn't stop that initial yelp.[57] Sucrose also reduces scores on the Premature Infant Pain Profile (PIPP), a commonly used scale called for measuring infant pain.[58, 59, 60] Interestingly, it's not so clear why.

Sugar may act via opioid receptors. At least one study showed that sugar's soothing effect can be reversed by a drug called naloxone, which blocks opioids, suggesting that sugar does work through the opioid system. Sugar also doesn't help babies who are born to mothers dependent on methadone, perhaps because the babies' opioid receptors are already full and thus unable to be stimulated further.[61]

But the magic in sugar as a pain reliever may not be attributable to an opioid effect at all. In fact, Britain's Maria Fitzgerald has shown that sucrose does not seem to act directly on pain circuits in the nervous system.[62]

Fitzgerald's team gave sucrose to 20 randomly selected newborns just before heel sticks, but gave sterilized water to 24 other newborns. She tracked brain activity in all of them with EEGs. Surprisingly, there was no difference on the brain tests. But the babies who got sucrose *did* have significantly better PIPP scores and didn't grimace as much as those who just got water. So, what's going on? Probably, it's that sugar has an emotionally calming effect on babies but is not strictly an analgesic in the sense of acting directly on pain nerves. Even if sugar acts only by blunting a child's emotional response to pain, that's still important— and well worth doing. And it may not even be the sugar itself that has a positive effect, says Celeste Johnston. It may be just the sweet taste, because artificial sweeteners work just as well.[63]

Other extremely benign interventions—especially pacifiers and breastfeeding—have also been shown to help control minor pain, particularly in newborns and tiny infants.[64, 65, 66] But perhaps the best infant pain reliever of all is the one that comes most naturally to mothers: "kangaroo mother care," basic holding and skin-to-skin contact.[67, 68] Research shows that skin-to-skin contact is more effective at reducing distress—as gauged by crying, grimacing, and heart rate increase—than swaddling a baby tightly in a crib during heel lance.[69] Familiar scents, especially that of the mother, also helps calm babies, as does simply the sound of the mother's voice.

With all this new knowledge, you might think that undertreatment of children's pain is a problem solved. Not so. In 1992, McGill's Johnston interviewed 150 randomly selected hospitalized children aged 4 to 14, and later, their parents, to assess children's pain experience in the hospital. The results were depressing. More than 87 percent of the children had had pain within the previous 24 hours, and 19 percent of them said their pain was severe. Only 38 percent had received analgesic medication in the previous 24 hours.[70]

In 2000, San Francisco researchers checked the medical records of hospitalized children who had been reported by nurses to be in pain. They found that opioid use was wildly uneven.[71] In 2002, other researchers studied 237 hospitalized children and found that more than 20 percent had significant pain.[72] In 2003, a Swedish nationwide survey of nurses and doctors showed that moderate to severe pain occurred in 23 percent of children who had had surgery and in 31 percent of children who had pain from other causes.[73] That same year, when researchers from Maine and Massachusetts examined the medical charts of 180 children aged six months to 10 years who were in emergency rooms for fractures or serious burns, they discovered that a whopping 65 percent of kids under 2 got no pain medication at all.[74]

Researchers from the Netherlands and the University of Arkansas studied 151 preemies and recorded all the potentially painful procedures they were subjected to in their first two weeks in intensive care—an average of 14 per child per day.[75] (To be sure, some of the procedures were relatively benign, like suctioning out the airway.) They found that preemptive analgesia was given to fewer than 35 percent of the babies. And 40 percent of the newborns never got any analgesia during their entire ICU stays.

Even today, serious undertreatment of children's pain persists, according to French pain researcher Ricardo Carbajal. In 2008, his team conducted a six-week study of 430 hospitalized preemies in and around Paris. He found that each preemie received an average of 16 painful or stressful procedures every day, though some of these procedures were minor. A whopping 79.2 percent of the time, the babies got no specific analgesia at all.[76] Carbajal himself was shocked. "It seems unbelievable how long it took the medical community to realize that newborns are able to feel pain," he wrote in a commentary. The problem, he said, is "the large gap that exists between published research results and routine clinical practice."[77]

Even in supposedly enlightened Canada, where pain treatment is arguably the best in the world, as recently as 2008, researchers found that only 27 percent of children in a leading hospital—the Hospital for Sick Children in Toronto—had any pain assessment in the preceding 24 hours. This was despite the fact that the children or their caregivers said the children had moderate to severe pain.[78]

Indeed, many hospitals and doctors still don't even do the little things to reduce pain, like providing sugar cubes and cuddling. One 2006 Australian study showed that only 23 percent of neonatal units used sucrose or other sweet-tasting solutions during minor procedures. Nor was breastfeeding used to offset pain when newborns were getting shots or having their veins or heels poked. The babies rarely got topical pain relievers, either.[79] Many doctors still don't give children local anesthetic creams like EMLA before injections.[80, 81, 82, 83, 84, 85] And many hospitals still do not have pain guidelines for children or attempt to assess infant pain.[86]

But here's the real heartbreaker—even children with cancer still die in pain. In 2000, Boston palliative care specialist Joanne Wolfe interviewed the parents of 103 children who had died of cancer between 1990 and 1997. According to the parents, 89 percent of the children suffered "a lot" or "a great deal" in their last month of life.[87] Wolfe campaigned for better palliative care for kids, then did a follow-up study in 2007 to see if things had improved. There was some progress. But not enough.[88]

Ultimately, I believe it will be up to parents, nurses, and the doctors who "get it" to convince those who still don't that (a) children do feel pain, (b) they can safely get opioids, and (c) little things like sweets and cuddling can relieve minor pain. Recently, a small cadre of doctors, a new group called "ChildKind," has begun waging a global campaign to combat untreated pain in children.[89] But the real pressure will have to come from consumers because doctors already know how to control pain in kids. They just don't always do it.

It has now been more than a quarter century since little Jeffrey Lawson's ordeal. Jill Lawson is now in her 60s and a widow. To her credit, she says she has "pretty much come to terms with" Jeffrey's death. "There's always a residue with me, the pain and the guilt. I don't think that's ever going to go away. But for the most part, it's okay now."[90]

It is fitting that the American Pain Society now presents an annual Jeffrey Lawson Award for Advocacy in Children's Pain Relief to a leading pediatric pain researcher. It is even more fitting that its first award went to Jill Lawson.

CHAPTER 6
The Mind–Body in Pain

OVERVIEW

Unless you're a Buddhist monk—or zonked out under general anesthesia—I guarantee that if you have serious pain, you will have some distinctly non-mellow feelings about it. And the longer your pain goes on, the more diffuse it is, and the more frustrated you get trying to find "the answer," the more intense your feelings will probably be. That is because—though you'd never know it from the way modern medicine is still divided into the "mental" and the "physical"—the mind and the body are truly, deeply, biologically one. It's inescapable. The International Association for the Study of Pain embeds that unity into its very definition of pain: an "unpleasant sensory *and emotional* [italics mine] experience associated with actual or potential tissue damage or described in terms of that damage."

Neuroscientist Jill Bolte Taylor puts it beautifully in her moving book about her own stroke, *My Stroke of Insight*:

Sensory information streams in through our sensory system and is immediately processed through our limbic system. By the time a message reaches our cerebral cortex for higher thinking, we have already placed a "feeling" upon how we view that stimulation—is this pain or pleasure? Although many of us may think of ourselves as *thinking creatures that feel*, biologically, we are *feeling creatures that think*.[1]

In other words, the meaning we give to pain is huge, as Henry K. Beecher, an anesthesiologist at Harvard Medical School, noted way back in 1956. He reported on a study comparing pain intensity and requests for narcotics in seriously wounded soldiers and male civilians with similar pain intensity. "The group of soldiers had very extensive wounds, were clear mentally and were not in shock; many had no morphine at all, yet less than one-fourth said, on being questioned, that they had enough pain to want anything done about it," Beecher wrote.[2] While only 32 percent of the soldiers studied wanted narcotics, 83 percent of the civilians did. Beecher's conclusion? "The intensity of suffering is largely determined by what the pain means to the patient."

More recently, in 2010, pain researchers at Oxford University conducted an experiment that dramatically confirmed the role that meaning plays in pain.[3] The team, led by neuroscientist Irene Tracey, asked 16 volunteers to lie in functional magnetic resonance imaging (fMRI) brain scanning machines. The volunteers were told that they were helping to test the safety of a laser that would zap their feet in six different spots. They were told that some of the spots had already been deemed safe, that some were not deemed safe yet, and that for some, safety was unclear. In actual fact, all the spots were safe. But the volunteers reported more pain when they were zapped on spots they feared were unsafe. Moreover, a specific part of the brain, the anterior insula, lit up on the brain scans even *before* the zaps hit the supposedly unsafe spots. This shows, the Oxford team says, that anticipation of pain—the mere threat of it—already primes the brain to feel pain.

At the most basic level of brain anatomy, an emotional response is intrinsic to pain. It's part of the deal. It's how we are hardwired. It's neurobiological. The parts of the brain that process emotions (the limbic system) are literally connected to the parts (the somatosensory cortex) that detect bodily sensations. In this chapter, we'll talk about the rich connections of the mind–body in pain. We'll see how "catastrophizing" and having significant fear of pain can lead to poorer functioning, less mobility, worse psychological distress, and more physical disability.[4] But we'll also see how boosting confidence in one's own ability to affect outcomes, a concept psychologists call *self-efficacy*, adopting good pain coping strategies, and, when appropriate, acceptance of the real limitations pain imposes can all help reduce pain.[5]

We'll see how specific psychological techniques—including those that aim to correct unhelpful thoughts (cognitions) and behaviors—can reduce the impact of pain. While no particular form of psychotherapy holds all the magic, several meta-analyses show that psychosocial interventions in general can often ease pain.[6] A key take-home lesson is this: The links between emotions and pain work both ways. "Negative" emotions like anger and sadness can make pain worse, whether you have a chronic pain condition or not.[7] And "positive" emotional states—like falling in love or being in a good marriage—can actually reduce pain.

Ponder this: Fifteen young, bonkers-in-love couples who had been together about nine months were brought into a brain scanning lab and asked to look alternately at pictures of their loved one or an equally attractive platonic friend, while undergoing moderate to painful heat stimulation. Pictures of the loved one, but not the friend, reduced pain significantly.[8] Among older people with arthritis, single people and those in bad marriages had more pain and disability; those in good marriages fared much better.[9]

I'm not saying pain is "all in your mind." Far from it. People with chronic pain are told that—and are rightly insulted—all the time. But pain *is* all in your brain. In fact, some areas of the brain, notably the insula and the anterior cingulate cortex, actually process both sensory and emotional aspects of pain at the same time. Even when people are just sitting in a lab *waiting* for a jolt of experimental pain, the insula, the anterior cingulate cortex, and the prefrontal cortex (where we make judgments and plans) all light up together.

All too often, though, modern medicine still doesn't get it. The more something complex like chronic pain defies simple diagnosis, the more doctors fall back on the psychogenic theory—the idea that if a physical problem can't be identified, the complaints must be emotional in origin. "If we cannot explain pain in terms of objective tissue pathology, Western biomedicine lures us to explain it in terms of patients' psychopathology," observes Harvard Medical School psychiatrist Ajay Wasan.[10] In the old days, doctors even believed there was such a thing as a "pain personality," according to Duke University pain psychologist Francis Keefe. Fortunately, that concept was eventually deemed as dubious as the "cancer personality."[11]

In the last few decades, a few brave souls have tried to change this antiquated, dualistic thinking, foremost among them, George Engel, a University of Rochester psychoanalyst. In a famous 1977 paper in

Science,[12] he argued for an end to mind–body dualism and for a more complex, sophisticated—and realistic—view, the *biopsychosocial model*. That's a mouthful of jargon, to be sure. But it captures what most of us would see as obvious—that health (or illness) is the interaction of biological, psychological, and social factors.[13]

Think of it this way. Sure, germs cause disease. But not everybody who is exposed to the common cold—or even the AIDS virus—gets sick or dies from it. A person's social situation, as well as cultural beliefs, sex, emotional makeup, genes, and overall health all play key roles in who will succumb to illness. It's been amply demonstrated, for instance, that lonely people get sick more than less lonely ones and are more prone to the type of overactive inflammatory response that can lead to cancer, heart disease, and neurodegeneration.[14] Culture plays into all this, too, with some cultures valuing stoicism in the face of pain, and others, expressiveness. Some cultures see pain as deserved punishment or a character-building opportunity, while others interpret pain as a harbinger of serious health problems. Even something as simple as a 0–10 scale for rating pain is not culture-free. When asked to rate their pain, some Native Americans choose a favorite or sacred number instead of the number that reflects their pain.[15]

The thing is, it's not just doctors who still get mired in this old dualistic thinking: it's people with pain, too. Like me. It took months for me to accept that my emotional response to my excruciating neck pain was part of the experience, not proof of some psychological inadequacy. It took even longer to believe that I could *do* something about my unhelpful thoughts and emotions without sliding down the slippery slope of thinking that if I could *change* my emotional response, it must mean that my emotions were the *cause* of my pain in the first place.

My severe neck pain had appeared suddenly, mysteriously, at a time when everything in my life was going well. I was also doing everything I could think of to help myself—exercises, physical therapy, acupuncture, massage, NSAIDs, acetaminophen, and opioids. Yet I was still in pain. When my first physician seemed to suggest that my pain was emotional, I flipped out. I was infuriated, which increased my suffering enormously. And needlessly.

Even the gentlest suggestion from Ken, a psychiatrist who was then my boyfriend and is now my husband, that I might be able to reduce my pain with psychological strategies such as meditation, cognitive behavioral therapy, or psychotherapy not only did not help: it enraged me! I interpreted these suggestions as his belief that the pain was all in my head. But slowly, fighting every inch of the way, I began to cooperate with Ken, who had long run mind–body groups at Newton-Wellesley Hospital near Boston for people with chronic medical conditions, including pain. (For the record, I met Ken *before* my neck pain started—I didn't choose him because of his expertise.)

Sometimes, he would just tell me to breathe through the worst pain attacks, like breathing during labor pains in childbirth. I began to see that my "pain panic" did make things worse. If I counted breaths and consciously got into a more comfortable physical position, like lying down with my head supported and neck muscles at least slightly relaxed, the pain eased a tiny bit, maybe from a 10++ on a 10-point scale to a 10. Hardly a slam dunk, but it was a start. Penney Cowan, head of the American Chronic Pain Association who has had fibromyalgia for 30 years, puts it this way: "If you listen to the waves, in that instant, you are not thinking about how much your back hurts. For that instant, you have reduced your suffering."[16]

As this chapter unfolds, we'll see how the mind can be tamed—a bit—and how that can offset pain. And we'll see that, even in the worst case—even if drugs, surgery, devices, exercise and other approaches can't do much for your underlying pain—you can learn to reduce your *suffering*. And that's huge.

THE POWER OF THE MIND: PLACEBOS

"Pain is the great illuminator of medicine," says Harvard Medical School's Ted Kaptchuk, an associate professor who is an expert in Chinese medicine and the placebo effect. "Pain tells us the truth—that we are not dealing only with biology, or only psychology. It's the interaction of biology, affect and meaning."

Nothing makes the power of the mind clearer than studies of the placebo effect: the idea that expectations of benefit can yield benefit, even when the "treatment" is a sugar pill or sham procedure. (Expectations, by the way, are a two-way street. The placebo effect has an evil twin, the *nocebo effect*, in which the power of suggestion causes harm, not benefit. This can happen if you focus too much about potential side effects of a treatment—you'll probably get some of them.[17])

Placebos—totally fake drugs or other treatments—have been shown to produce improvements in 30 to 60 percent of people with everything from arthritis to depression.[18] The mechanisms by which placebos work their magic in the brain are many. Placebo medications, for instance, have been shown to help people with Parkinson's disease by boosting levels of the neurotransmitter dopamine,[19] and to help people in pain with release of endorphins. Placebos—pure fakes—can reduce levels of adrenaline, calming people with heart disease. Placebo medications are so effective against depression that drug companies must struggle to prove their concoctions are superior. Placebo medications have even been shown to change metabolic activity in certain brain regions.[20]

In fact, one famous study reviewed outcomes of 6,931 people who had participated in efficacy studies of five interventions that are no longer used: a type of surgery for asthma, gastric freezing for ulcers, and three treatments for herpes simplex viral infections. A whopping 70 percent of the patients said they had good to excellent results, despite later evidence showing that these treatments did absolutely no good medically.[21]

Interestingly, the person with pain is not the only one to be influenced by the placebo effect—it can impact people close to that person, too, a relative, or even the doctor. And the "placebo by proxy" effect can work both ways, note Kaptchuk and his colleague, David Grelotti.[22] Family members may think a treatment is working even when there is no physiological benefit, or they may think it's not when it is. And the family member's view may differ from that of the person with pain. A spouse's expectation of benefit, for instance, may encourage a person with pain to hang in more optimistically through treatment—but also could encourage him or her to hang in too long with a treatment that really isn't working.

Powerful as it is, though, it's wise to keep in mind that the placebo effect has its limits. "Placebos don't shrink tumors," Ted Kaptchuk told me, "or help a person with a severed spine walk. They do, however, make a person feel less pain, anxiety, nausea and they can improve sleep."[23]

While the placebo effect can influence many things, its potential effect on pain "is one of the most robust."[24] A recent review from the Cochrane Collaboration, an international group that analyzes medical data, pooled results from 202 placebo studies involving 60 different clinical outcomes.[25] Although the review found that placebo interventions were not effective overall, the results were more encouraging in studies of pain.

Until recently, the dogma was that the placebo effect works only when the person is deceived into thinking that a pill or procedure is the real stuff. But in a well-designed, paradigm-shattering study in *PLoS One* in 2010, Kaptchuk's team showed that the placebo effect works *even when patients are told the pills they are getting are fake.*[26] The study involved 80 people with irritable bowel syndrome (IBS). Half were randomly assigned to take fake pills presented as "placebo pills made of an inert substance, like sugar pills, that have been shown in clinical studies to produce significant improvement in IBS through mind-body self-healing processes," and the other half received no treatment but the same amount of time interacting with supportive providers.

Guess who got better. The placebo folks. At the very least, a delighted Kaptchuk told me, the study should "give people more courage to pay attention to the non-material parts of illness and health. It shows the interpersonal relationship is a powerful part of therapy."[27] That kind of healing relationship is, as other researchers note, a "genuine psychobiological event."[28] In 2012, another Harvard team including Kaptchuk showed that placebo and nocebo responses can occur even outside conscious awareness.[29]

Put more mechanistically, placebos work by creating changes in the brain that reduce the experience of pain. In general, placebo analgesia appears to work at three different stages of pain processing: anticipation of pain, changing the actual perception of pain, and changing pain ratings after stimulation.[30] Here's a fascinating case in point. At Oxford University in England, pain researchers applied heat to the legs of 22 volunteers, who were also hooked up to IV drip machines so that a powerful pain reliever, remifentanil, could be secretly administered— or not. They were also placed in fMRI brain scanning machines.[31, 32] At baseline, the volunteers rated their pain a 66 out of 100 on average. Without their knowledge, they were given a dose of the pain reliever, after which their pain ratings dropped—to 55. They were then told they were getting a powerful pain reliever and their scores dropped even more dramatically—to 39. Then—here's the cool part—they were told the pain reliever had been withdrawn, though in reality, it hadn't been. Their scores soared—to 64, nearly up to baseline. The changing pain scores were reflected in changing brain scans, too. Powerful stuff, these expectations.

So, what's going on in the brain? Positive expectations have been linked to *decreasing* activity in pain-sensitive areas of the brain, including the thalamus, insula, and anterior cingulate cortex.[33, 34] And to *increased* activity in the prefrontal cortex—where cognition and judgment occur. This might explain why expecting less pain—anticipation of comfort—can act against pain before pain even hits, as fMRI studies from North Carolina and Italy suggest.[35, 36] Positive expectations may also act on reward areas of the brain such as the nucleus accumbens, according to Randy Gollub, a Massachusetts General Hospital neuroscientist and brain scanning expert. Positive expectations may also work by decreasing anxiety.

Mechanistically, one theory is that the placebo effect accomplishes all this through endogenous opioids that we all make in our bodies, the endorphins. Functional MRI brain scanning technology has shown that positive expectations of a drug or treatment trigger the release of endogenous opioids (endorphins). This flood of endorphins then acts directly on *descending* pathways (from the brain down the spinal cord) to mute pain signals heading up to the brain from the rest of the body.[37]

True healers have probably known, or suspected, the power of placebos for centuries. But in the research world, the first breakthrough in understanding placebos and pain came in 1978, when University of California researchers showed that naloxone, a drug that blocks opioids, also blocks the placebo effect.[38] The implication was clear: If the pain-relieving effect of placebos can be turned off with naloxone, it must mean that the placebo effect works, at least in part, via opioids, or more precisely, through the brain's own natural opioids, the endorphins. Numerous other studies have confirmed that placebos work through the opioid system.

In one study in 2002, Swedish researchers, using positron emission tomography (PET) scans, showed that placebo analgesia—pain relief—involves the same areas of the brain (notably, the anterior cingulate cortex and the brainstem) that are involved in analgesia triggered by real opiate drugs.[39] In other important studies published in 2005 and 2007, University of Michigan researchers led by Jon-Kar Zubieta used PET scans to study people who had been given a placebo and told it would reduce their pain.[40, 41] Several brain areas immediately "lit up" on the scans, showing an increase in endorphins acting on mu receptors, a particular type of opioid receptor. Tellingly, while their brains were lighting up, the patients also reported that they felt less pain. A year later, the Michigan team found that placebo-induced pain relief also works by changing a person's emotional—affective—experience.[42]

But what really blows me away is that placebos can have different effects in different parts of the body. In a 1999 study, Italian researchers induced pain in volunteers (by injecting capsaicin, which causes burning pain) in four parts of the body: left hand, right hand, left foot, and right foot.[43] They also induced specific expectations of pain relief. They rubbed a cream on one area, say, the left foot, and told the volunteers it was a powerful pain reliever. The cream was actually fake—a placebo. Amazingly enough, the volunteers said that while the other three body parts hurt, their left feet, which got the cream, didn't. When the experiment was repeated so that the volunteers got injections of naloxone (the opioid blocker), the placebo response disappeared completely. Pretty strong evidence that placebos work, at least in part, via endogenous opioids.

Buttressing the opioid theory is research showing that, just like real opioids, which can slow breathing (a potentially dangerous side effect), endogenous opioids triggered by the placebo effect can do the same thing.[44] Placebo-induced pain control can also slow the heart rate, just like real drugs, though, of course, it's the drug-induced respiratory depression that is dangerous.[45]

But there's at least one other pathway by which placebos can lead to pain relief—the endocannabinoid system. (Endocannabinoids are marijuana-like substances made naturally in the body that can reduce pain. For more on marijuana, see Chapter 10.) In 2011, Italian researchers showed that if they block a receptor called CB1 for endocannabinoids with a drug (rimonabant), they also block placebo analgesia.[46] The researchers first recorded how long healthy subjects could stand the pain of a tight tourniquet and then were given a nonsteroidal anti-inflammatory drug (NSAID), which allowed them to tolerate the pain a bit longer. When the researchers substituted a placebo in place of the NSAID, the subjects still did well, a kind of conditioning effect. But when they were given rimonabant, which blocks receptors for endocannabinoids, the placebo effect disappeared and the subjects felt pain again. By contrast, rimonabant had no effect on opioid placebo response. This is good evidence that the cannabinoid system, as well as the opioid system, is involved in the placebo effect.[47]

Interestingly, some research suggests that the placebo effect may wear off over time.[48] But that may be just a lab, not a real-world, phenomenon. In real pain patients over long periods of time, says Harvard's Kaptchuk, "placebo effects last as long as any drug effect."[49]

PAIN AND DEPRESSION

Like philosophers of old debating how many angels could fit on the head of a pin, modern psychiatrists, psychologists, and neuroscientists have spent decades on this one: Which comes first, chronic pain or depression? The question arises because millions of people suffer from both, as numerous studies, including a large 2003 study of 18,980 people randomly picked from the general European population, have shown.[50] Sadly, though, many, if not most, psychiatrists are woefully ill-equipped to deal with people who have both pain and depression because they, like other physicians, know so little about pain. "Psychiatrists appear to be inadequately trained in pain medicine and to consequently perceive their work with patients who have chronic pain as ungratifying," noted David Borsook, a Harvard Medical School neurologist and senior author of a 2010 paper called "The Missing P [for Pain] in Psychiatric Training."[51] If psychiatry residents "received training in pain, they would be more adept and less fearful of handling these patients," he said.

The overlap (*comorbidity*, in medical jargon) between pain and depression is "huge," Harvard Medical School psychiatrist Ajay Wasan told me.[52] By some estimates, mood disorders are two to three times more prevalent in people with chronic pain. And the more physical pain symptoms a person has, the more likely he or she is to also have mood or anxiety problems.[53] Some estimates of depression in people with pain may actually be low because primary care doctors often focus on the pain symptoms, not realizing that the person may also be depressed. And patients often don't acknowledge that they're depressed, preferring to focus on their physical pain.

Overall, epidemiological evidence suggests that in the general population, at least 20 percent of people in chronic pain have a serious mood problem. The good news is the flip side: 80 percent don't. In other words, mood problems are not inevitable. Among people in pain in primary care clinics, the number is higher: about 40 percent. And of those going to pain clinics, it's even higher: 60 to 75 percent.[54] This still means that one-quarter of people in miserable pain don't get seriously depressed or anxious.

For years, psychiatrists and psychologists, wedded to the theory of *somatization*—that is, the tendency to express emotional distress in terms of bodily symptoms—leaned heavily toward the view that depression comes first and gets expressed as chronic pain later. And to some extent, they're right. Being depressed can lead to more pain, as an unusual study (that I'm glad I did not volunteer for) showed.[55] Researchers from Oxford University and Harvard Medical School gathered 20 healthy volunteers. Each rated his or her mood on standard scales, then underwent a standardized (so-called Velten) mood-induction procedure. This meant that the volunteers read depressing statements such as "I feel worthless" while listening to depressing music (Prokofiev's "Russia Under the Mongolian Yoke," played at half speed no less). In the alternate condition, they read neutral statements such as "Cherries are fruits" and listened to slightly cheerier music (the largo movement from Dvorak's "Symphony from the New World"). During all this, the hardy volunteers lay in fMRI scanners and were given painful (heat) stimulation.

Here's what happened. During the down moods, the volunteers had more negative thoughts and rated their pain as significantly more unpleasant. Part of depression, after all, involves negative and pessimistic thoughts. The volunteers' brain scans reflected this, too: increased activity in the prefrontal cortex, anterior cingulate cortex, and hippocampus. Clearly, being depressed can make the pain experience worse.

But the emerging view today is that in most cases in which people have both pain and depression, it's the chronic pain that comes first, and mood problems, later. "We are pretty sure that depression doesn't cause chronic pain," says Harvard Medical School psychologist Robert Jamison. "There was a notion for a while that if people were depressed, that's why they had pain. That, fortunately, has not been supported."[56]

There have been many studies aimed at this chicken-and-egg question, but one of the most clear took a close look at people with disabling occupational spinal injuries. The researchers found that psychiatric disorders were much more likely to develop *after* the onset of the work injury, which shows that the injuries are probably the initiators, not the consequences, of mood problems.[57] Another prime example is a 2012 Boston study showing that women who have had migraine headaches are 40 percent more likely than women without a history of migraines to develop depression.[58] In other words, most of the time, depression *follows* the onset of chronic pain and is not preceded by it.[59] Even when this isn't true, there is little clinical benefit to be gained by debating which came first. This makes sense. When people have chronic pain, an invisible disorder, and "every time they get up and move, they hurt, they can't be as active, they can't do their job, they can't sleep, their friendships have disappeared, that naturally contributes to being depressed and anxious," Jamison told me. And this can obviously become a vicious cycle: the more depressed and anxious you are, the worse your pain gets—a phenomenon that brain scan studies have repeatedly shown.[60]

Indeed, neuroimaging studies show that different parts of the brain—notably, the anterior cingulate cortex, the insula, and the dorsolateral prefrontal cortex—all work together in ways that can amplify pain.[61] When these areas are activated, our natural pain relievers, the endogenous opioids (endorphins) become less effective, evidence that negative affect can make pain worse. Negative affect can make exogenous opioids—drugs *prescribed* for pain—less effective, too. Opioid drugs simply do not work as well for people with higher levels of depression and anxiety as for those with fewer psychological symptoms.[62]

So, the real question becomes, not which comes first, pain or depression, but what to do if you have both, or, as Kurt Kroenke, a professor of medicine and pain researcher at Indiana University, puts it, what to do if you have a "double hurt."[63] The answer, backed by a huge body of research, is not surprising: Treat both.[64] If you just treat the depression, says Kroenke, pain may get a bit better, but not as much better as the depression.[65] Many physicians, however, still hold to this misconception.[66]

There are, as we'll see in a minute, many non-drug treatments for the double-whammy of pain and depression. But for the moment, let's zero in on the *pharmacological* approaches—with a word of warning: Many researchers who study drugs get financial support from drug companies, a potential conflict of interest that can skew results. In many cases, researchers turn to pharmaceutical funding because there is so little funding available from the federal government. I have chosen not to get into such conflicts here because that could be a book in itself. (And indeed, it already *is* a book.[67]) The main rule of thumb for treating pain and depression together is, in addition to using opioids if necessary, using antidepressant medications that have independent analgesic (pain-relieving) effects as well—that is, antidepressants specifically designed to work on pain symptoms as well as mood.[68]

There are different classes of antidepressants. The class known as selective serotonin reuptake inhibitors (SSRIs) and serotonin and norepinephrine reuptake inhibitors (SNRIs) work against depression by boosting levels of these neurotransmitters in the brain. These drugs, especially the SNRIs, can also somewhat damp down pain signals traveling up to the brain from the peripheral nerves and spinal cord.[69] SNRIs that work against the "double hurt" of pain and depression include duloxetine (Cymbalta), venlafaxine (Effexor), and milnacipran (Savella).

Older-style antidepressants called tricyclics can also help with both pain and depression. These include nortriptyline, amitriptyline, and desipramine, better known as Pamelor, Elavil, and Norpramin, respectively. In some cases, the analgesic features of tricyclics may kick in at lower doses than that needed for the antidepressant effects. An additional benefit of tricyclics is that they can also enhance sleep, which is often disrupted in people with chronic pain.[70] Other classes of drugs may also help with both pain, particularly neuropathic pain, and depression. One example is the class of drugs called anticonvulsants (antiepileptics), such as Neurontin, though this is more powerful at pain relief than mood improvement. Similarly, antipsychotic drugs such as olanzapine (Zyprexa) might help with both pain and mood problems, but this is controversial, and the US Food and Drug Administration has so far not approved any antipsychotics for pain relief.[71]

But sorting out exactly how well the different drugs work is not easy. For instance, one 2009 review by Australian researchers for the Cochrane Collaboration pooled data from six studies and separately examined data from two other studies. They concluded that antidepressants (of several different types) were not effective at relieving low back pain.[72] That same year, however, a team from the United Kingdom also did a Cochrane review.[73] They asked specifically whether the antidepressant duloxetine (Cymbalta) relieves the pain of diabetic neuropathy or other chronic pain. They came to a more encouraging conclusion. At 60 milligrams a day (but not at a lower dose, 20 mg), they found that Cymbalta is effective against both diabetic neuropathy and fibromyalgia, although side effects from the drug forced 16 percent of patients to stop taking it.

A third Cochrane review looked at 61 randomized controlled trials of 20 different antidepressants in 3,293 people with neuropathic pain.[74] This review concluded that tricyclic antidepressants such as Elavil are somewhat effective against pain, as is venlaxafine (Effexor). The review found only "limited evidence" for the SSRIs such as Prozac.

Kurt Kroenke, the Indiana University pain researcher mentioned earlier, also combed through mountains of pain data, disease by disease. For irritable bowel syndrome, for instance, he found that the tricyclic antidepressants reduce pain but the SSRIs do not.[75] For back pain, the tricyclics were moderately effective but, again, not the SSRIs. For headache, once again, tricyclics seemed to help, especially as preventives, and the SSRIs didn't help at all. For fibromyalgia, tricyclics were beneficial for sleep problems as well as pain.

The best evidence for treating pain and depression together comes from another Kroenke study, the SCAMP trial. This was a randomized, controlled, 12-month study of people with chronic low back, hip, or knee pain who were also depressed.[76] Half of the people were taught self-management skills such as coping with negative emotions, knowing what situations trigger pain flare-ups, increasing physical activity, deep breathing, muscle relaxation, and so on. Each person also got individualized antidepressant medications, with the researchers trying different doses and different medications until something worked. Overall, the people who got this "optimized" antidepressant drug therapy plus the self-management training saw substantial improvements in depression and moderate reductions in pain severity and disability.

"CATASTROPHIZING"

One of the worst things you can do if you are in chronic pain is to catastrophize. *Catastrophizing* is a maladaptive cognitive and emotional habit that leads to focusing obsessively on pain, imagining all sorts of worst case scenarios and generally believing that the pain will be endless, life-wrecking, horrible, and unfixable.

Believe me—I know whereof I speak. Like many women, I was a big catastrophizer. Studies show that women *do* catastrophize more than men, and that, if it weren't for this tendency, the gap between men's and women's reported pain might be significantly smaller. Nobody knows *why* women catastrophize more, but researchers suspect it may be that girls, more than boys, pick up verbal and nonverbal catastrophizing cues from their mothers, as UCLA pediatric anesthesiologist Lonnie Zeltzer, among others, has found.[77] With osteoarthritis, for instance, both men and women live in considerable pain. And many people in pain, but particularly women, also tend to be depressed. But when researchers look more closely at men and women with osteoarthritis pain, it turns out that catastrophizing, not depression, accounts for much of the difference in pain experiences of men and women.[78]

The same seems to be true with experimental pain. At Johns Hopkins, researchers tested 198 healthy young people (115 of them women) in the lab, triggering pain by heat, cold, and ischemia (applying a tight tourniquet). When they asked men and women to react to the pain, the women catastrophized more than men, as gauged by self-reports. In other words, in this study, too, it was not mood or depression, but catastrophizing that was linked to women's reports of greater pain.[79]

To be honest, when you're in terrible pain, it's almost impossible *not* to catastrophize. After all, chronic pain *can* hugely impact your life, your mood, your well-being, your work, and your relationships. And, quite often, there really is no obvious medical fix. Even the pros catastrophize, as Russell Portenoy, a pain and palliative care specialist at Beth Israel Medical Center in New York and a leader in pain research, confessed to me a while back as we chatted in his office. "Years ago," he told me, "I woke up at 1 or 2 a.m. with a pain in my cheek, near my eye. I am a neurologist. So clearly, it was a brain tumor! Or cluster headaches. Should I go to the ER? Wake my wife? It was distressing. What did it mean? How serious was it?" The next morning he called his brother, a dentist, who solved the problem: an abscessed tooth, with referred pain to the eye.[80]

But catastrophizing does make a bad situation worse. And you *can* learn to reduce it—especially with cognitive behavioral therapy (CBT), which we'll get to soon.

There are several ways to tell how much you may be catastrophizing, including the 13-item Pain Catastrophizing Scale.[81] The scale is designed to measure the intensity of a person's tendency to ruminate, to magnify things, and to feel helpless. To take it, simply assign each item a number from 0 (not at all) to 4 (all the time), and then add up the score. Here are the statements:

1. I worry all the time about whether it will end.
2. I feel I can't go on.
3. It's terrible and I think it's never going to get any better.
4. It's awful and I feel that it overwhelms me.
5. I feel I can't stand it anymore.
6. I become afraid that the pain will get worse.
7. I keep thinking of other painful events.
8. I anxiously want the pain to go away.
9. I can't seem to get it out of my mind.
10. I keep thinking about how much it hurts.
11. I keep thinking about how badly I want the pain to stop.
12. There's nothing I can do to reduce the intensity of the pain.
13. I wonder whether something serious may happen.

Healthy, pain-free adults usually get catastrophizing scores in the single digits. If your score is in the mid-teens, you're a moderate catastrophizer. As your score creeps up toward 52, the highest possible, you're a serious catastrophizer. People with fibromyalgia, for instance, often score in the mid- to high 20s. Not surprisingly, people with chronic low back pain and arthritis also tend to have relatively high scores. Being a high catastrophizer is not just miserable, it's a bad prognostic sign. Catastrophizing can interfere with your ability to cope: It can amplify the way your nervous system processes pain, and it can actually get in the way of benefiting from treatment.[82]

Consider this: Rob Edwards, a staff psychologist at Boston's Brigham and Women's Hospital, and his team invited 42 healthy volunteers to the lab to take a pain catastrophizing questionnaire and get their blood drawn for baseline levels of cortisol, a stress hormone, and interleukin-6 (IL-6), a natural, pro-inflammatory chemical that plays a role in inflammatory diseases such as arthritis. The volunteers then underwent standardized pain testing—with hot, cold, and unpleasant mechanical stimuli. Not surprisingly, both cortisol and Il-6 rose during the painful stimulation. But cortisol went back down to baseline an hour later. Il-6, which can boost inflammatory pain, did not. It stayed up. And the greater a person's tendency to catastrophize, the more Il-6 went up and stayed up.[83]

With fibromyalgia, University of Michigan researchers found that high catastrophizers, when given the same objective pain stimuli in the lab as low catastrophizers, show greater brain activity on fMRI scans in parts of the brain that control anticipation of pain (medial frontal cortex and cerebellum), attention to pain (anterior cingulate cortex and prefrontal cortex), and emotional response to pain (an area called the claustrum, which is near the amygdala, a fear-processing center).[84] Moreover, the effects of catastrophizing held true regardless of whether the people with fibromyalgia were depressed or not, another strong clue that catastrophizing is an independent variable. Similar brain responses have been found in healthy people, too, not just people with chronic pain. In a study at the University of Toronto, researchers used fMRI scans and showed that catastrophizing had no effect on the purely sensory processing of experimental pain, but it did make affective regions of the brain light up.[85]

In my experience, it's comparatively easy to catch yourself when you're catastrophizing (as opposed to noticing when more subtle, harmful thoughts kick in). Catastrophizing thoughts often contain words like "always" and "never." In other words, you should "always" be on the lookout for these and "never" succumb to their seductive, but misplaced, logic.

And now, some good news. In recent years, a number of psychologists and psychiatrists have developed specific non-drug coping techniques to help people with chronic pain. If you practice these, chances are you will not only feel better emotionally, but your pain and ability to function may improve as well.[86] Based on numerous research findings—and an abundance of common sense—the approach has 10 steps, which have been shown to work.[87, 88] Many pain clinics now offer versions of this approach, but you may wind up putting together your own program (as I did).

The first step, which you've already done if you've read Chapter 2, is to understand how pain works, including the idea (dubbed the *gate control theory*) that pain perception occurs when small fibers carrying their pain signals flow up (as if through an open gate) to the brain, through the dorsal horn in the spinal cord. Inhibitory signals travel down from the brain to the dorsal horn, damping down pain (as if closing the gate). The idea is to use various mental techniques to boost these pain inhibition signals.

Once you understand basic pain biology, the goal is to practice specific techniques. The most basic is relaxation. (Read Herbert Benson's classic, *The Relaxation Response*, if you haven't already.[89]) A corollary here is the technique of *progressive relaxation*, in which you lie or sit comfortably and focus on parts of the body in succession—the fingers, the hands, the forearms, upper arms, and so on—and then try to relax each set of muscles in turn. The mere fact of paying attention to parts of your body that don't hurt can distract you from your pain, and the muscle relaxation also directly eases tension and thereby, some components of your pain.

But it's not just about calming yourself down. It's also about changing your behavior—increasing *adaptive* responses to pain, like exercise, and decreasing the *maladaptive* ones. For instance, it can help a lot to pace yourself throughout the day: to alternate activity and rest. I was at a conference not long ago with Cindy Steinberg, the woman you met in Chapter 1 who has been in constant pain for years since a heavy filing cabinet fell on her, ruining her back. At the conference, she calmly gave her speech from her seat on the panel, then quietly got up and went to lie down on the floor in the corner of the room for the next hour or so as other people spoke, then went back to her seat to participate in the animated general discussion. Nobody batted an eye. And I suspect we all admired her ability to quietly take care of herself.

Setting reasonable goals is important, too: Given the limitations that chronic pain imposes, it's crucial to set goals that you can realistically expect to accomplish. Acceptance—a slippery concept—fits in here, too. "The struggle to control persistent pain can become so all-encompassing that patients neglect other valued aspects of their lives such as family, friends, work, and leisure," Duke psychologist Francis Keefe has found. "In such instances, a balance of change and acceptance efforts might be particularly useful; change is used where it is likely to work, and acceptance is used when change efforts are not likely to succeed."[90]

Finally, add pleasant activities to your day, and make sure to schedule in the time for them so they don't get lost in the shuffle.

COGNITIVE BEHAVIORAL THERAPY

Of all the coping skills shown to help people with certain chronic pain conditions, cognitive behavioral therapy (CBT) is among the most effective.[91, 92] In fact, CBT is one of the biggest success stories of modern psychotherapy. Instead of focusing on deep, underlying emotional issues stemming from childhood (which also can be useful), CBT is very here-and-now oriented. It may not change your underlying pain per se. If you have rheumatoid arthritis, for instance, it may not make your joint inflammation better. But it can ease your emotional *distress* about pain, which in turn can reduce your suffering. As with other treatments—even opioids—CBT is not a magic bullet. But it can help.

The CBT approach grew out of the work of psychologist Albert Ellis, sometimes dubbed the grandfather of CBT. It was developed further by psychiatrist Aaron Beck and has been popularized still further by psychiatrist David Burns. (If you're unfamiliar with CBT, I strongly recommend reading *Feeling Good: The New Mood Therapy*, by Burns.[93]) CBT emphasizes becoming aware—even keeping diaries—of your thoughts, feelings, and behaviors as they connect to significant events in daily life. The idea is that "thoughts, beliefs and expectations play a key role in the perception of pain and how people adjust to pain."[94]

Once you have noticed and identified these thoughts (which is not easy, given that thoughts fly by in a nanosecond), you then critique them, asking yourself how realistic or true they are. For instance, if you're thinking, "I'm a total loser," chances are you'll feel terrible. If you notice this thought, hold it in your mind for a moment, and replace it by a more accurate one, you might think, "I mess up sometimes, but often I'm pretty good at things." The result is that you will probably feel better. Similarly, if you're thinking, "The pain will always be this intense forever," you might look at your diary and, hopefully, see that in fact your pain fluctuates somewhat during the day, so it won't be at its max all the time.

In a study of people with temporomandibular joint disorder (TMD), for instance, those who had had four sessions of CBT training experienced impressively less pain—and less interference with daily activities—than similar patients who had received only education about TMD. The results also appeared to endure, lasting at least one year.[95] CBT has been shown to reduce the pain of other specific syndromes, too: fibromyalgia, chronic fatigue syndrome, irritable bowel syndrome, back pain, and, as a preventive strategy, headache as well.[96]

In a massive 2006 review of 16 rigorous meta-analyses—each meta-analysis itself a compilation of data from other studies—CBT was found very effective for psychiatric problems such as depression that is not part of manic-depressive disorder, generalized anxiety disorder, panic disorder, social phobia, posttraumatic stress disorder, and childhood depressive and anxiety disorders. CBT was effective for pain, too, though the evidence was not as strong as that for the psychiatric disorders.[97]

An earlier meta-analysis of 25 studies by British researchers led by clinical psychologist Stephen Morley at the University of Leeds found that CBT and biofeedback were effective at reducing the overall experience of pain, though the improvement was modest.[98] More recent research by Morley found that between one in three and one in seven patients using CBT achieved "clinically significant gains" on such "endpoints" as pain experience, interference in daily life, and emotional distress, though it's often tricky, he cautions, to know exactly what these measures mean in real life.[99, 100, 101] Cognitive behavioral and other psychological therapies also work for children and adolescents, a 2009 review showed.[102]

More recently, Harvard Medical School researchers pooled results from 11 studies of CBT in which people with chronic pain learned the technique online. They found that even web-based CBT can help reduce pain, though again, the improvements were small.[103] CBT, by the way, can also be helpful against the depression that often accompanies pain.[104] And CBT seems to be especially effective in people who catastrophize. People in pain who learn to change their negative beliefs and reduce catastrophizing wind up with less physical disability, fewer depressive symptoms, and lower pain intensity, according to work by researchers from the University of Washington.[105] Moreover, CBT reduces catastrophizing, even among people who have been in pain a long time—as long as 12 years.[106]

DISTRACTION

Distraction has long been known to help divert attention, at least in the short term, from minor moments of pain, and even not-so-minor ones. In a meta-analysis involving pooled data from 51 studies with nearly 4,000 pain patients, for instance, music was shown to reduce pain and the need for opioid drugs. The effects were small, but good enough to take the edge off.[107] Distraction works in animals, too. In one study, Irish researchers distracted rats by putting them in a novel environment or giving them a novel object, after which the animals showed reduced responses to painful stimuli.[108] But distraction is now going high-tech for people in pain, particularly as a way to pry attention away from excruciating medical procedures such as burn debridement—the frequent changing of burn dressings and cleaning of wounds to prevent infection.

Among the leaders in this movement is a team of psychologists from the University of Seattle—Hunter Hoffman, Mark Jensen, and David Patterson—who wondered whether distraction using virtual reality, complete with very cool goggles, might help during burn treatments.[109] They tried it on one of their early patients, a 40-year-old man with deep burns on his legs, neck, back, and buttocks who needed constant opioids just to get through the day. When his wounds were being cared for, the drugs barely touched the extreme pain. But virtual reality helped significantly. Granted, it does look a bit weird. The burn patient sits hooked up to a goggle apparatus as a nurse cuts away the bandage on one hand, while the patient grips a computer joy stick with his other bandaged hand. He wears a headset and maneuvers his way through a make-believe place called SnowWorld. You can't see his face, but his body language suggests he's into the game.

Virtual reality is "very immersive," Patterson told me. With goggles on their eyes and sounds coming in through earphones, "people fly around shooting snowballs at igloos" in an engrossing, imaginary world that takes the person's attention away, at least somewhat, while nurses and doctors do their job. It gives users the sense that they are somewhere else.[110] By drawing attention away from wound care, the researchers believe, virtual reality leaves less attention available to process incoming pain signals.[111, 112, 113] In one study of experimentally induced pain, the Seattle team tested the virtual reality technique in healthy young people. They divided 77 volunteers into three groups before subjecting them to pain (heat). One group used a high-tech virtual reality helmet, the second got a lower-tech one, and the third group got no distraction at all. The high-tech group had significantly less pain in the "worst pain" tests, experienced less "pain unpleasantness," spent less time thinking about pain—and had more fun.[114]

In a study of 12 real pain patients, the patients rated a virtual reality experience called SpiderWorld better at pain control than opioids.[115] And pain patients not only *say* they feel less pain, their fMRI brain scans corroborate it, the Seattle team has found. In one experiment, when the team compared virtual reality analgesia to no virtual reality, the technique reduced activity in five brain areas known to be activated with pain: the anterior cingulate cortex, primary and secondary somatosensory cortex, the insula, and the thalamus.[116]

To be sure, not all people with pain have access to virtual reality equipment. But the distraction principle is a good one: Drawing attention away from pain can help.

Researchers from University Medical Center Hamburg-Eppendorf in Germany showed that distraction can actually reduce the transmission of pain signals from the spinal cord to the brain. Using a group of 20 male volunteers, the researchers, led by neuroscientist Christian Sprenger, used two different forms of a memory task to distract the volunteers during pain tests using a heat stimulus on the arm. During the tests, the volunteers were placed in fMRI machines that tracked neural activity in their spinal cords. The easy memory test proved too unchallenging—it wasn't enough of a distraction to block ascending pain signals. The harder test, however, did block pain signals significantly—at the level of the spinal cord, an astounding discovery.[117] As an extra measure, the scientists then injected either a placebo or an opioid blocker (naloxone) to see whether distraction blocked pain signals partly by generating endogenous opioids. It did. When given naloxone, distracted subjects were not able to block pain signals as efficiently.

BIOFEEDBACK

Biofeedback is a fascinating technique that provides yet more proof—as if any were needed—of the instantaneous, and intricate, mind–body connection. If you want a simple demonstration of basic biofeedback, get a blood pressure monitoring kit from the drugstore, go home, lie down, and take your blood pressure. Then consciously relax your muscles and, to the extent you can, your thoughts and your emotions. Take your blood pressure again a few minutes later. Chances are, it will have gone down. It can work the other way, too. If your blood pressure is high the first time and you freak out about it, chances are your second reading will be higher. Officially, *biofeedback* is defined as "a process that enables an individual to learn how to change physiological activity for the purposes of improving health and performance."[118] And pain reduction is becoming one of the main uses of biofeedback, as German researchers, among others, have shown.[119, 120]

There are several different ways to do biofeedback. One is with *surface electcromyography* (sEMG). In this technique, surface electrodes are placed over certain muscles to detect signals called *action potentials* that trigger muscle contractions. This type of biofeedback is used for a number of pain problems, including headaches, chronic pain, neck spasms, and TMD.[121] A fancier technique uses electrodes placed on the scalp to detect electrical activation in the brain. Scientists are just beginning to explore how well this technique, using electroencephalography (EEG), may help reduce pain.[122]

But the most exciting type of biofeedback for pain comes from the lab of neuroscientist Sean Mackey, director of the Stanford Systems Neuroscience and Pain Lab. It's technically called neurofeedback with real-time functional magnetic resonance imaging (rtfMRI). Unlike traditional biofeedback, which monitors *downstream* processes like heart rate, blood pressure, temperature, and the like as a way to sense and reduce the arousal of the autonomic nervous system in general, rtfMRI neurofeedback focuses *upstream*, on particular brain areas that act earlier in the experiential process. In a pivotal experiment published in 2005, Mackey's team had volunteers—both healthy people who agreed to undergo experimental pain and people with chronic pain—lie in fMRI scanners and watch and control their own brains in real time.[123]

Mackey was interested in one section of the brain in particular, the anterior cingulate cortex (ACC), a structure that is well known to have many functions, including working memory, focusing attention, orienting attention to pain, encoding the intensity of pain, and emotional regulation of pain. The ACC, in other words, is a key pain processing center. "Our question," Mackey told me, "was to see if people could learn how to control isolated regions of the brain—in this case, the anterior cingulate cortex—and if they could, would that lead to increased control over pain."[124] The answer to both was *yes*.

The first part of the experiment involved healthy young people (20 men and 16 women whose average age was 23). The researchers taught them various cognitive strategies that would lead to increased or decreased brain activity in the ACC—such as focusing attention, distraction, and reappraisal (e.g., telling themselves the pain was not so bad or not dangerous). As Mackey's volunteers practiced, they watched a computer screen that was getting signals from the ACC. The computer displayed the incoming information visually in several ways, such as having a flame look hotter or cooler depending on the messages from their ACCs. The volunteers got pretty good at controlling their ACCs. "Some people found it fun, others had a hard time," says Mackey.

The volunteers were subjected to heat stimulation on their arms, ranging from mild to fairly painful, as they learned to consciously control the activity of the ACC. Amazingly, they were able to amplify or damp down at will their own perceptions of pain using the techniques they had been taught. Using several control groups, the researchers were able to show that this learned control over pain was due to control over the ACC in particular, not to a generalized autonomic relaxation. And they showed that the learned ability to control pain held true only when the volunteers were focusing on the ACC, not on other parts of the brain. "We discovered that directed control can be learned and that this does lead to specific changes in the perception of pain," says Mackey.

The team then did much the same experiment with eight people who were long-term chronic pain patients; in this condition, the researchers did not subject the patients to experimental pain. Like the healthy volunteers, the real pain patients learned to control their ACC—with dramatic results. They reported a decrease in pain intensity of 64 percent on a standardized pain questionnaire and a 44 percent decrease on another measure of pain. The next step, says Mackey, will be further experiments to see how rtfMRI neurofeedback, mindfulness meditation, cognitive behavioral therapy, and acupuncture work to control pain and the common and distinct brain systems that are affected.

MEDITATION

If you haven't yet discovered mindfulness meditation, or think it's too new age-y, Eastern, or weird, it's time to put aside such prejudices and give it a try. It's fairly easy to learn. It's free. It's available 24/7. And it works. Granted, meditation won't levitate the Pentagon, or cure cancer. But in 20–30 minutes a day, it can quiet the mind through what some call moment-to-moment nonjudgmental awareness. Conceptually, mindfulness meditation is different from a more generalized practice such as Herbert Benson's famous "relaxation response." But meditation has been linked to some of the same responses as the relaxation response, which has been shown to lower blood pressure, heart rate, and respiration; reduce anxiety, anger, hostility, and mild to moderate depression; help alleviate insomnia; and reduce some types of pain.[125, 126, 127, 128, 129]

There are lots of different meditation techniques, many of them based on thousands of years of Buddhist tradition. But the basic idea is to sit quietly and focus your mind on the present, becoming aware of your thoughts and feelings without judging them or spinning out "cognitive elaborations" of them. Many people count breaths; others silently repeat the word "calm" on the in breath and "relax" on the out breath. Some stare at a burning candle. Others listen to a pleasant sound, like waves or rain in a forest. (Many people do yoga and tai chi, too, both of which have strong meditative elements; we will discuss those in Chapter 13.) In terms of dealing with chronic pain, mindfulness meditation is essentially a way to stop fighting with the pain and learn to work with it.

I'm reminded of a conversation I had recently in the ladies' locker room after one of my swim team practices. I was speaking with another swimmer, chatting about this book, and she told me about a friend, a potter, who had been in terrible pain and had found relief at a pain clinic at a prominent Boston hospital.

"What worked?" I asked, intrigued.

My friend stopped getting dressed, smiled and pointed to her head. "They taught her that pain was her friend," she said.

"Really?"

"Well, not quite," she answered. "But they convinced her it was not her enemy."

That's the key, experts concluded at a workshop not long ago on acceptance and meditation sponsored by the American Pain Society.[130] The goal, they stressed, is to become more psychologically flexible, to not stay stuck in feelings and beliefs that just make the pain worse. This means loosening your preoccupation with the past or the future and your own storyline (especially if you are the star of your story—the tragic hero or heroine). It means, quite literally, changing your mind.

There have been countless studies documenting meditation's myriad positive effects. But the groundbreaker—the first to show how meditation changes activity in the front of the brain and the first to document positive changes in immune function—was done in 2003.[131] The leaders were meditation guru Jon Kabat-Zinn, a former molecular biologist who created the widely used eight-week mindfulness-based stress reduction program at the University of Massachusetts Medical School, and neuroscientist Richard Davidson, director of the laboratory for affective neuroscience at the University of Wisconsin.

The basic idea is that in people who are stressed, the right cortex (the more emotional side) of the brain is overactive and the left cortex (the more analytical side), underactive. Stressed-out people also show heightened activity in the amygdala, a key center for processing fear. By contrast, people who are habitually calm and happy typically show greater activity in the left frontal cortex relative to the right, and tend to pump out less of the stress hormone cortisol. Davidson and Kabat-Zinn recruited stressed-out volunteers from the Promega Corporation, a high-tech firm in Madison, Wisconsin. At the outset, all volunteers were tested with electroencephalograms (EEGs), in which electrodes were placed on the scalp to collect brainwave information. The volunteers were then randomized into two groups—25 in the meditation group, which got Kabat-Zinn's eight-week course, and 16 in the control group.

At the end of eight weeks, all the volunteers got another round of EEG tests and a flu shot. They also got blood tests to check for antibody response to the shot. Four months later, all got EEG tests again. By the end of the study, the meditators' brains showed exactly what the researchers had hypothesized, a demonstrable shift toward the left frontal lobe, while the nonmeditators did not. The meditators also had more robust immune responses to the flu shots.

In 2005, using more modern scanning technology, magnetic resonance imaging (MRIs) instead of EEGs, neuroscientists Sara Lazar and Bruce Fischl at Massachusetts General Hospital in Boston studied 20 volunteers who were experienced meditators.[132] The volunteers were serious meditators and yoga practitioners who had been meditating for years for an average of 40 minutes a day. The scientists compared their brain scans to those of 15 nonmeditators. The results? Strong evidence that meditation can produce long-term changes in the brain. Indeed, meditation was linked with increased cortical thickness all over the brain, but specifically in parts of the brain associated with attention, interoception (paying attention to internal, bodily stimuli, like noticing that your stomach is in knots or your neck is tense), and sensory processing. This was the first structural evidence for experience-dependent brain plasticity associated with meditation practice.

Similarly, researchers from the University of Montreal studied 17 long-term meditators and 18 controls using MRI and found lower pain sensitivity in the meditators and greater thickness in pain-related brain regions, including the anterior cingulate cortex, the parahippocampal gyrus, and the anterior insula.[133] The researchers suspect that one way in which meditation helps is by "decoupling" the sensory component of pain from the cognitive-evaluative component.[134]

Other studies have since poured out of labs all over the world. In fibromyalgia patients, a mindfulness-based stress reduction course reduced depression and overall sympathetic nervous system arousal.[135] A quasi-randomized 2007 study came to similar conclusions, including reduction of pain.[136] A 2011 study similarly found that an eight-week mindfulness meditation course reduces reactivity to the threat of pain.[137] Another study of a similar stress reduction course at University for the Humanistics in Utrecht, the Netherlands, was a bit more disappointing—only modest improvement for fibromyalgia patients.[138] And in a 2011 study using brain scans, researchers from Marquette University in Milwaukee and Wake Forest University showed that mindfulness meditation—even with just four days of training—reduced scores of pain unpleasantness and pain intensity by 57 percent and 40 percent, respectively.[139]

With experimentally induced, as opposed to chronic, real-life pain, even very short-term meditation practice seems to help. After meditating for just 20 minutes a day for three days, a 2010 study showed, volunteers' ratings of experimental pain dropped sharply.[140] And after you learn the basics in a mindfulness-based stress reduction course, the more you practice meditating at home, the more relief you will get, according to a 2010 Drexel University study.[141] In a lab at the University of Manchester in the United Kingdom, researchers compared long-term meditators to nonmeditators as they administered painful stimuli with laser beams, with the same level of pain stimulation for both groups.[142] The meditators perceived the pain as less unpleasant than the nonmeditators, and the more meditation experience they had, the less pain they perceived.

The standard eight-week mindfulness-based stress reduction course has also been shown to increase gray matter—brain density—in the hippocampus, a center for memory in the brain, and to decrease gray-matter density in the amygdala, a center for processing fear and stress. In one study, researchers Sara Lazar and Britta Holzel in Boston, studied 16 volunteers before and after the eight-week meditation course and compared them to 17 people who did not take the course. The study documents the underlying changes in brain structure that occur with—and probably account for—the improved mental health of people who learn mindfulness meditation.[143] Specifically, the research showed an increase of 1 to 3 percent in the brain's gray matter in areas responsible for learning, memory, and emotional regulation. This has implications for empathy, as well, because the brain regions involved help a person see things not just from his or her own point of view but that of others as well.

In a different 2011 paper, Lazar, along with Tim Gard, a colleague at Mass General, and colleagues from Germany, found that meditators, but not nonmeditators, were able to reduce "pain unpleasantness" in experimental pain labs by 22 percent, and anticipatory anxiety by 29 percent, when they were in a "mindful" state.[144] The fMRI scans of the volunteers also hinted at that "decoupling" effect: The meditators' brains were able to separate out the sensory aspect of pain from the affect part. "It makes sense," says Lazar, who took up meditating herself several years ago. "When you meditate, you just note sensations, you don't try to change them, you don't elaborate on them. So the sensory experience is more intense, but it doesn't bother you as much. You accept it. You separate out the affect from the sensory experience."[145]

HYPNOSIS

Hypnosis and self-hypnosis are similar to other techniques we've talked about in that they involve deep relaxation and focused attention. The big difference is that hypnosis also involves "suggestions" for a person to experience something different (for instance, something pleasurable rather than painful) or to do something different when "cued" (such as reach for a stick of gum instead of a cigarette). Experts define *hypnosis* as a social interaction in which one person responds to suggestions offered by another person, the hypnotist, for experiences involving alterations in perception, memory, and voluntary action.[146] In this sense, hypnosis is also similar to interactive guided-imagery, a technique in which the patient and therapist work together, in a less hierarchical way than traditional hypnosis, to focus attention on images that are healing. In self-hypnosis, the patient learns to do this for himself or herself.

There are numerous types of "suggestions" that hypnotherapists can use to help offset pain. Sometimes it works to suggest that the pain is changing, perhaps diminishing or turning to numbness, or to imagine a growing sense of comfort. Sometimes the therapist can suggest that a stabbing pain be imagined more as vibrations; other times, the suggestion might be that the pain is ever so subtly moving from, say, the abdomen to a leg. A person in pain can also try to imagine being dissociated from the body—moving into another, more pleasant place.

To be sure, in some circles, hypnosis still has something of a bad rap. "It was not so long ago that a predominant image associated with hypnotic phenomena was that of a mustachioed, dark-eyed man, focusing with a fixed stare upon a vulnerable, young woman, conveying by the intensity of his stern visage the plan to coerce and perhaps harm this helpless young person," wrote Joseph Barber, a psychologist at the University of Washington.[147] But in reality, hypnosis can be a useful nonpharmacological tool for reducing the impact of pain, and dramatic when it works. "To observe the tranquil face of a patient undergoing a painful medical procedure, with no anesthetic agent except words, is a remarkable, perhaps even unbelievable, experience," as Barber put it.

In 2011, University of Washington psychologist Mark Jensen and colleagues reported on a study of 33 adults with chronic pain, finding that those using a combination of self-hypnosis and cognitive restructuring were better at reducing pain than those using either technique alone.[148] Jensen's team also showed that self-hypnosis decreased daily pain in people with spinal cord injuries.[149] Hypnosis also helps reduce pain in children undergoing painful procedures such as lumbar puncture and bone marrow aspiration.[150]

Research studies, including some using neuroimaging, suggest that hypnosis, at least in lab experiments, can block pain signals from reaching the somatosensory cortex in the brain and can also modulate emotional response to pain in the limbic (emotional processing) system.[151] No one is quite sure how it works. But it "is not magic," says Jensen.[152] "It's pure physiology. When you focus your awareness on one object, the brain calms down. When the brain calms down, it hurts less." Like many of the other mind techniques we've talked about here, hypnosis will probably not eliminate your pain. But it can help reduce *suffering* so that you can feel more in control and more relaxed and, hopefully, can sleep better as well.[153]

EMPATHY

So far, we've been talking about mind–body interventions that may help ease pain, or at least the emotional suffering that accompanies pain. Empathy—the ability to feel another person's feelings, including pain—is different.

While empathy can be one of the most healing things that a physician can offer, it is obviously not something that a patient can force a physician to have. When healthcare providers lack empathy, it's not that they are intrinsically mean, according to psychologist Kenneth Prkachin of the University of British Columbia.[154, 155] It's more that doctors and nurses tune out and become numb to other people's pain to protect themselves precisely because they do see so much pain every day. Even the Dalai Lama, who embodies "an unusual capacity to respond with empathy," as James Austin notes in his book *Selfless Insight*,[156] might buckle under the pressure of seeing people in pain all day long in a stressful, time-sensitive managed care system.

Not surprisingly, doctors who themselves have experienced serious pain are more likely to be empathic. In general, doctors who have undergone treatment for serious medical problems tend to be nicer—they acknowledge when they've kept patients waiting, they listen carefully to patients' concerns and complaints, and they're more attuned to the nonverbal aspects of care, Harvard Medical School psychologist Robert Jamison told me.[157]

From an evolutionary point of view, it's interesting that empathy even exists. Why would we mammals be so programmed to feel one another's pain? Nobody really knows, but empathy might have survival advantages if it prompted healthy members of a tribe or herd to take care of their wounded members. But that raises more questions: Where in the brain does empathy lie? And how does it work?

It's clear that when you observe pain in others, the same regions in your own brain react as though you yourself were feeling the pain.[158] A leading hypothesis involves mirror neurons—nerve cells first discovered in macaque monkeys that fire both when an animal itself performs an action and when it observes the same action performed by another animal. In animals, mirror neurons were first found in and near the premotor cortex and later in the parietal lobe. This discovery set off quite a buzz among scientists because these mirror neurons were bimodal—that is, they acted both like sensory neurons and like motor neurons—a striking degree of neuronal flexibility. It's not clear yet whether mirror neurons exist in other parts of the brain. But Harvard Medical School neuroscientist Marco Loggia suspects, on the basis of brain scanning studies, that they do.[159]

Supporting the mirror neuron theory of empathy is a growing body of evidence suggesting that dysfunctional or missing mirror neurons may be involved in the lack of affect in cold-hearted people and people with autism, another clue to the potentially important role these cells may play in empathy.[160, 161, 162, 163, 164, 165]

Empathy comes naturally to most of us. By age five or six, most kids can empathize when they look at facial expressions of pain in others, psychologist Prkachin told me. And most of us get better at it as we get older.[166] Empathy is strongest in married couples who really like each other, too. In a study by researchers at the University of Virginia and the University of Wisconsin, 16 married women were subjected to the threat of an electric shock while their brains were being scanned with fMRIs. The women were sometimes allowed to hold the hand of their husbands, sometimes the hand of an anonymous male experimenter, and sometimes no hand at all. The scans showed that a woman's neurological response to the threat was significantly lower—she remained calmer—when she held her husband's hand than when she held the stranger's. And the better the marriage, the calmer the woman remained.[167]

Wonderful as empathy can be, though, and as much as we may crave it, it can take a toll on both the empathizer and the person being empathized with. "Empathy hurts," concluded one team of McGill researchers who studied 48 healthy human volunteers.[168] A different McGill team found much the same thing in mice: When one member of a pair of mice observes its cage-mate in pain, its own sensitivity to pain increases.[169] Some people—called "extreme empaths" or "pain synaes-thetes"—have such exaggerated reactions to other people's pain that they sometimes can't tell whose pain they are feeling: their own, or someone else's.[170]

And too much empathy, if you're the one being empathized with, can sometimes make your own pain worse. In one study several years ago, Australian researchers put dozens of young adults, men and women, through experimental pain tests in the lab. During the tests, women did not seek out interaction with an empathic person any more than men did. But when they did, the empathic interactions had generally nega-tive effects on pain perception and coping, the researchers found.[171] The same thing can happen within marriages, too. If a partner becomes overly solicitous of the spouse in pain, the spouse may feel even more pain, more psychological distress, and more physical disability.[172]

As for the toll of empathy on empathizers? It's real. In 2004, University of London neuroscientists Tania Singer, Chris Frith, and their team assessed brain activity in volunteers receiving experimental pain stimuli and compared this to their brain activity while they watched a loved one receiving a similar pain stimulus. The same brain areas—the ante-rior insula, anterior cingulate cortex, as well as the brainstem and cer-ebellum—"lit up" in both conditions.[173] In other words, they really did feel their loved one's pain. Similarly, Prkachin and his team showed on brain scans that the same brain areas (notably the anterior cingulate cortex and the insula) light up when a person reacts to facial expres-sions of pain in someone else and when they're experiencing their own, experimentally induced pain.[174]

But it turns out that whether you empathize with someone in pain may also depend on how much you like them. Singer and colleagues asked male and female volunteers to play a kind of economic game in which confederates of the researchers (stooges, if you will) played the game either fairly or unfairly. The team then scanned the brains of the volunteers while they watched the confederates receiving experimental pain. Both men and women's brains lit up in empathy with confeder-ates who had played fairly. But men (though not women) changed their tune abruptly—shutting off empathy completely—when they were watching pain being inflicted on unfair players.[175]

So where does all this leave us? There seems to be an optimal amount of empathy that can be helpful and comforting to a person in pain yet not cause too much distress in the empathizer. Ideally, this delicate balance could be taught in medical schools. Since most medical students are young and may not yet have experienced serious pain in their lives, it could be useful, as part of their education, for them to be subjected to small, controlled experiences with intense pain so they could be more empathic with patients. Indeed, researchers at Johns Hopkins have been trying just this approach.

CHAPTER 7

Opioid Wars, Part I

The Problem

OVERVIEW

Hyrum Neizer would be dead today if his wife hadn't walked in on him with the gun in his mouth. He was in unremitting pain. Because of the pain, and the drugs he took trying to control it, he had lost his job as a Salt Lake City truck driver. Without his $80,000 income a year, he quickly lost his house. Then his car and, along the way, his self-esteem, his role as husband and father of two young teenagers, and his manhood.[1] With no place to live, Hyrum and his wife Dena, a cake decorator, reluctantly turned to her mother, who lent them the money to rent a truck to move their furniture—and their lives—to her house. The thought that passed through his mind just before his wife caught him with the gun was: "If I die, who will move all this stuff?"

Hyrum is a solid, decent human being, a "proud person," in his words, a man who never wanted anything that he didn't earn or deserve. Yet his life was ruined not just by his chronic physical pain but by the very people who were supposed to be helping him—doctors: They eventually made him believe that, because he relied on pain relievers, he was a drug abuser. He was not. He was simply, like 100 million other Americans, a person in chronic pain. "All I wanted was to get back to normal, to get rid of the pain," he told me one chilly autumn morning several years ago in his doctor's office at the University of Utah.

Until the headaches started, more than a decade ago, Hyrum said he had been enjoying a great life. He had always relished his physical prowess—he's six foot five, 290 pounds. While taking courses in criminology and police science at the University of Washington, he played football for the Huskies and tried to go pro. When that didn't pan out, he moved to Salt Lake City to help his grandmother, who had fallen ill. Shortly after he arrived, he met Dena and married her less than a year later. Married life started well. He initially wanted to get a job in law enforcement in Salt Lake, but the pay was too low. So he became a teamster, driving trucks for $18.50 an hour. After the kids were born, Hyrum would often do extra runs: "When my kids wanted stuff, I worked even more."

But then, the headaches started. "Really bad ones, twice a week," he recalled. Initially, the doctor gave him pain relievers. But the pain did not abate. He went to the emergency room, again and again. It was humiliating. It was always the same. "I sat there for frickin' ever. It was killing me. There were tears in my eyes. I'm a big guy, but I was crying." The doctors began to suspect that he was just trying to get drugs. He went to another doctor, who gave him the same prescription. But that doctor, too, eventually disbelieved him and said, "No more pills." Doctor after doctor assumed he was lying about his pain.

"They had me convinced I was a drug abuser." He was devastated. "It was so bad I checked into a neuropsychiatric hospital," he said. "Everybody was telling me I had a drug problem. When you hear you are a drug abuser for so long, you start to believe it." He went to Narcotics Anonymous meetings, even though he didn't fit the profile of a drug abuser. "Everybody was telling their story. My heart felt for them. But their stories weren't my story. I didn't have the desire to sell a kidney for drugs. I didn't want to rob pharmacies for OxyContin." All he wanted was for his pain to stop.

After the first suicide attempt, there were others, and, in his words, "major, major depression." He tried to throw himself in front of a train, hoping to make it look as though he just slipped. Luckily, he failed. He considered rolling the car off a mountain pass. "Just something to make the pain go away." Even Dena, like frustrated spouses of other people in pain, began to doubt whether his pain was real. One night, he recalled bitterly, "She threw me an icepack and said, 'Just suffer.'" So he did, lying down in the other room. But the pain soon drove him out again. He begged Dena to take him to the hospital. "I felt like my head would explode."

Finally, these doctors believed him and ran tests looking for the cause for his pain, something his previous doctors, assuming he was a drug seeker, had not bothered to do. It turned out he had two aneurysms—ballooning arteries in the brain. He was operated on that night for one and several months later for the other.

COLLIDING EMERGENCIES: PAIN PATIENTS VERSUS STREET ABUSERS

While stories of prescription drug abuse dominate the headlines, stories like Hyrum's almost never do. And that is a big problem.

The reality is that there are *two* public health emergencies—*epidemics*, if you will—in the United States today, and they are on a collision course. One is the emergency of undertreated pain due in some measure to limited access to opioids. Access to opioids is often difficult for pain patients because of exaggerated fears of abuse and addiction, even though most pain patients never become addicts.[2] (By some estimates, as many as a third of chronic pain patients who need opioids don't get them.[3]) The other emergency is abuse of opioid (formerly called narcotic) drugs such as OxyContin and Vicodin for illegal, nonmedical purposes, though whether the term *epidemic* truly applies here is debatable.[4]

The result of these colliding patterns is what some call the *opioid conundrum*—people with chronic pain (often older people with no history of substance abuse) can't get the opioids they need and could probably use responsibly, while street abusers, often young people, get them all too easily.[5, 6] This conundrum is at the heart of the opioid mess in America, and discovering the truth—or truths—is difficult indeed, for patients, for doctors, for policymakers, and for journalists like me. For the record, I have no ties to and receive no money from either "side" in these opioid wars. Like many others, I have struggled to figure out what to believe—and whom.

Complicating this struggle is the fact that many respected pain researchers and professional organizations receive funding from pharmaceutical companies that make opioids. That clearly raises red flags for potential conflict of interest, though it obviously does not mean their information is automatically invalid, as the mainstream press seems to think. At least there *is* some transparency about industry funding on the websites for some of these not-for-profit groups, through tracking services such as GuideStar.org, and on the IRS website.[7] On the other hand, there is little transparency about funding for the major group on the other side, Physicians for Responsible Opioid Prescribing (PROP), which is opposed to what it views as excessive prescribing of opioids for long-term use.

The group says on its website that it gets no funding from drug companies. According to the group's leader, the group simply "passes the hat" among members for cash.[8] Unlike many other pain organizations, it's not legally categorized as a not-for-profit organization, although it uses the ".org" tag on its website (www.supportprop.org), which in the public mind often connotes not-for-profit. The group at one point tried to join a larger organization that does have not-for-profit status, but that arrangement did not happen.[9]

I want to be clear up front. The complex truth is that opioids, especially opioids for long-term use in chronic non-cancer pain, are probably both underprescribed for some patients and overprescribed for others. I'm also not suggesting that opioids are *the* answer for people in severe pain. Many people with terrible pain can get significant help from nonopioid treatments, including mind–body approaches (see Chapter 6), exercise (see Chapter 13), and alternative remedies (Chapter 11). Like opioids, these approaches are also hugely underutilized. Nor am I suggesting that opioids are wonder drugs even when they *are* needed and *are* prescribed appropriately. Overall, they reduce persistent pain only 30 to 40 percent. And, as we'll see later in this chapter, it's far from clear how well they work over the long term. Opioids, in other words, may be necessary, but they are rarely sufficient. What I *am* saying is that government drug policy seems to be lopsided, politicized, stacked against legitimate pain patients, and fueled by public hysteria over abuse of prescription pain relievers. That hysteria, in turn, is fueled by often-misleading media coverage.[10, 11]

That said, prescription pain reliever abuse is unquestionably a major problem. "Enough prescription painkillers were prescribed in 2010 to medicate every American adult around-the-clock for a month," as the Centers for Disease Control and Prevention put it in November 2011. "Although most of these pills were prescribed for a medical purpose, many ended up in the hands of people who misused or abused them."[12, 13, 14] By 2009, drug "poisoning" exceeded fatal motor vehicle accidents as a cause of death.[15, 16]

In 2010, about 12 million Americans aged 12 or older reported non-medical use of prescription pain relievers in the past year, according to government figures. Prescription pain reliever overdoses in 2008 were three times higher than in 1999.[17] Even newborn babies get swept up into the opioid abuse problem because of opioid-abusing mothers. The illicit drug use rate is 16.2 percent among pregnant teenagers and 7.4 percent among pregnant women aged 18 to 25, with the result that more and more babies are being born with neonatal abstinence syndrome, or drug withdrawal, according to a 2012 study in the *Journal of the American Medical Association*.[18] Indeed, between 2000 and 2009, the incidence of neonatal abstinence syndrome grew from 1.20 in every 1,000 hospital births per year to 3.39, with healthcare costs soaring in tandem. There's also no question that drug makers have spurred—and profited from—all this, by shamelessly promoting their drugs while underplaying the risks, as we'll see in a minute.[19]

But I am *also* saying that we have to put this into perspective. Twelve million people abusing opioids is bad. But the denominator in this equation is never mentioned, and it is huge. That same year, 2009, *200 million* prescriptions for opioids were filled nationwide, according to the SDI Vector One National database, a privately owned prescription and patient-tracking service.[20] And here's another important comparison. According to the federal Centers for Disease Control and Prevention, there were 16,651 deaths in 2010 involving opioid pain relievers (more than cocaine and heroin combined).[21, 22, 23] Obviously, that's 16,651 too many.

But what the media rarely mentions is that the same CDC data also show that only 29.4 percent of those deaths involved opioids alone.[24] Many of these prescription pain reliever deaths, roughly 30 percent, involved benzodiazepines. Alcohol, too, was also involved in many overdose deaths. When opioids get vilified, people in pain may take the hit.

And consider this: Yes, there were 16,651 opioid-related deaths in 2010. But 443,000 American adults die every year from cigarette smoking, and more than 80,000 die annually from excessive alcohol use.[25, 26] Even nonsteroidal anti-inflammatory drugs (NSAIDs) like ibuprofen are linked to almost as many deaths as opioids—an estimated 7,000 to

10,000 American adults a year.[27] In fact, a 2012 report by University of Rochester researchers who analyzed data from new registry called the Toxicology Investigators Consortium (ToxIC) found that nonopioid analgesics and psychotropic agents are more likely than opioid analgesics to be associated with drug poisoning overdose.[28] The most common types of drugs linked to poisoning cases were, in order, sedative-hypnotics/sleeping pills, nonopioid analgesics, opioids, antidepressants, stimulants, and alcohol. In other words, when it comes to drugs, our collective thinking is out of whack.

In fact, many people of varying political persuasions now believe that the war on drugs has been "a failure," imprisoning people who really need treatment, as New Jersey governor Chris Christie, a former prosecutor, proclaimed in July 2012, according to the *New York Times*.[29] That was also the conclusion of the Global Commission on Drug Policy, an elite group that included former heads of state, Kofi Annan (the former secretary-general of the United Nations), Paul Volker (former chairman of the Federal Reserve), and George P. Shultz (former US secretary of state).

"The global war on drugs has failed," the commission reported in June 2011. Vast expenditures on criminalization and repressive measures directed at producers, traffickers, and consumers of illegal drugs have clearly failed to effectively curtail supply or consumption, it said.[30, 31] When the United Nations Single Convention on Narcotic Drugs came into being 50 years ago and when President Nixon launched the US government's war on drugs 40 years ago, policymakers believed that harsh law enforcement action against those involved in drug production, distribution, and use would lead to an ever-diminishing market in controlled drugs such as heroin, cocaine, and cannabis, and the eventual achievement of a drug-free world. "In practice, the global scale of illegal drug markets—largely controlled by organized crime—has grown dramatically over this period," the commission concluded.

* * *

At root, I see the prescription pain reliever controversy as a *culture war*, a highly emotional struggle in which much of the "debate" is driven not by scientific facts but by dueling anecdotes of horror. This should not be surprising. We humans get mixed up about risks all the time. Women often think breast cancer is their biggest health risk, when it's really heart disease. We think the nuclear power industry kills more people than the coal industry, when it doesn't.[32] We think our big health problem is toxic stuff in our air, water, and food, and ignore the huge health risks from sedentary lifestyles.

"Risk is not just a statistic. It is an idea and a feeling, a perception informed not just by the reasoning of the thinking cortex that humans have more recently developed, but by all the emotional and instinctive cortical systems we have had since pre-human times, long before we developed the relatively recent ability to think and reason," writes risk expert David Ropeik.[33]

New York Times columnist David Brooks makes a similar point in his book *The Social Animal*.[34] Emerging research in neuroscience, he writes, shows that we are not primarily the products of our conscious thinking. "We are primarily the products of thinking that happens below the level of awareness"—in other words, gut feelings, prejudices, fears, and emotions. This emotionally laden processing skews the opioid debate, with genuinely tragic stories of dead drug abusers—like 23-year-old Jaclyn Kinkade of Florida, whose slide into abuse was chronicled in 2012 by the *Wall Street Journal*—trumping the hidden suffering of pain patients in the public mind.[35]

"Who could fail to be moved by the death of a young person from schoolyard Percocet?" University of Washington pain researcher Jane Ballantyne asked not long ago in a piece for the International Association for the Study of Pain. "Yet suffering from untreated pain is equally real, if less visible."[36] In terms of sheer numbers, there are more people with chronic pain than people addicted to all drugs, licit and illicit, according to clinical psychologist Robert Twillman, policy director at the American Academy of Pain Management.[37] Even the word *opioid* itself, though not quite as emotionally laden as *narcotic*, has become a dirty word, stigmatizing abusers and pain patients alike. The patient–doctor relationship has taken a beating, too. "The sanctity of the doctor-patient relationship is being destroyed by federal bureaucrats, who have turned the drug war into a war on pain relief," as former presidential candidate and Texas Republican Representative Ron Paul put it in a 2004 column.[38]

None of this is new. Historically, Americans have been ambivalent about opioids for decades, with the pendulum of public opinion swinging back and forth, as the late Yale University medical historian David Musto has amply chronicled.[39] Opioids were used fairly freely until the beginning of the 20th century, when the government began introducing regulations to put the brakes on opioid use and physicians' opioid prescribing, as Ballantyne has written.[40]

These restraints triggered a pendulum swing the other way, prompting doctors, especially those trying to ease the suffering of dying cancer patients, to protest. Eventually, their complaints were heard, and advocacy effectively restored opioid treatment for pain.[41]

Along the way, opioids began to be used (properly, in my view) not just for dying cancer patients but for people with intractable pain from non-cancer causes. Pain itself began to be seen as the "fifth vital sign," a measure that should be assessed regularly in hospitals, along with a patient's pulse, temperature, respiration, and blood pressure. Medical ethicists, too, began to argue that pain relief should be viewed as a fundamental human right—and the lack of adequate pain relief as akin to malpractice, even torture.

All of which, of course, was music to the ears of the pharmaceutical industry, which jumped enthusiastically into the development of newer, longer-lasting opioids, most famously, OxyContin. (Other extended-release pain relievers are in the works, and also causing concern, among them Zohydro, not yet FDA approved, as of March 2013.[42, 43]) OxyContin had a built-in time-release mechanism that, the marketing hype suggested, could actually reduce the risk of addiction, a pitch that made doctors more comfortable in prescribing it. What happened, though, was that abusers found it all too easy to defeat the time-release mechanism by simply chewing or crushing the drug, thus getting all at once a dose that was supposed to last for hours.[44]

The marketing of OxyContin was unquestionably aggressive—and misleading. So much so that in 2007, three executives with the American operation of Purdue Pharma pleaded guilty in a US federal court to misleading regulators and the public about the addiction potential of OxyContin, agreeing to pay $634 million in civil and criminal fines.[45, 46] In its statement, the company defended itself by saying it had not advertised OxyContin on television and promoted the medicine only to healthcare professionals, not to consumers.[47] The company did admit that its "fraudulent conduct caused a greater amount of OxyContin to be available for illegal use than otherwise would have been available."[48]

But don't cry for Purdue. OxyContin is still doing well financially. It garnered $3.1 billion in sales in 2010, the latest year for which figures are available through IMS Health, a healthcare information company that tracks markets.[49]

Pharmaceutical industry money—the third rail in the tense world of opioid politics—has recently triggered another firestorm. In the wake of investigative reporting from ProPublica, an online investigative news organization, the US Senate in May 2012 launched an investigation into drug industry funding of a number of pain patient advocacy groups, including the American Pain Foundation, which got 90 percent of its money from industry.[50, 51] The pain foundation immediately shut down, citing irreparable economic circumstances. (For the record, I have asked for and received conflict-of-interest disclosures from many of the scientists I quote.) Industry funding is a complex problem. The underlying assumption is that if industry pays for research, the results are necessarily tainted. Industry money *should* raise red flags. But some industry-funded research is relatively hands-off, so it's hard to know when the *appearance* of a conflict of interest is a *real* conflict.

In any case, with all the industry marketing hype, it's no surprise that prescriptions for opioids, both long- and short-acting formulations, have soared.[52, 53] Between 1997 and 2005, prescriptions for oxycodone rose 588 percent; for methadone, 934 percent; for fentanyl, 423 percent; for morphine, 154 percent; for hydrocodone, 197 percent; and for hydromorphone, 224 percent.[54] Today, opioids are among the most commonly prescribed medications in the United States.[55] Importantly, however, there are early signs that opioid prescriptions may be slowing. In 2012, they dipped slightly for the first time in years, according to new data from IMS Health, the drug market research firm.[56]

By the same token, soaring opioid use has spurred an enormous federal bureaucracy to combat abuse, a bureaucracy that extends from the "drug czar," Gil Kerlikowske, at the White House–based Office of National Drug Control Policy (ONDCP), on down through an alphabet soup of other agencies. It's difficult to put a dollar figure on the federal effort to combat opioid abuse because the federal drug control budget does not break out opioids from other drugs that can be abused.[57]

But many agencies are involved. Within the Department of Health and Human Services (HHS), drug-focused agencies include the Substance

Abuse and Mental Health Services Administration (SAMHSA), under which are the Center for Substance Abuse Treatment (CSAT) and the Center for Substance Abuse Prevention (CSAP). Also under HHS is the US Food and Drug Administration (FDA), which approves opioids for marketing but does not prosecute abusers. Also within HHS is the Atlanta-based Centers for Disease Control and Prevention (CDC), which tracks drug overdose deaths, and the National Institute on Drug Abuse (NIDA), which is part of the National Institutes of Health (NIH). Even Medicare and Medicaid, also part of HHS, do some drug monitoring as part of their monitoring of "appropriate care."

Then there's the Department of Justice, which includes the Drug Enforcement Administration (DEA), which goes after suspected drug pushers and abusers, and the National Drug Intelligence Center (NDIC), which collects data from law enforcement sources. The Federal Bureau of Investigation (FBI) investigates things like pharmacy robberies.[58] The military gets involved, too, in part because illicit drug use increased from 5 percent to 12 percent among active duty service members between 2005 to 2008, primarily because of prescription drug abuse.[59] And that's just the federal piece. Most states today have prescription drug monitoring programs that track doctors' prescribing patterns and pharmacies' prescription dispensing patterns. (How well these programs work is a big question, as we'll see in the next chapter.) Even though these are state programs, the federal DEA is a strong supporter of them.[60]

Because the issue of drug abuse is so heated and the emotions it generates so raw, the rhetoric often becomes extreme. Some law enforcers have likened doctors to terrorists and the Taliban and have called OxyContin in particular a "seductive, deadly menace," says University of Maryland legal scholar Diane Hoffmann.[61, 62]

It's unclear whether this polarized mentality will change. In May 2010, drug czar Kerlikowske signaled a possible shift when he said federal policy would treat illegal drug use more as a public health issue and put more resources into prevention and treatment. And on April 19, 2011, the Obama administration said that "any policy in this area must strike a balance between our desire to minimize abuse of prescription drugs and the need to ensure access for their legitimate use."[63] But given the government's paltry investment in pain research (roughly 1 percent of the NIH budget) compared to its huge bureaucratic commitment to the "war on drugs," it remains to be seen whether this announced shift is real.

In fairness, doctors who prescribe opioids are not always angels, either. Consider the infamous Massachusetts doctor Joseph P. Zolot, who was indicted, along with his nurse practitioner, Lisa M. Pliner, in March 2011. This pair caused the overdose deaths of at least six people they knew to be drug-addicted by systematically prescribing them unnecessary pain relievers in order to make a profit. This has become one of the most significant cases of medical misconduct to reach a criminal court anywhere in the United States, law enforcement officials told the *Boston Globe*.[64]

There have been other stunning coups for law enforcers, too. On February 23, 2011, in a maneuver called "Operation Pill Nation," DEA agents and local police swept through South Florida after a yearlong investigation into "pill mills"—shady operations often advertised as pain clinics in which unscrupulous doctors hand out prescriptions for opioids to people who claim to be in pain. Florida has had a particularly disastrous drug problem and accounts for a sizable share of all oxycodone pills prescribed in the United States.[65, 66] In the massive raid by 400 law enforcement officers, 20 people, including five doctors, were arrested.[67] In a subsequent action, dubbed "Pill Mill Nation II," DEA officials arrested 22 people in Orlando and Tampa, including five doctors and two pharmacists.[68]

My hat's off to these law enforcers. At the same time, though, the zeal of the DEA and other federal, state, and local law enforcers has had what some physicians feel is a chilling effect on good doctors and real pain patients. The rhetoric gets heated on this side, too, with some doctors voicing fears of the "government jihad" against them and their patients.[69]

In reality, physicians' fears may be somewhat exaggerated. The DEA insists that "doctors have nothing to fear from DEA" in the legitimate practice of medicine. Practitioners, the DEA says, have a longstanding requirement under the law to prescribe controlled substances only for legitimate medical purposes in the usual course of professional practice. This, the DEA contends, should not cause any physician to be reluctant to provide legitimate treatment.[70] Nor does the DEA think, as some physicians do, that it is on a campaign to target physicians who prescribe controlled substances for the treatment of pain. The DEA argues that only a tiny fraction of US doctors have been taken to task for alleged improper opioid prescribing.

That view is supported by a 2005 study from Weill Medical College of Cornell University in which researchers showed that the actual risk of a US doctor being disciplined by a state medical board for treating a patient for a genuine pain condition was "virtually nonexistent."[71] Another study, published in *Pain Medicine* in 2008, also found that only a tiny fraction of US doctors annually have been prosecuted or administratively sanctioned for improperly prescribing powerful pain medications.[72]

The study was done by researchers from the Center for Practical Bioethics, the National Association of Attorneys General, and the Federation of State Medical Boards. It found that only about one in 1,000 physicians was tried or sanctioned—725 physicians out of nearly 700,000 practicing physicians in the United States. On average, the DEA investigates only four to five doctors in each state every year for possible criminal offenses linked to prescription pain medications.[73] But physicians say that even if that rate is accurate, it's still 250 doctors a year, more than enough to cause them to think twice before prescribing opioids.

And while some investigations of physicians have been fair and legitimate, others have not, notes Maryland legal scholar Hoffmann.[74] One of the most famous of these cases was that of William Hurwitz, a Virginia pain specialist with a medical degree from Stanford University and a law degree from George Mason University School of Law. He was aggressively prosecuted for prescribing high doses of opioids to pain patients. Sadly, some of his patients did abuse the drugs and redistribute them on the black market.

In 2004, he was convicted of 50 counts of distribution of narcotics—opioids—and was sentenced to prison. Hurwitz argued that he had prescribed the drugs in good faith. Nonetheless, "the outcome sent chills through the pain treatment community and was criticized by a number of prominent journalists," Hoffmann says.

Hurwitz's conviction was overturned by an appeals court in 2006. He was retried in 2007, found guilty on some but not all counts and was sentenced to 57 months in prison. He is now free, according to the lawyer who defended him, Richard Sauber.[75] But the memory of Hurwitz's case still hovers over the practices of pain doctors.

There is increasing scrutiny by regulatory people, according to Lynn Webster, a pain physician who heads CRI Lifetree Clinical Research in Salt Lake City and is president-elect of the American Academy of Pain Medicine.[76] His focus now is research, but until recently, because of his reputation as a physician who will take on difficult cases and prescribe high doses of opioids if necessary, Webster had a big practice. Which meant regulators were all over him. "They want to audit our records. That process alone intimidates most physicians. Without doubt, it has a chilling effect," he told me. He has had to hire attorneys to be sure he is protected. Most physicians, he told me, would stop prescribing for fear they would end up like Hurwitz if they experienced this type of oversight.[77]

UNDERTREATMENT OF PAIN

Opioids are kind of like airplane food: not that great—but for some people with pain, impossible to get enough of. That's the dilemma faced by many people with chronic pain who wind up undertreated because they—or their doctors—are afraid of addiction, getting in trouble with the law, or both. A related problem is that, because doctors know so little about treating pain, they often fail to take advantage of *multimodal treatments*, that is, using different classes of medications in combination so as to maximize pain control while minimizing side effects.[78] (In this book, I will focus primarily on opioids for chronic, non-cancer pain because that's where the controversy lies. Hardly anyone these days questions the use of opioids for acute pain in surgical patients.[79, 80, 81] And few raise serious objections to giving opioids to cancer patients dying in pain.)

Nobody knows for sure how many Americans in chronic pain are undertreated. But it's probably about 30 percent, according to Webster of Utah. (Undertreatment, of course, means not just barriers to opioids but insufficient use of many other treatments, including non-drug approaches.)

It's estimated that about 8 million Americans with chronic pain *do* get opioids, says epidemiologist Michael Von Korff of the Group

Health Research Institute in Seattle.[82, 83] But think about the numbers. There are 100 million American adults in chronic pain, and many, perhaps a third, or 30 million of them, have such severe pain that they are disabled by it.[84, 85] If Webster's estimate is right, there could be millions who are not getting the help they need. Among those millions are people with persistent back pain, headaches, joint pain, and cancer, says the New York–based Mayday Fund, a foundation dedicated to alleviating human physical pain. Undertreatment is even worse for minorities and the poor, 2009 Mayday figures show.[86] In one nationwide survey, for instance, 1,204 people were randomly selected from the general US population and questioned during a single week in April 2005. Thirty-one percent said they had experienced moderate to very severe pain in the past two weeks. Only half of those who sought medical attention said they got significant pain relief.[87]

Why? To be sure, many doctors shy away from prescribing opioids because they don't know how to use them safely, don't know how opioids might interact with other drugs the patient is taking, or don't know how to assess a patient's risk of substance abuse. Doctors also worry about costs, though, in fact, suboptimal pain care can actually cost more because frustrated patients go from doctor to doctor and get lots of diagnostic tests.

And, let's face it. People in pain—myself included—can *be* a pain. If you've gone from doctor to doctor, hearing over and over that the pain is all in your head, you inevitably arrive at the next doctor with a chip on your shoulder.

But the biggest reason for underuse of opioids is probably fear of regulatory scrutiny.[88] There is abundant evidence that patients justifiably fear undertreatment of distressing symptoms, wrote palliative care specialists Timothy Quill of the University of Rochester and Diane Meier of Mount Sinai School of Medicine in 2006 in the *New England Journal of Medicine*.[89] To be sure, lack of proper training and overblown fears of addiction contribute to such undertreatment, Quill and Meier concluded, but "physicians' fears of regulatory oversight and disciplinary action remain a central stumbling block."

Serious undertreatment of pain is not just an American problem, either. It's rampant worldwide. And has been for decades. In 2010, researchers looked at availability of opioids for cancer patients in 21

Eastern European and 20 Western European countries, and found huge access problems because of costs and regulatory barriers. In some countries of Eastern Europe such as Lithuania, Tajikistan, Albania, Georgia, and Ukraine, certain essential opioid medications were virtually unavailable, creating what the researchers call a "public health catastrophe."[90]

Way back in 1961, the world community adopted an international agreement called the Single Convention on Narcotic Drugs, which said, among other things, that narcotic drugs were indispensible for the relief of pain and suffering, according to Human Rights Watch, an advocacy group that considers pain control a top priority.[91]

Yet today, 50 years later, the promise of that agreement remains largely unfulfilled, the rights group says, noting that 80 percent of the world's population still doesn't have adequate access to treatment for serious pain.[92] In India, for instance, many major cancer hospitals don't give patients morphine, even though more than 70 percent of their patients are believed to need it. A February 2009 report from the World Health Organization confirms that dismal conclusion. WHO estimates that 5 billion people live in countries with little or no access to controlled medicines and have insufficient or no access to treatment for moderate to severe pain.[93] A 2010 editorial in *Palliative Medicine* concurred, saying there continue to be ongoing problems with access to opioid analgesics for relief of pain globally.[94]

Worldwide, millions of people still suffer because of lack of availability of opioids related to government fears of opioid abuse. Both WHO and the International Narcotics Control Board, an independent, quasi-judicial body set up by the United Nations, stress that while preventing drug abuse is important, this should not hinder pain patients' ability to get the care they need. But it does. Human Rights Watch puts it this way: There is still "a shocking willingness by many governments around the world to passively stand by as people suffer."[95]

THE REAL RISKS OF ADDICTION
(AND A DRUG ADDICT'S STORY)

At the heart of the opioid controversy is the widespread but often exaggerated fear of addiction. One of the main factors feeding this

fear is confusion over the terms *addiction, physical dependence, tolerance,* and *abuse.* Almost everybody—patients and doctors alike—gets
these terms mixed up. As a group of 25 leading pain specialists put it
in a 2010 report, the general public and many healthcare professionals
"frequently overstate" the risk of addiction or fail to differentiate addiction from physical dependence or tolerance.[96] The important point is
this: Physical dependence is a normal response to taking opioids long
term, but it is not necessarily harmful. Addiction, abuse, and misuse, on
the other hand, are *not* normal and certainly *not* inevitable.

Because it's so important to keep all this straight, consider the official
definitions.[97]

Substance misuse is the use of any drug in a manner other than that
indicated or prescribed.

Substance abuse is the use of any substance when such use is
unlawful or detrimental to the user or others. *Abuse* is also defined as
self-administration of a medication for a non-medical purpose, such as
to get "high." Both real pain patients and nonpatients can be abusers.

Addiction is a disease—a primary, chronic, neurobiological condition characterized by impaired control over drug use, compulsive
use, continued use despite harm, and craving.[98] In 2011, the American
Society of Addiction Medicine released a new definition of addiction as
a chronic brain disease, a controversial move if the goal was to remove
stigma.[99, 100, 101]

Physical dependence is a state of adaptation manifested by a withdrawal syndrome triggered by abrupt cessation, rapid dose reduction, decreasing blood levels of the drug, or by administration of an
antagonist, or drug blocker, such as naloxone, in the case of opioid
dependence.

Withdrawal symptoms may include flulike symptoms, sweating,
muscle aches, joint pain, stomach cramping, increased heart rate, goosebumps, diarrhea, muscle aches, and irritability. (Sometimes withdrawal
can be prolonged, notes Wisconsin pharmacologist June Dahl, and pro-
tracted withdrawal can be linked to considerable suffering, including
anxiety and insomnia, that can persist for six months.[102])

Tolerance is a state of adaptation in which the drug's effects diminish
over time, prompting a patient to need more of the drug to control pain.
Tolerance is not an inevitable consequence of chronic opioid therapy.

Aberrant drug-related behavior is behavior suggestive of a substance abuse or addiction disorder or both. This can involve selling prescription drugs, prescription forgery, stealing or "borrowing" drugs from others, injecting *oral* formulations, obtaining prescription drugs from nonmedical sources, multiple episodes of prescription "loss," repeatedly seeking prescriptions from different clinicians, deterioration in function at work or home, or repeated resistance to getting help despite clear physical or psychological problems.

Recently, a group of physicians (PROP) who take a dim view of long-term opioids has argued that the attempt to conceptually—and clinically—separate opioid dependence from opioid addiction may constitute a distinction without a difference.[103] Perhaps, they suggest, *addiction*, at least in chronic pain patients, should be called "complex persistent opioid dependence." But it must be said that Andrew Kolodny, the leader of this group and a psychiatrist at Maimonides Medical Center in Brooklyn, New York, adheres to a radically different—and significantly expanded—definition of *addiction* compared to other groups:

> Addiction doesn't mean you will start stealing radios and breaking the law. That is not how we define "addiction." That is how the opioid industry defines it. Addiction is much easier to understand this way—if I put you on a medicine that decreases your quality of life, yet you continue taking it, that is addiction. You spend all day vegged out on the sofa, with no quality of life, with everyone who knew you and loved you saying you are gone, that person has a problem. The person may not see it, and may continue to take opioids. But I would say that person is addicted.[104]

Pinning down the risk of actual addiction, as opposed to physical dependence, is tricky, as we'll see in a minute. But when genuine addiction does occur, it's a nightmare, a horror that no litany of statistics alone can capture. One cold spring morning, I went to a methadone clinic for drug addicts in Somerville, Massachusetts, to see for myself the ravages of addiction.

There, I met a woman who spoke to me freely.[105] She is in her mid-40s with an open, Irish face, long reddish hair, and freckles all over. Finally clean after years of struggle, she was wearing a long, gold chain around her neck, a diamond on the ring finger of her left hand, and her heart on her sleeve. The wedding was just a few months away. When I asked if I could use her full name, she paused for a few minutes, then agreed, looked me straight in the eye and proclaimed, "I don't have nothing to hide." Later, after conferring with her counselor, she changed her mind.

Her story came out in bits and pieces. She has bipolar disorder, though it took years of popping the wrong pills and masking her troubles with heroin before she got the right psychiatric diagnosis and the right treatment. The losses in her young life began piling up early. Her father died of a neurological disorder when she was three, leaving her mother alone with eight kids. She was the youngest girl. Home was not exactly peaceful. By 17, she fled from the family house and married a man who turned out to be violent and who abused her repeatedly.

At 18, she and her husband were struck head on by a drunk driver going the wrong way. Her neck and back have never been the same. Even now, more than 20 years after the accident, her pain is often a 4 on a 0-to-10 scale. She became one of the pain patients doctors dread most—a person with significant, chronic pain AND a person at high risk for drug abuse. After the accident, she was given Percocet for the pain, her first brush with what she now disdainfully calls "pain management." She loved her "Percs." So much that she began taking not only the 90 pills a month the doctor prescribed, but "lots more," from friends and anybody else she could find hanging out on street corners. She had a baby, and her troubles began to grow. The baby died of sudden infant death syndrome (SIDS). Within months, her mother died, too. She had three more babies. (Her sons are now in their mid-20s.) While her children were still toddlers, her life—and her husband's— became so unmanageable due to drugs and abuse that family members got involved and took custody of the children.

Finally, she summoned the nerve to leave her abusive husband. But she quickly fell into another abusive relationship with a man she sarcastically calls "Mr. Wonderful." Her losses multiplied further. Her four brothers died, one by one, because of drugs. One died of an apparently accidental overdose. The three others were intravenous drug users, all of whom contracted AIDS and died. Along the way, she lost a sister to lymphoma. "Very sad," she said, her voice trembling. "A lot of deaths." She began increasing her use of drugs, some of which, like the benzodiazepine Klonopin, were prescribed specifically for her. But many others were not. Eventually, her beloved "Percs" stopped working for the pain and she no longer experienced the "happy feeling." So she began sniffing heroin. "I never used IV," she said, a bit proudly, her voice shaking. "But I was on the edge of it. I was freaked out because needle use and death was all around me. I was young, in my late 20s. I had three kids. I watched four brothers die. I had a lot of panic attacks. I wasn't sleeping. After my last brother died, I was at rock bottom. I was going to die next if I didn't get help."

Mercifully, she found her way to a detox program in a nearby town. Instead of the expected five days, she opted to stay for 30. She was horribly "dope sick," with vomiting, diarrhea, leg cramps, wild mood swings, runny nose, goosebumps, and severe sweating, all at once. "It was gross. It was just miserable," she said. It was also the beginning of a better life. Clean and now on methadone maintenance, she was finally diagnosed with bipolar disorder. Initially, she had trouble with the bipolar medications. Now, she's taking effective medications for bipolar disorder and anxiety, along with her daily methadone.

As I listened to her story, I was stunned, impressed as much by her courage as by her suffering. Despite all she went through, she looked relatively composed, clearly thrilled about her upcoming marriage, and proud of the new life she has struggled so hard for.

"I used to be angry, with a lot of mood swings. I was very loud, mean," she said. "Now I'm not like that."

I believed her. She is still working hard on herself, she said. She takes no opioids other than methadone. "I struggled through hell and high water to get clean. It's not just staying clean, I have to do things like go to meetings and deal with the inside of myself and peel away the layers. If you don't work this program, it's not going to work. If I go back, I will end up on opiates. I've been clean this long, I don't want to go back." I told her what I'd been learning, about the stigma of opioids, and how abuse of opioids by street addicts gives both opioids and genuine pain patients who need them a bad name. She agreed. "There are some people who truly need the opioids, who can tolerate them and not get addicted," she said. "Unfortunately, I am not one of them. I've been on both sides," she said. "I know what it's like."

* * *

Stories like this young woman's are common, and becoming ever more so as growing numbers of young people abuse prescription opioids. But the actual risk of addiction for the general population is still far less than all the sensational headlines might suggest.

To illustrate that point, Russell Portenoy, a leading pain specialist at Beth Israel Medical Center in New York, loves to tell this story. During the Vietnam War, about half of the American enlisted men who were stationed in Vietnam tried opioids, and at least half of these were regularly abusing the drugs.[106] After they got back home, however, fewer than 10 percent continued to exhibit behaviors consistent with addiction. That suggests, Portenoy says, that the base rate of susceptibility to addiction in the general population is probably about 10 percent.[107] Howard Heit, a pain and addiction specialist at Georgetown University, also pegs the addiction risk at about 8 to 10 percent for the general population.[108] Indeed, there is probably a genetic propensity for addiction in some people, with as many as 30 different genes likely underlying this risk.[109] A 2006 study by researchers from Yale University School of Medicine and the University of Connecticut looked at 393 families in which at least one member abused opioids. By studying the family members' DNA, the team found that two sites on chromosome 17 were strongly linked statistically to the risk of opioid addiction.[110]

But teasing out the real risk of addiction becomes tricky, and the figures can vary, depending on how accurately researchers define *addiction* (as opposed to *abuse*, *dependence*, and so on), and on the specific population being studied, cautions Lynn Webster, the pain researcher in Salt Lake City, Utah.[111]

The federal government acknowledges that it doesn't really know what the risk of opioid addiction is because reports range from 2.7 to 30 percent, depending on a variety of factors.[112] A recent systematic review of 17 studies involving 88,235 people by Italian researchers reported a similar range and concluded that opioids are not associated with a major risk of opioid dependence syndrome, defined as including loss of control over use. But again, it was difficult to find high-quality studies.[113]

In 1992, for instance, psychiatrists at the University of Miami led by David Fishbain tried to make sense of the data by reviewing 24 studies.[114] Only seven of the studies used acceptable definitions. Within these seven studies, the incidence of abuse, dependence, and addiction was in the range of 3.2 to 18.9 percent. These rates are "significant," the researchers said. "However, there is little evidence in these studies that addictive behaviors are common within the chronic pain population." A subsequent Fishbain study in 2008 looked at 67 studies of opioids in thousands of people with chronic pain.[115] Overall, the risk of abuse or addiction was only 3.27 percent, a strikingly low number. For patients with no prior or current drug abuse or addiction problem, the rate was even lower, 0.19 percent.

That's very good news. It means that if a person with chronic pain has never been a substance abuser before, he or she is unlikely to become addicted when taking opioids for pain. Long-term opioid use *"will* [italics mine] lead to abuse/addiction in a small percentage of chronic pain patients," the Fishbain team concluded. But even this risk can be lowered if physicians screen out patients with current or past substance abuse problems, the team found.

Other researchers have come to similar conclusions. Lynn Webster's research shows that the risk of addiction among pain patients is 2 to 5 percent, much less than the risk of abuse (20 percent) or misuse (40 percent).[116] And if you survey only low-risk patients seeing doctors in primary care clinics, he says, the prevalent addiction rate is less than 2 percent. In other research, scientists from the University of Wisconsin and the University of British Columbia looked at 801 pain patients in primary care practices, all of whom were taking opioids daily. Few became addicted. Considering the potential benefit to improving the lives of patients with chronic pain, they noted in a 2007 paper, "a 3.8 percent rate of opioid addiction is a small risk compared with the alternative of continuous pain and suffering."[117]

That's also the conclusion reached by a group of 25 leading pain specialists writing in 2010. If a person does not have a history of substance abuse, they said, the risk of addiction is between 3 and 5 percent.[118] And it might even be lower. In a 2010 meta-analysis for the Cochrane Collaboration, in which data on 4,893 patients from 26 studies were pooled, signs of opioid addiction were found in only 0.27 percent.[119] In fact, far from being drug seekers or constantly upping their doses, people in chronic pain with no history of addictive behaviors—49 percent in one study—tend to *undermedicate* themselves, frequently stopping or cutting down on their opioids.[120]

But some pain researchers, among them Seattle-based Michael Von Korff, worry that studies like these may paint too rosy a picture. He argues that some of the studies that find low addiction rates are methodologically flawed. Credible estimates of those who become addicted range from 5 to 25 percent, "which is not a low risk," he told me.[121]

That's pretty sobering. But you can also flip those numbers around. Even if the risk of addiction is a whopping 25 percent, that still means that 75 percent of people are probably *not* at risk and should therefore not let the fear of addiction keep them from taking opioids if they need them.

That said, it's also true that addictive disorders are often underdiagnosed, partly because most physicians who prescribe pain medications have little or no training in identifying and treating addictive disorders, according to pain and addiction specialist Jan Kauffman, who runs the addiction treatment program in Somerville, Massachusetts, where the young woman I interviewed is being treated.[122] Kauffman argues that pain and addiction should be taught together, both to medical students and to doctors already in practice, because most don't know enough about either.[123] Doctors could also do a much better job of screening pain patients for substance abuse risk and psychiatric problems before prescribing opioids. In the real world of busy doctors' offices, screening for addiction risk is often cursory, notes Von Korff.[124]

But screening *is* possible. In an important 2007 study, Harvard Medical School researchers looked at 228 people in chronic pain and gave them all a series of questionnaires designed to spot psychiatric problems and the potential for misusing drugs.[125] The tests were the Screener and Opioid Assessment for Pain Patients (SOAPP), Current Medication Misuse Measure (COMM), and Drug Misuse Index (DMI). The SOAPP test, for instance, has been shown to be a reliable measure of the risk for substance misuse; it correlates well with a history of substance abuse, legal problems, craving, smoking, and mood disorders in chronic pain patients. In this study, the questionnaires reliably raised red flags for more than half the group. The 55 percent of patients who were flagged as having more psychiatric problems were indeed at higher risk of misusing drugs and were more likely to have abnormal urine drug tests. This doesn't mean these people shouldn't get opioids for their pain, but it does suggest that once they are on opioids, they should be monitored closely. Another Harvard study by psychologist Robert Jamison showed that close monitoring plus brief cognitive behavioral counseling can help reduce opioid misuse.[126]

But there's also an important twist to this story. In a crucial 2009 Harvard study, the researchers found that people in chronic pain who are at higher risk for drug abuse may actually be experiencing more pain.[127] The Jamison team gave the SOAPP test to 110 chronic pain patients who also kept diaries of their pain levels, mood, how much their pain interfered with normal life, medications, and side effects for 10 months.

Pain intensity, not psychiatric history, turned out to be the best predictor of opioid misuse. In other words, the pain patients at the greatest risk of misusing their drugs are often those who experience the most subjective pain. This is crucial. The new data, the Jamison group said, do not point to psychopathology or a mood disorder as accounting for the differences among patient groups over time. Rather, the primary difference between groups was pain intensity. In theory, the bottom line seems simple. Opioid addiction is a low risk for most chronic pain patients. And to reduce it even further, doctors should ask their patients about prior substance abuse before they write opioid prescriptions.

DEPENDENCE (AND A DOCTOR'S STORY OF PAIN, NEAR SUICIDE, AND THE STRUGGLE TO GET OFF OPIOIDS)

"By definition, all mammals who take opioids for a long period of time become [physically] dependent and experience withdrawal symptoms when the opioid is discontinued," says Harvard psychologist Jamison. Mild withdrawal symptoms can begin within a week of stopping opioids. In other words, physical dependence, as opposed to addiction, is intrinsic to the way opioids work. The body reacts and exhibits withdrawal symptoms if the drugs are stopped, particularly if they are stopped abruptly.

But the important point is that many people in chronic pain do just fine when they're physically dependent on opioids. They do their jobs, raise their kids, live their lives, maintain stable doses, and achieve reasonable pain relief for years. Physical dependence and tolerance do not necessarily implicate a maladaptive pattern of substance abuse among chronic pain patients receiving medically prescribed opioids, as Seattle pain researcher Michael Von Korff puts it.[128]

Indeed, the fear of dependence on pain treatment "is largely unfounded, as almost all patients are able to stop their opioid-medication at the end of their treatment with no long-lasting effects," according to the World Health Organization.[129] But if a person tries to go cold turkey, or tries to taper off opioids too fast, withdrawal can be horrific.

As Paul Konowitz can attest. He is 53, a lovely man, a warm, compassionate physician who works as an ear, nose, and throat specialist at one of Boston's oldest and most prestigious medical institutions—the Massachusetts Eye and Ear Infirmary. His wife, Laurie, 53, is also kind, articulate, and outgoing and works as a neonatologist at Tufts-New England Medical Center in Boston. If any couple should have been prepared, with all those years in medical school, to deal with a chronic pain nightmare, it should have been Paul and Laurie.

But their battle with Paul's sudden, excruciating pain and his resulting physical dependence on opioids left them feeling as helpless as anyone else coping with pain, pain relievers, and the medical system. Paul contacted me shortly after reading the column I wrote on my own severe neck pain in the *Boston Globe*.[130] So, one warm Sunday afternoon, I visited Paul and Laurie in their home in a Boston suburb. Sitting side by side, looking at each other often, they tossed details of dates, medications, and memories back and forth, reconstructing their ordeal for me.

In April 2004, Paul, then 46, came down with pemphigus vulgaris, a rare autoimmune disease in which, for unknown reasons, a person's own antibodies start attacking the proteins that hold the two layers of mucous membranes together. The attack caused deep, widespread blisters—in his mouth, nose, tongue, eyes, and larynx. He stopped eating, quickly losing 25 pounds. "It was horrifically painful," he said. For a few months, Paul hung in at work, even as the pain steadily worsened. "I was doing sinus and thyroid surgeries," he recalled. "I couldn't even take Percocet. I did all my work, but it wasn't easy."

Then in August, all hell broke loose. To calm down his overactive immune system, doctors had given him high doses of prednisone and intravenous immunoglobulin. They also put him on another drug, Rituxan, which kills the cells that make antibodies. It worked, sort of.

The pemphigus began to abate. But the immune suppression left him susceptible to new problems, including a severe herpes infection in his esophagus.

That, too, became excruciating. "It was searing, unbelievable, indescribable, constant, unrelenting, unmanageable pain," he said. "It was hard to be around him," Laurie told me softly. Making matters worse, the prednisone was making him temporarily psychotic and unable to sleep. One episode in particular stands out in Laurie's mind. "I was on call at the hospital. The kids were at camp. I was paged at 6 a.m. on a Sunday. Paul was not making any sense. He was not rational. I called someone to relieve me and I took him to the emergency room."

The horror continued. Despite opioids, including fentanyl patches, Paul's agony lasted for another three months. The herpes infection eventually went away, only to be replaced by yet another problem—postherpetic neuralgia, an extremely painful condition that often follows herpes infections. "He was suicidal," said Laurie.

"I didn't actually have a suicide plan," Paul added quietly. "But I would hope that I would not wake up in the morning. You think you'd rather be dead. That's how bad it was. I thought death would be better. I would think, 'If this doesn't go away, I can't live my life.' Every day was the same. There was no end in sight. It never stopped."

As a physician, he told me that he used to feel reluctant to prescribe pain relievers "because you can be punished." His own severe pain changed all that. He has learned that when doctors are faced with patients in severe, chronic pain, they should "give people the benefit of the doubt. Unless you have some other clue that they are drug-seeking, you have to err on the side of the patient." He also came to the same insight that became emblazoned in my own psyche after my excruciating neck pain: "You can't understand pain unless you've had it."

Eventually, Paul's pain did abate. But then he faced yet another hurdle: getting off opioids. "I knew I had to get off," he recalled. But, because few doctors are taught about pain in medical school, much less about the intricacies of opioids and opioid withdrawal, none of his doctors or doctor friends knew what to do. "Doctors don't do pain well," Paul concluded. "They don't understand addiction, physical dependence, withdrawal. We had to figure it out for ourselves, and we had an advantage—we had the background and people to talk to."

One doctor suggested tapering off opioids over the course of a week. That was way, way, way too fast. "I quickly discovered I couldn't do that," said Paul. "The withdrawal symptoms were almost as horrific as the pain itself. I felt like I was crawling out of my skin. I didn't know what to do with myself. It truly was such an overwhelming, awful feeling. I was on antianxiety medications, antidepressants."

He kept trying to cut back, but still tried to taper too fast. Each time, the withdrawal agony would come back. "He would become nervous, anxious, nauseous," recalled Laurie. Finally, realizing he had to taper off baby step by baby step, he very gradually reduced his doses. It took two or three months, but he became drug-free and went back to work. The moral of his story is clear: If and when the time comes to quit opioids, get help, from a pain and addiction specialist if necessary, and cut back very, very slowly. Many people are wrongly labeled drug seekers because they can't stand the withdrawal symptoms like anxiety and insomnia, which can be disabling.

Today, Paul is much better. "I don't even think about what I went through." His wife Laurie looked at him quietly and murmured, "I do."

THE RISKS OF OVERDOSE AND DEATH FROM OPIOIDS

Of all the risks associated with opioids, the scariest—for good reason— is overdose. Overdoses, intentional and accidental, fatal and nonfatal, can occur both with street abusers who take opioids for nonmedical purposes and with pain patients, though overdoses happen more often with the former.

Figures vary on the exact rate of opioid-related overdose deaths. Overall, the rate is not high for people taking lower doses, especially considering how many opioid prescriptions are filled every year— about 200 million, according to a nationwide tracking service.[131] But even one overdose is one too many, and the grim numbers are on the rise as opioid prescriptions soar.

As we saw earlier in this chapter, there were 16,651 opioid-related deaths in 2010, according to the federal Centers for Disease Control and Prevention. But, as we also noted, many of these deaths involved at least one other drug, including benzodiazepines, cocaine, and heroin. And many involved alcohol.[132] These deaths, in other words, can't be blamed solely on opioids.

There have been other attempts to gauge the risk of opioid overdose. In 2009, a government team from the National Drug Intelligence Center (NDIC), part of the Justice Department, reported on the period 2001 through 2005. They found that unintentional opioid-related deaths increased during that time from 3,994 deaths per year to 8,541.[133] A different team, reporting in 2010, was led by Richard Chapman of the University of Utah. His group of 25 researchers looked at the period 1999 through 2002 and found a 91.2 percent increase in deaths due to what they called "opioid poisoning."[134] Yet another team conducted the Consortium to Study Opioid Risks and Trends (CONSORT) study. Led by Michael Von Korff, a senior investigator at the Group Health Research Institute in Seattle, the team looked at 9,940 people who received multiple opioid prescriptions for conditions such as back pain and osteoarthritis between 1997 and 2005.[135]

Not surprisingly, the CONSORT team found that patients getting the highest doses of opioids were more likely to overdose than those on low doses. But most of the overdose cases actually occurred among people taking low or moderate doses because so many more people are on those lower doses. So what were the risks, at least in this study? For people taking fewer than 20 milligrams of opioids per day, the annual risk was tiny: 0.2 percent. For those taking 50 to 99 milligrams per day, it was higher: 0.7 percent. And for those taking more than 100 milligrams per day, it was more worrisome: 1.8 percent. Still, it's worth nothing that the total number of overdoses was small: 51 out of the entire sample. And, thankfully, not all were fatal: Only six of the 51 overdoses in this study resulted in death.

A more recent study published in the *Journal of the American Medical Association* in 2011 supports the CONSORT findings. This 2011 study found that the unintentional fatal opioid overdose rate among patients on opioid therapy was quite low, 0.04 percent, but again, the risk rises with increasing dosage.[136] This study looked at 750 overdose deaths out of a sample of 154,684 pain patients on opioid therapy. Similarly, another 2011 study also found the risk of death rose with increasing dosage.[137] Obviously, people in pain on high doses of opioids need to be very careful not to exceed the prescribed dosage. But by and large, it's people who take opioids for nonmedical reasons—the abusers—not pain patients, who are more likely to fatally overdose.

In a revealing 2008 study from West Virginia, which experienced the nation's largest increase in drug overdose mortality between 1999 and 2004, researchers looked at every single person—295 in all—who died of unintentional overdoses in that state in a single year, 2006.[138] Two-thirds of the deaths—63 percent—involved *diverted* drugs (mostly opioids), in other words, drugs prescribed for someone else. Most of the people who died from diverted opioids were also young—8 to 24, with the prevalence of diversion dropping steadily with older and older age groups. In addition to receiving diverted drugs, young people are also often the ones *doing* the diverting. A 2011 University of Maryland study of 192 people aged 21 to 26 found that a quarter said they diverted their analgesics to others.[139]

* * *

There's another important piece of the opioid fatality problem: methadone, the synthetic opioid developed in Germany as an alternative to morphine during World War II.[140] "Methadone is a unique actor," says June Dahl, a professor of neuroscience at the University of Wisconsin. It has a long and very variable duration of action and its adverse effects last long after the pain relief it provides.[141]

"Methadone is a wonderful medicine used appropriately, but an unforgiving medicine used inappropriately. Many legitimate patients following the direction of the doctor have run into trouble with methadone, including death," says pain specialist Howard Heit of Georgetown University.[142]

Methadone, the staple of drug rehab programs, is used to treat both opioid withdrawal, also called *abstinence syndrome*, and to directly treat pain. When used for abstinence syndrome, it is usually given once a day; for pain, it is usually prescribed for use two to four times a day.[143] One of the problems with methadone, says Tufts University anesthesiologist Daniel Carr, is that it can cause potentially dangerous heart arrhythmias. This is not a run-of-the-mill opioid side effect: It's distinctive to methadone, he told me. Methadone can prolong the *QT interval*, the time the heart muscle stays contracted before it relaxes again in the next heart beat. Prolonged QT interval can lead to arrhythmias.

In one study of 20 unintentional opioid-related deaths, for instance, methadone accounted for half the deaths, Utah pain specialist Webster told me. Strikingly, three-quarters of these deaths were attributable to errors by the prescribing doctor, not misuse by patients. Nationwide, methadone is probably responsible for one-third of all opioid-related deaths, a staggering number.

The problem with methadone is that it is highly attractive drug because it's very cheap—just pennies a dose. But it's also extremely difficult to prescribe safely. Most doctors simply don't know how to prescribe it, and most patients don't know how to use it. Webster paints this common scenario, using a fictitious patient:

> Mary Jane Smith finally found a doctor who was sure he could really treat her chronic pain. The methadone he would prescribe was different: It was cheap, it would work and it wouldn't have the side effects of other narcotics she tried. (She thought methadone was only for drug addicts, but the doctor said otherwise.) She left the office with a prescription and a return appointment for two weeks. The doctor said she only had to follow the directions: One pill, four times a day. She could do that! But she didn't. She hurt so bad when she got home that she took a double dose of methadone. After two hours, there was no pain relief, so she took another pill. She had a glass of wine with dinner; she was feeling better. She wasn't high, but she was sleepy. She told her husband she was going to bed early. She took one more pill to hold her through the night. She fell asleep snoring.
>
> She never woke up.[144]

The harsh truth, Webster has found, is that "if you start someone on too high a dose of methadone, they will die." That's because the drug's analgesic effect lasts a fraction of its *half-life*—that is, the time it takes for half the dose to be eliminated from the body. The pain-relieving effect of methadone lasts only four to six hours, which means a person wants to take it again at that point for continued pain relief. But the drug isn't cleared from the body—and can continue to adversely affect breathing, liver function, and cardiac rhythm—for up to three days, which means taking it every four to six hours is dangerous. It was because of this very problem that the US Food and Drug Administration issued a public health warning in November 2006.[145]

With methadone, the key is to start slow and go slow, according to Janice Kauffman, a nurse, addiction specialist, and vice president at the North Charles Institute for the Addictions in Somerville, Massachusetts.[146] It's important not to shy away from methadone if you are working with a doctor who knows how to use it. Many pain patients—not to mention recovering drug addicts—derive enormous benefit from methadone. But it's important to be aware of the dangers, too.

Recently, insurance companies in Washington State, worried about the expense and abuse potential of OxyContin, required doctors to prescribe methadone instead. What happened was a dramatic rise in unintentional overdose deaths.

In fact, reporters at the *Seattle Times* won the 2012 Pulitzer Prize for their reporting on the methadone mess there.[147] The *Times* investigation showed that at least 2,173 people in Washington State had died between 2003 and 2011 after accidentally overdosing on methadone, which for eight years was one of the state's two preferred pain relievers for Medicaid patients and recipients of workers' compensation. In its citation, the Pulitzer committee honored *Times* reporters Michael J. Berens and Ken Armstrong for their investigation of how a little-known governmental body in Washington State "moved vulnerable patients from safer pain-control medication to methadone, a cheaper but more dangerous drug, coverage that prompted statewide health warnings." And it was poor people who suffered most. While Medicaid recipients make up only about 8 percent of Washington's adult population, they accounted for 48 percent of the methadone deaths.

OTHER OPIOID PROBLEMS: HORMONE CHANGES, *INCREASED* PAIN, AND FALLS

Besides addiction, physical dependence, and overdose, there are other potential problems with opioids, including serious side effects that limit their usefulness. These include hormonal dysfunction, immune suppression, and *increased* pain from a phenomenon called opioid-induced hyperalgesia, according to an analysis by a blue-ribbon task force in

2010.[148] In fact, the culture war over opioid abuse and diversion has been so prominent in the media that too little attention has probably been paid to these and other side effects, which can be serious.[149]

One of the most overlooked risks, especially in older people, is falling and breaking a hip or the pelvis. In one study of 2,341 people taking opioids for non-cancer pain, the risk of fracture was double that of non-opioid users.[150] Among people taking moderate to high doses (50 mg a day or more), there was an almost 10 percent per year chance of fracture. While fractures may sound trivial compared to overdoses or addiction, they're not. There is a 24 percent risk of death in the first year after a hip fracture for people over 50.[151]

With chronic use, opioids may also suppress the immune system and may lower testosterone levels in men.[152] In fact, the longer a man takes daily opioids, the more likely he is to have hypogonadism (impaired production of testosterone).[153] Chronic opioid therapy can also lead to menstrual irregularities in women.[154] Opioids can also exacerbate depression and cause serious constipation, including fecal impaction. They may also decrease cognitive function.[155, 156, 157] One of the most baffling problems is opioid-induced hyperalgesia (OIH). Nobody is sure what triggers it. But in certain people, opioids seem to rev up the nervous system (a process called central sensitization) instead of calming it down.[158] Opioids may also increase pain, at least in rats, by acting on that glial cell receptor, TLR-4.[159]

The fact that opioid pain relievers can actually *increase* pain complicates the already complicated opioid prescribing problem. When a person in pain takes opioids and keeps experiencing worse pain, the obvious assumption is that the dose should be increased. But that's precisely the wrong thing to do if the problem is opioid-induced hyperalgesia. Switching to different opioids can sometimes help.[160]

THE DIVERSION PROBLEM: WHERE *DO* STREET ADDICTS GET THEIR DRUGS? (IT'S NOT WHERE YOU THINK)

I was stunned to discover, in the course of researching this book, that the drug abuse problem in this country is partly my fault. Well, not mine alone. Yours, mine, and that of everybody else whose medicine cabinet is full of unused opioids. In my case, I found bottles of leftover oxy-codone and fentanyl patches from my late husband's prostate cancer, pain relievers from my own, long-forgotten dental work, not to mention more recent prescriptions for my neck pain. I wasn't even taking this stuff. But I didn't know what to do with it, either. If an abuser had broken in to my house, he or she would have stumbled upon a pharma-cological gold mine.

Contrary to widespread belief, roughly 70 percent of the drugs that wind up on the street come from initially legitimate sources, not from bad doctors writing too many prescriptions. According to the government's 2009 National Survey on Drug Use and Health, here's where Americans 12 and older got their pain relievers the most recent time they abused them:

55.3	percent from a friend or relative for free
9.9	percent bought from a friend or relative
5.0	percent from a friend or relative without asking
17.6	percent from one doctor
2.0	percent from more than one doctor ("doctor shopping")
4.8	percent bought from a dealer or other stranger
0.4	percent bought from the Internet
0.2	percent wrote a fake prescription
0.5	percent stole from a doctor's office, clinic, hospital, or pharmacy
4.2	percent some other way[161]

Which raises the obvious question: What are people supposed to do with all the drugs, especially opioids, so ripe for the stealing? I eventu-ally flushed my inadvertent stash down the toilet so I could write this book in good conscience. But, as I found out later, that's not the best solution because of potential environmental harm to fish, trees, and other living things.

The government, through the Drug Enforcement Administration, does have a solution, albeit a weak one. The DEA designates a specific time period (actually four *hours* in 2012—September 29, 2012, from 10 a.m. to 2 p.m.) during which people are supposed to take unused drugs to a designated disposal place.[162] In four previous take-back days, the response *was* impressive—people disposed of 774 tons of unwanted prescription drugs. But four hours a year seems microscopic compared to the enormity of the problem, although some local communities are beginning to make drug drop-off boxes more available. There are other solutions as well. The best I've seen is from the American Pharmacists Association.[163] They suggest mixing old pills in a sealable plastic bag with water, then adding kitty litter, sawdust, or coffee grounds to make it too gross for kids and pets to eat, and then putting the sealed bag in the regular trash. (For your own privacy, it's a good idea to remove your name from the now-empty bottles before you toss them.)

But it's not just friends and relatives who innocently contribute to the drug abuse problem. Thefts from doctors' offices, clinics, hospitals, pharmacies, and other parts of the "supply chain" are a growing part of the problem, too. Though pain patients and doctors are often blamed, these drugs get stolen *after* prescriptions are written and *before* they reach pain patients. Which raises another obvious question: If the government is so eager to catch drug abusers, why does it focus so much on doctors instead of putting more energy into chasing obviously illicit dealers, abusers, and drug thieves?

Researchers at the University of Delaware who wondered the same thing went straight to drug abusers for answers. In an intriguing 2007 study, they conducted focus groups with people from ethnically diverse, illicit-drug-using populations in Miami. These were club drug users, street drug users, methadone maintenance patients, and HIV-positive people—recreational users for whom the drug culture was a way of life.[164] These people got their drugs all over the place—from physicians, pharmacists, parents, relatives, "doctor shopping," leftover supplies in medicine cabinets, personal visits to Mexico, South America, and the Caribbean, direct sales on the street and in nightclubs, thefts from pharmacies and hospitals, under-the-door apartment flyers advertising telephone numbers to call, and, as the researchers note, "grandma's medicine cabinet."

"While doctor-shoppers, physicians and the Internet receive much of the attention regarding diversion, the data reported in this paper suggest that there are numerous active street markets involving patients, Medicaid recipients and pharmacies as well," the University of Delaware team found. In addition, they said, there are other data suggesting that the contributions of residential burglaries, pharmacy robberies and thefts, and "sneak thefts" to the diversion problem may be understated. In other words, news headlines about abuse and diversion make it seem as though doctors and pain patients are the problem. But often, they are not.

HOW EFFECTIVE *ARE* OPIOIDS LONG TERM? (A DYING CANCER PATIENT'S STORY)

Throughout most of this book, I focus on people with chronic non-cancer pain because that is where most of the controversy lies. But even people in the final stages of cancer often die in unnecessary pain, in part because opioids are simply not as effective as everyone wishes.

The result is that even in hospice and palliative care programs, pain is common. One-third of people in hospice report pain at the last hospice care visit before death, an Institute of Medicine report found.[165] A recent study from the University of Texas MD Anderson Cancer Center found much the same thing—one-third of cancer patients and cancer survivors had untreated or undertreated pain.[166] That's better than 18 years ago, when Texas researchers found that 42 percent of cancer patients had inadequately treated pain.[167] But not much.

Just 11 weeks before his death from esophageal cancer, I sat down at Memorial Sloan-Kettering Cancer Center in New York with Tom Fersch, 48, and his father, Stephen, who had come out from Arizona to be with him.[168] Tom walked in slowly, almost staggering under his burden of sadness, pain, and despair. As he peered out from his glasses, his bearded face was solemn. He had been diagnosed with cancer 15 months earlier and had soldiered through chemotherapy, radiation, and extensive surgery. To little avail.

"I have several months to live," he told me flatly, though his doctor, with whom I would speak later that day, doubted he would even make it to his next appointment in a month. Speaking in a whisper because doctors had nicked a vocal cord during surgery, Tom was hanging on by a fingernail to his job as director of sales for the New York Mets. "I will have to give it up soon," he said sorrowfully. A solitary man, his only social connections, aside from family scattered across the country, were his work friends. They want to help, he said, but he has refused their offers. "I don't want to be a charity case," he said. "I'm self-conscious of that." This afternoon, as usual, his overriding problem was pain—all over—in his stomach, his chest, and his back. The cancer, originally in the esophagus, was spreading relentlessly.

Surely, if anyone knew how to treat Tom's end-of-life pain, it would be the doctors here at Sloan-Kettering, a worldwide pioneer in pain management for cancer patients. But Tom's doctor, palliative care specialist Paul Glare, was running into the same harsh limits of modern medicine that frustrate all physicians trying to help people in unrelenting pain. Tom was already on every drug that Glare thought might help—three simultaneous, high-dose fentanyl patches, oral hydromorphone (Dilaudid), and oxycodone, plus two antidepressants. The drugs weren't cutting it.

"On a scale of zero to 10," I asked Tom, "how bad is your pain right now?"

"Eight," he said. Better than a 10. But nowhere good enough.

"The truth is, opioids only reduce pain by about 30 to 40 percent. There isn't anything out there that's 100 percent," Harvard psychologist Robert Jamison told me.[169] And some studies suggest the pain relief is not even that good.[170] In other words, opioids usually do not *eliminate* pain—even in the high doses that Tom Fersch and other cancer patients take at the end of life, when concerns like addiction, dependence, and abuse become irrelevant.

So what does the research show on long-term efficacy of opioids? [171] It's an incomplete and somewhat discouraging picture.

Some researchers, among them Forest Tennant, who runs a pain clinic in West Covina, California, believe opioids can be used safely and effectively for very long periods of time. In a 2010 article in *Practical Pain Management*, Tennant informally reviewed outcomes for 100 non-cancer pain patients whom he and three other doctors had treated with opioids for 10 years or more. This was purely anecdotal evidence, not a clinical trial. Nonetheless, most patients appeared to be doing well and almost half had not had to increase their dosages for at least three years.[172]

Recently, a small observational study of nearly 60 people with chronic non-cancer pain found that when low doses of opioids are administered intrathecally—that is, directly into the space around the spinal cord—both "worst" pain and "average" pain is reduced significantly.[173]

More scientifically solid studies on long-term opioid effectiveness are hard to come by. In fact, there is a conspicuous deficit of good evidence on long-term opioid use under real-world conditions, although, of course, absence of evidence is not evidence of absence.[174, 175] (Part of the reason for the lack of long-term data is that pharmaceutical manufacturers are not required to do long term studies.) Still, this knowledge gap has far-reaching consequences. "Because the long-term benefits are poorly defined and essentially undocumented, evidence of the *harms* [italics mine] of opioid pharmacotherapy tends to dominate the impressions of policy makers and the general public," concluded 25 pain specialists in a 2010 report.

The need for a stronger evidence base is urgent, the group said, adding that it takes studies that follow patients for a long time, not just a few weeks or months, to gauge long-term effectiveness. (In addition, the maximum doses of opioids used in randomized controlled trials are often lower than that used in clinical practice, which may also contribute to the impression of limited long-term efficacy.[176]) Citing one of the best studies that do exist, the group noted that on average, fewer than 40 percent of patients reach the criterion of 30 to 35 percent improvement in pain control, with even less evidence for improvement of function."[177]

Seattle pain researcher Michael Von Korff and his colleagues in Physicians for Responsible Opioid Prescribing (PROP), bemoan the lack of solid data on long-term opioid effectiveness, adding that, for many people, the efficacy of opioids may not be maintained over time.[178] For these and other reasons, Korff et al. say physicians should err on the side of caution when prescribing opioids long-term.[179]

In 2008, Pennsylvania researchers reviewed 17 studies involving 3,079 non-cancer patients taking opioids for more than six months.[180] Their depressing finding was that many patients were so dissatisfied with adverse events or insufficient pain relief from opioids that they withdrew from the studies. The dropouts included one-third of patients on oral opioids who couldn't stand side effects such as nausea, constipation, and upset stomach, and 12 percent on oral opioids for whom the drugs weren't helping. Opioids did reduce pain— somewhat—in the relatively small proportion of people who were able to keep taking them.

In 2010, the Pennsylvania group did another review of long-term opioids, this time analyzing 26 studies involving 4,893 patients.[181] Once again, they found huge dropout rates due to adverse side effects or insufficient pain relief. Twenty-three percent of oral opioid users dropped out for the former reason, and 10 percent for the latter. Their dismal conclusion? Opioids can provide pain relief in some patients, but the evidence is "weak."

Dropout rates were high in another analysis, by the 25-member team led by Richard Chapman in Utah. When they pooled results from many studies, they found the dropout rate was about 45 percent for people taking oral opioids, 25 percent for people using transdermal (skin) patches, and 17 percent for intrathecal opioids (infusions into the space around the spinal cord).[182] Patients dropped out mostly because of insufficient pain relief, adverse side effects, or both. A Danish study is even more discouraging. Researchers from Copenhagen conducted one of the first population-wide epidemiological studies of opioid therapy in chronic pain patients. (Denmark, which has an unusually liberal policy for opioid prescriptions, has the highest per capita usage of prescription opioids, mostly for non-cancer pain, in the world.[183, 184]) The researchers compared people in chronic pain who were taking opioids to similar people who weren't. The opioid users actually reported more severe pain, worse health, and lower quality of life than the nonusers. This pattern persisted even after controlling for pain severity.

A subsequent population-based Danish study in 2010 by some of the same researchers came to a similar conclusion: "The odds of recovery from chronic pain were almost four times higher among individuals *not* [italics mine] using opioids compared with individuals using opioids."[185] Even "when opioids are widely used to treat chronic pain, as they are in Denmark, a substantial number of patients do not achieve the chief goals of treatment to improve pain, function and quality of life," comments University of Washington pain specialist Jane Ballantyne.[186] It's enough to discourage the hardiest of patients and the most concerned doctors. Some discouraged physicians, such as San Francisco's Michael Katz, have lost so much faith in opioids that they advise setting limits— a maximum dose—on opioids, a recommendation with which other leading pain specialists vigorously disagree.[187, 188]

Meanwhile, as the researchers write papers, people like Tom Fersch, the Mets salesman with esophageal cancer, still suffer. Not long after I saw him, Tom Fersch died, despite his doctor's best efforts to control his pain and the best drugs so far available. Tragically, he died in pain.

BOX 7.1 CONTROLLED SUBSTANCES BY CSA SCHEDULE

The federal government, via the 1970 Controlled Substances Act, has outlined five "schedules" for classifying prescription drugs that have the potential to be abused.[189, 190]

Schedule I: These drugs have a high potential for abuse and have no currently accepted medical use in treatment in the United States. Drugs in this category include the opioid heroin, as well as non-opioid drugs such as MDMA (Ecstasy), GHB (gamma hydroxybutyrate), LSD, marijuana, peyote, methaqualone, psilocybin (magic mushrooms), and many others.

Schedule II: These drugs also have a high potential for abuse but do have currently accepted medical use in the United States. Opioids drugs in this category include opium, codeine, fentanyl, hydromorphone, levorphanol, meperidine, methadone, morphine, oxycodone and oxymorphone, as well as the combination of oxycodone plus acetaminophen (Percocet).

Schedules III, IV, and V: These drugs have a lower potential for abuse relative to the drugs in Schedule II and have currently accepted medical uses in the United States. Schedule III drugs include the opioids hydrocodone and codeine in combination with nonopioids. Hydrocodone plus acetaminophen is Vicodin, Lortab, Lorcet, and others. Codeine in combination with acetaminophen is Tylenol with Codeine. Buprenorphine is in Schedule III. There are no opioid or opioid combination drugs in Schedule IV; drugs in this schedule include the benzodiazepines such Valium, Ativan, and Xanax, and sleep medications such as Ambien. Schedule V drugs include codeine-cough syrup and Lyrica (pregabalin).

Table 7.1 FEDERAL SCHEDULES FOR CONTROLLED SUBSTANCES

Schedule Number	Potential for Abuse	Examples	Availability and Restrictions
Schedule I	No currently accepted medical use in the United States. High potential for abuse.	Hallucinogenic substances (e.g., LSD); heroin and certain other opioids; methaqualone, marijuana.[a]	Available for research, instructional use, and chemical analysis purpose. Marijuana available for a few patients.
Schedule II	Currently accepted medical use in the United States. High potential for abuse. Severe liability to cause psychological or physical dependence.	Opium, morphine, codeine, hydromorphone, oxycodone, oxymorphone, methadone, fentanyl, tapentadol, dextroamphetamine, methamphetamine, methylphenidate, amobarbital, pentobarbital, secobarbital, nabilone.	Written prescription required except in emergencies; however, written prescriptions may be transmitted by fax in some instances. No refills.
Schedule III	Potential for abuse less than for drugs in Schedules I and II. Abuse may lead to moderate or lower physical and psychological dependence than substances in Schedules I or II.	Combination products of codeine or hydrocodone with aspirin, acetaminophen, or ibuprofen; certain sedative drugs such as thiopental; buprenorphine; dronabinol; anabolic steroids.	Oral prescription orders allowed. Prescription orders valid for six months. Five refills allowed in six months.
Schedule IV	Lower potential for abuse than drugs in Schedule III. Limited physical or psychological dependence.	Benzodiazepines,[b] zaleplon, zolpidem, zopiclone, phenobarbital, certain sedative drugs, butorphanol.[c]	Same restrictions as for Schedule III.
Schedule V	Potential for abuse is less than for drugs in Schedule IV.	Pregabalin,[d] lacosamide, pyrovalerone, and antitussive and antidiarrheal preparations containing moderate quantities of opioids.	May be dispensed without a prescription order. Antidiarrheals that contain low doses of difenoxin and diphenoxylate. In some states, antitussives with codeine are prescription drugs.

Note. Tramadol and carisoprodol (Soma) are controlled substances in some states. Data compiled with assistance from J. Dahl (personal communication, April 22, 2011).

[a] New Marijuana is in Schedule I; thus it is against federal law to prescribe it as medicine. Nevertheless, many states have passed medical marijuana laws to make the substance available for medical use. The Justice Department has decided not to prosecute people in the states who grow, sell, and use marijuana. Note also that dronabinol (a Schedule III drug) contains THC in sesame oil.

[b] Benzodiazepines are in Schedule II in New York.

[c] Butorphanol and nalbuphine are mixed agonist-antagonist opioids. However, butorphanol is in Schedule IV and nalbuphine is not scheduled.

[d] Pregabalin is in Schedule V, but gabapentin, which has an essentially identical mechanism, is not scheduled.

CHAPTER 8

Opioid Wars, Part II

Proposed Solutions

NALOXONE FOR EVERYBODY: THE ANTIDOTE TO OPIOID OVERDOSES?

The worst risk of opioids, obviously, is overdose, whether intentional or not. An astonishingly elegant, simple, and apparently effective idea is now emerging to safeguard against this: Give pain patients taking opioids a supply of naloxone, an opioid antagonist, to have on hand at home in case of overdose.

Naloxone (Narcan) is a standby in emergency rooms. In fact, drug addicts who overdose are routinely injected with naloxone to reverse potentially fatal breathing problems. Naloxone is also available as a nasal spray. In both forms, naloxone rapidly knocks heroin and other opioids off opioid receptors, potentially triggering instant withdrawal but also restoring breathing and thus saving lives. It has virtually no abuse potential and a favorable safety profile.[1] In the *harm-reduction* scenario researchers are now exploring, pain patients would simply get a prescription for naloxone from their doctors along with their opioid prescription. Naloxone is not a controlled substance and hence could be prescribed by any doctor and many advanced practice nurses. Better yet, some say, given its good safety profile, naloxone could be made available over-the-counter.[2]

In Wilkes County, North Carolina, in a community-based effort called the Lazarus Project, free, intranasal naloxone has been central to successful efforts to combat opioid overdose deaths.[3] Preliminary data, published in 2011 in *Pain Medicine*, show that, though Wilkes County initially had one of the highest drug overdose death rates in the nation, the Lazarus Project was linked to a reduction in deaths from 46.6 per 100,000 in 2009 to 29.0 per 100,000 in 2010.[4] The Lazarus Project involved both substance abusers and pain patients. (Pain patients on long-term opioids are actually less likely than substance abusers to develop respiratory depression because they often become tolerant to the drugs.[5])

In Boston, Massachusetts, the city's public health commission reported in April 2011 that deaths from overdoses among abusers of heroin and other opioids plunged after the city began distributing Narcan kits to addicts in 2006.[6] Overdose deaths dropped by 32 percent between 2007 and 2008 alone, the city said. The success of the Boston program has spurred Massachusetts to begin a larger, statewide program to distribute Narcan in hopes of reducing overdose deaths.[7] When sprayed into the nose, Narcan is "safe, easy to administer and has no potential for abuse," the state says.

At the national level, the federal Centers for Disease Control and Prevention announced in February 2012 that community-based programs using naloxone have prevented the opioid overdose deaths of 10,171 people since 1996. As of October 2010, there were at least 188 such programs in the United States, the agency said.[8] Perhaps in part because of that success, the US Food and Drug Administration is now considering approval of wider distribution and use of naloxone.[9] While both the injectable and nasal spray forms of naloxone work well, a big advantage of the nasal formulation is that rescuers don't need to draw up naloxone in a needle and inject it, says anesthesiologist Daniel Carr of Tufts University.[10] Using a nasal spray also eliminates the potential problem of infections from needles.

But there is an obvious drawback to the naloxone "rescue" idea. For it to prevent death in someone who has overdosed, there must be other people around—friends, relatives, or emergency medical personnel—who recognize when someone is in trouble and know how to administer naloxone.

THE IRONY: USING DRUGS TO TREAT DRUG DEPENDENCE

In addition to preventing deaths from opioid overdoses, doctors and scientists are trying to find ways to help people in pain who become physically dependent on or even addicted to opioids to withdraw from them safely. This can get tricky. While on opioids, a person may think he or she is no longer in pain. But if the pain is still present, it may get worse again if the opioids are decreased or stopped, making it a delicate balancing act to manage the symptoms of opioid withdrawal while controlling the pain. It's more difficult still to treat chronic pain in people who also have a history of substance abuse.

Understandably, many pain patients want nothing more than to get off opioids the minute they think their pain is better. If drugs are the problem, the thinking goes, why not just get all that bad stuff out of your system as fast as possible, hope that the underlying pain is really gone, and get on with life? And it often *is* that easy. "Tens of millions of people per year are started on some dosage of opioids and all pretty much get off. As the need diminishes, they just taper the dose. It happens all the time and people don't think about it," Carr of Tufts told me.[11] This is especially true for people taking opioids for a few weeks or so after surgery.

But as we saw with Paul Konowitz, the Boston physician and pain patient we met in Chapter 7, getting off opioids can sometimes be more difficult, in part because many doctors don't know how to help people do it. The simplest way, says Carr, is to taper very, very slowly, cutting the dose of opioids by about 10 percent a week. "That's super gentle," he said, and usually avoids symptoms of withdrawal, also known as opioid abstinence syndrome.

Some people, very eager to get off drugs, don't do it quite that slowly. Keosha Johnson, an editor/producer at WBUR.org in Boston was one of them.[12] After spinal fusion surgery, she was discharged from the hospital and told to take oxycodone, which worked very well to control her pain. In fact, it made her feel normal. About six weeks later, she decided she didn't need it anymore. "I did know I was supposed to taper off," she says. "I was told that when I was in the hospital, and given paperwork that said to call my doctor when I was ready to get off to get specific instructions on how to do it. I just forgot. Plus, I figured I could quit cold turkey because I was no longer in pain—it never occurred to me that I would experience severe withdrawal after taking it for six weeks."

But she did. Within a day of taking her last dose, she lay in bed "practically twitching, as an intense jittery feeling spread through my upper torso. I tossed and turned until dawn, breaking a sweat as I repeatedly stretched one arm, then the other, as something akin to having consumed several cans of Red Bull continued to wreak an internal havoc inside of me." She called her doctor, who told her to taper more slowly, which she did, with few problems. Now she is opioid-free.

For people who *do* encounter opioid withdrawal symptoms, it's reasonable to counteract those symptoms with judicious use of other drugs, Carr says. Granted, it may sound crazy to think of taking *more* drugs to combat the effects of the initial drugs. But done properly, it can be a safe, temporary fix to allow the body to get its biochemistry back to normal. One drug that can ease the agitation of opioid withdrawal is clonidine, a blood pressure medication that reduces the jittery feelings that are triggered when the body overproduces the stress hormones epinephrine and norepinephrine during opioid withdrawal. Clonidine also blocks excessive epinephrine and norepinephrine production. Another option is a sedating antidepressant medication such as Trazodone, which blunts the tendency of the heart to race and blocks some of the agitation and anxiety triggered by withdrawal. If opioid withdrawal triggers intense anxiety, benzodiazepines such as Ativan can also help. (Dependence and addiction can be a problem with Ativan, but to a lesser extent than with some other drugs.[13]) Antiemetics can also be used to combat nausea and vomiting, antidiarrheals to treat diarrhea, and quinine to help with skeletal muscle cramps.[14]

The reason it can be hard to get off opioids is that once you have been taking them regularly, opioid receptors in the nervous system get used to being occupied. And they don't like it when they're suddenly empty. If you stop cold turkey, opioid receptors start "screaming because they are no longer full. You get pain, sweating, chills, abdominal cramps, muscle aches. That's where the expression 'kicking the habit' came from—people kick their legs to relieve the muscle cramps," explains Carol Garner, an addiction specialist at Boston's Faulkner Hospital.[15] That's why tapering very, very slowly is key.

But what if you have become, not just physically dependent on opioids, but addicted? And what if, in addition, you still have a legitimate problem with chronic pain? What if, in other words, you are both a pain patient and a person with addiction? This is a difficult problem for patients and doctors alike, but even here, there are options.

One is methadone, a substitute opioid that can be used as a maintenance drug. That is, it fills up opioid receptors to reduce symptoms of withdrawal from and craving for other opioids while also providing pain control.[16] Instead of needing an opioid every three to six hours, a person can take methadone once a day and still avoid withdrawal symptoms, says Jan Kauffman, an addiction specialist at the North Charles Institute for the Addictions in Somerville, Massachusetts.[17]

When used primarily for pain, as opposed to addiction, methadone is often given two or three times a day.[18] It can be taken for years if necessary. Another benefit of methadone is that it can be taken orally instead of by injection. As long as a person stays on methadone, it reduces the risk of addictive behaviors like injecting drugs, which can lead to more problems, including AIDS and hepatitis from dirty needles.[19, 20, 21]

A possibly better, though more expensive, option for pain patients who have become addicted to opioids may be buprenorphine, which is also an opioid, but one that binds to some opioid receptors less strongly than other opioids.[22] (Buprenorphine is sold as Suboxone and Subutex. Pure buprenorphine is Subutex; if the opioid blocker naloxone is added, it's Suboxone.)

When an opioid hits its receptor, the receptor changes its physical shape, which triggers a cascade of chemical events inside the cell that, ultimately, leads to pain relief. But tiny changes in the shape of an opioid can make it fit more or less securely into the receptor. Morphine, for instance, binds very well to opioid receptors or, to put it more technically, has a high "affinity" for these receptors. Buprenorphine keeps opioid receptors occupied, but not fully.[23] In theory, buprenorphine binds just enough to keep withdrawal symptoms away, and to provide some pain relief as well. Often, for someone who has both persistent pain and addiction, a doctor trained in both pain and addiction medicine will "cross-taper" regular opioids and buprenorphine. It's a pretty complicated regimen,[24] but involves slowly *decreasing the* dose of the standard opioid and gradually *increasing* the dose of buprenorphine.

Buprenorphine doesn't seem to have the same overdose risk of other opioids, and also appears less likely to produce respiratory depression and tolerance. (Tolerance means a person needs more and more of a drug to achieve the desired effect.[25, 26]) In the buprenorphine-plus-naloxone formulation, there's also a built-in anti-abuse feature. If someone tries to crush the tablets, mix the powder with water, and inject it to get high, the naloxone will kick in and block the effects of buprenorphine, triggering withdrawal.

In 2011, researchers at McLean Hospital and Harvard Medical School conducted the first randomized large-scale clinical trial at 10 sites nationwide with 653 people who were physically dependent on prescription opioids. Almost half were people who also had chronic pain. The researchers tested the effectiveness of Suboxone for different amounts of time and with different amounts of counseling added.[27] Short-term Suboxone treatment did almost no good—only about 7 percent of patients randomized to a two-week treatment followed by a two-week tapering off period were able to get off and stay off their prescription opioids. In the group that took Suboxone for 12 weeks, followed by a four-week taper, however, almost half the group (49 percent) successfully got off prescription pain relievers. (The group that had the longer treatment were those who had failed with the shorter treatment.) The amount of counseling made no difference in outcomes. But here's the bad news: Once Suboxone treatment was stopped, there was a high rate of relapse.

Buprenorphine can also be used under the tongue, transdermally (through a patch on the skin),[28] and via implants. In a study led by researchers from the University of California, Los Angeles, doctors at 18 medical centers around the country studied people with opioid dependence recruited from addiction centers. They randomized the patients to get implants of buprenorphine or implants of a placebo medication. (The study did not include people with chronic pain requiring opioid treatment.) All were followed for six months, and they provided regular urine samples as they went along. The results were impressive. The buprenorphine group had significantly more "clean" urine samples, meaning they had not taken illicit drugs, during the study than the placebo group. The buprenorphine group also had fewer withdrawal symptoms and less drug craving.[29] If confirmed by further studies, the new findings would represent a major advance.[30]

Implantable buprenorphine has the additional advantage that once it's placed under the skin, it can't be tampered with, so it is less likely than an oral formulation to be abused. A study of transdermal buprenorphine in 1,160 people, this time, in people with chronic back pain, also yielded encouraging results.[31] On the downside, taking buprenorphine is no walk in the park. It can cause nausea, vomiting, constipation, head-aches, leg swelling, and insomnia.[32]

Methadone and buprenorphine are not the only drugs used to treat opioid dependence and addiction. In 2010, the FDA approved an extended-release form of naltrexone (marketed as Vivitrol), which acts by blocking opioid receptors but is not itself an opioid, as buprenor-phine is. Janet Woodcock, director of the FDA's Center for Drug Evaluation and Research, praised Vivitrol's approval as "a significant advancement."[33]

OPIOID ROTATION

Opioid rotation is another approach to managing opioid problems, par-ticularly tolerance and opioid side effects. One of the leaders in modern opioid rotation is Perry Fine, a pain specialist in Salt Lake City, Utah. Fine grew up wanting to be a professional cellist and composer, became "addicted" to soccer while going to high school in France, then swerved to science and finally medicine, because, he said smiling, he wanted "to be of service and have a meaningful life."[34]

He certainly has had that. When the Olympics took over Salt Lake City in 2002, Fine, who had been the sideline trauma physician for the University of Utah football team, was there at the ice center, watching Sarah Hughes win the gold in figure skating and tending to the other athletes' aches and pains. But his real passion has become helping people in chronic pain and teaching doctors how to use opioids more safely and effectively. To that end, Fine, along with Russell Portenoy, the New York pain specialist, Roger Chou, a pain specialist at the Oregon Health & Science University and a handful of others, have fine-tuned a systematic way of rotating opioids to minimize *tolerance*—the body's adaptation to opioids that results in needing higher doses to get the same reduction in pain. The idea is to rotate opioids without triggering new bouts of pain.

Opioid rotation formulas have been around for 40 years and are slowly being revised as pain specialists learn more about the drugs.[35, 36, 37, 38] The goal, says Fine, is to use "equianalgesic tables" to estimate what dose of the opioid to be tried is equal in pain relieving capacity to the old one that is no longer working or that has too many side effects. This is stated in *mor-phine equivalents*. In other words, the prescribing doctor mathematically calculates the daily dose of the old opioid as an equivalent dose of morphine, then uses the tables again to convert from morphine to the new opioid; the doctor then reduces the dose of the new drug slightly to avoid overmedication. Ideally, the doctor does a second assessment soon after the patient changes to the new drug, and lowers or raises the dose accordingly. The patient's job is to be alert to increases or decreases in pain and side effects. It sounds easy. But in practice it becomes very tricky, partly because each person responds differently to any given drug. Certain drugs (especially fentanyl and methadone) are especially complex. Things also get complicated changing from an oral drug to an IV formulation or from long-acting to short-acting, or vice versa.

In fact, one of the biggest problems in opioid rotation is prescriber mistakes, which can occur because of insufficient training and the use of inaccurate dose conversion tables, conclude Fine and Utah colleague Lynn Webster, medical director of Lifetree Clinical Research in Salt Lake City. In 2012 papers,[39, 40] Webster and Fine describe a new paradigm for a patient who needed to be changed from extended-release oxycodone to extended-release hydromorphone. They slowly decreased the oxycodone while slowly increasing the hydromorphone. The key was to provide enough fairly fast-acting rescue opioid to handle breakthrough pain and stop acute withdrawal symptoms. Webster's and Fine's technique involves three steps—reducing the original opioid dose by 10 to 30 percent while starting the new opioid at the lowest available dose, then further reducing the original opioid by 10 to 25 percent per week while increasing the new opioid by 10 to 20 percent. All the while, it's important for the patient to use rescue opioids occasionally as needed if pain becomes too intense. Most patients can be rotated safely to the new opioid in about a month. But it takes a careful doctor and a careful patient to keep track of three different medications (the old opioid, the new one, and the rescue drug) on a specific schedule.[41]

NEW ABUSE-DETERRENT OPIOIDS: ANOTHER ANSWER?

One of the holy grails for researchers has been to create versions of opioids that are harder to abuse—so-called abuse-deterrent, tamper-resistant, or tamper deterrent formulations of existing drugs.[42, 43] These are drugs that are designed to be harder to tamper with or to use improperly, such as by crushing the drugs in order to snort or inject them. (Obviously, determined abusers can still *swallow* abuse-deterrent drugs in excessive quantities to get high.)

Importantly, the abuse-deterrent formulations are made with *abusers*, rather than responsible pain patients, in mind. But these drugs can indirectly help pain patients if they reduce abuse and the resulting stigma attached to opioids.

Abuse, of course, can happen with both long-acting and short-acting oral opioids. But long-acting opioids are particularly worrying because, if abusers crush or chew them, they get the full dose of the opioid all at once, not, as is supposed to happen, over many hours. At high enough doses, this form of abuse can be fatal.[44]

In August 2010, Purdue Pharma began selling an abuse-deterrent formulation of OxyContin that is harder to crush. (In Canada, it's sold as OxyNeo, according to Purdue spokesman Jim Heins.[45]) The new version breaks into chunks rather than a powder, as Katherine Eban explains in 2011 in *Fortune*.[46] If water is added, "the result is a gelatinous goop. So far, the new OxyContin appears to be withstanding attempts to crush, snort or inject it."

Which is precisely the deterrent effect the manufacturer hoped for. The street price of the abuse-deterrent formulation—the price abusers are willing to pay on the black market—has dropped from 73 cents per milligram to 52 cents, Eban reported. Data from the Researched Abuse, Diversion and Addiction-Related Surveillance (RADARS) System, a program funded by Purdue, also show that abusers, as hoped, do not like the new OxyContin.[47, 48, 49]

But there's downside to this apparent success. Early signs show that determined abusers are switching to other opioids, including heroin. In a July 2012 letter to the *New England Journal of Medicine*, researchers from Washington University reported that the percent of drug abusers who chose OxyContin as their primary drug of abuse dropped from 36 percent *before* the release of the new abuse-deterrent formulation to 13 percent today. In the same time period, abusers reported that their use of heroin almost doubled.[50, 51] Besides OxyContin, other harder-to-crush opioids are now on the market, including Exalgo (by Covidien),

Opana ER (by Endo), and Nucynta ER (by Janssen). It's too soon to tell what the abuse-deterrent effect of these formulations will be. But abusers who are now shying away from OxyContin do seem to be turning to Opana as well as heroin.[52]

Coming up with strategies for abuse-deterrent opioids has not been easy, and some seemingly good ideas have fallen by the wayside. One idea was the cleverly designed Embeda, an extended-release combination of morphine and naltrexone. Morphine was placed around the outside of the pill, with naltrexone, an opioid blocker, sequestered on the inside. If you swallowed the pill as intended, you would get the long-lasting, pain-relieving effects of morphine; the naltrexone would not be absorbed and would just pass right through your system, doing nothing. If, however, you crushed or chewed Embeda, the naltrexone would be released all of a sudden, which would keep the morphine from binding to opioid receptors. This would prevent a high, and would also bring on sudden, potentially dangerous, withdrawal, making the drug decidedly unattractive to abusers. Unfortunately, safety problems temporarily doomed Embeda and in March 2011, King Pharmaceuticals recalled all dosages of it.[53]

Drug makers have tried other abuse-deterrent strategies—like adding something noxious to opioids such as niacin, a vitamin that, in high doses, produces uncomfortable flushing. A potential drug in this category was Acurox, oxycodone plus niacin. But the FDA rejected it on the grounds that niacin was not a powerful enough deterrent.[54] The agency also rejected another abuse-deterrent product, Remoxy.[55] Currently, researchers are also testing other ways to reduce abuse. One strategy is to create *prodrugs* that become active only when the body metabolizes them. The chemical process of metabolism converts the opioid from an inactive to an active form.[56] Still another idea is an anti-opioid vaccine, which, in theory, could protect against both heroin and HIV. Pieces of the heroin molecule would be attached to the tetanus bacterium to stimulate antibodies against heroin. So far, it has not been tested in the real world, but is being studied at the Walter Reed Army Institute of Technology, sponsored by the National Institute on Drug Abuse.[57]

OTHER WAYS TO COMBAT ABUSE: MEDICATION CONTRACTS AND TESTS

Increasingly, pain specialists are requiring patients to sign *contracts*, or the term many pain specialists prefer, *agreements*, which spell out the opioid doses to be taken, the risks of misusing the drugs, a list of rules and obligations, and signs of side effects and potential improvement to be recorded.

It sounds reasonable. But some analysts and ethicists worry that the contracts can be insulting and stigmatizing for patients. After all, we don't force people with other medical problems to sign such things. The agreements may be a decent educational tool for informing patients about the risks and benefits of opioids. There's certainly no harm in making sure people understand the risks and benefits of any drugs they're taking, opioids included. And there's no harm in reminding people not to try to refill prescriptions too early, not to increase doses on their own, and not to drink alcohol with medications.

The trouble is, it's not clear how effective such documents really are. Moreover, they can potentially do more harm than good by interfering with the essential trust between patient and doctor. Some agreements actually border on the offensive, like those that say, "You will be on time for appointments," or "You will be respectful to me and my staff."[58] (As far as I know, agreements don't specify that doctors be on time or be respectful toward patients.) More important, medication agreements often miss the point. What pain patients really want from their doctors is pain relief, not a discussion of the public health problems of opioid misuse. In other words, contracts essentially shift the locus of concern from helping pain patients to protecting providers against the perceived risk from regulatory and law enforcement agencies, says Myra Christopher of the Kansas City–based Center for Practical Bioethics. In essence, she says, medication contracts address a *social* problem—the drug abuse epidemic—rather than a *clinical* problem, as if every pain patient were a potential criminal.

In a paper in 2010, Christopher and a team of leading ethicists and pain specialists argue that contracts don't really address the problem of opioid drug *diversion*. As federal statistics show, the main way opioids get into the wrong hands is not by bad patients trying to scam their doctors but from friends and family—including home medicine cabinets from which opioids can easily be taken. Intentional diversion by patients, the Christopher team notes, is potentially quite small. Compelling patients to sign medication agreements, in other words, not only focuses on a comparatively trivial part of the diversion problem, but it stigmatizes patients and corrodes patient–doctor trust.[59]

A much better approach, the bioethicists say, is to use standard informed consent forms that spell out potential risks, as is done for surgical procedures. Some major medical organizations—including the American Academy of Pain Medicine and the Veterans' Health Administration, as well as the Federation of State Medical Boards—do say that physicians should consider medication contracts for patients at high risk for medication abuse on the grounds that such contracts may be helpful for patients having difficulty managing their medications. But curiously, when the US Food and Drug Administration in 2009 first introduced its idea for a different drug-control program (REMS, which we'll get to in a minute), it endorsed these "prescriber–patient agreements." But in June 2010, after public hearings, the FDA issued its final recommendations for REMS and no longer required the universal use of opioid contracts or agreements.[60]

In any case, it's not clear how effective medication agreements are. The research is ambiguous.[61] A 2010 review by researchers from New York, Boston, New Haven, and Philadelphia, for instance, looked at 11 studies and found only relatively weak evidence supporting the use of patient contracts along with urine testing.[62] And there are potential harms. The New York team, led by Joanna Starrels of Albert Einstein College of Medicine, worried that patients might feel so stigmatized by the contracts that they might forgo pain treatment. On the other hand, some respected pain specialists, like Harvard Medical School's Robert Jamison, think the contracts are valuable if they encourage communication between the patient and the doctor, and reinforce to patients that they should not "doctor shop" or use up their pills faster than prescribed. But they're certainly not a panacea, he adds, because "folks who misuse [drugs] will agree to anything."[63]

Medication contracts may clarify patient and physician responsibilities, noted California public health guru Mitchell Katz. "But when you create a contract, and the patients do not follow their part of the bar-gain, what do you do next?"[64]

The contracts may also be unenforceable for a number of reasons, writes commentator Mark Collen in the *Journal of Law, Medicine & Ethics*.[65] An opioid contract, he says, may be considered an "unconscio-nable adhesion contract," which means it is, in essence, a contract pre-pared by one party (a doctor) to be signed by a party (the patient) in a weaker position. Given the asymmetrical power distribution in the doctor–patient relationship, such a contract may be intrinsically unfair because it does not involve meaningful choice for the patient. And there's one last concern: Opioid contracts are often written at such a high level as to not be fully understood by the patient.

* * *

Another tactic to try to make sure pain patients don't abuse opioids is urine testing. Indeed, many opioid contracts stipulate that patients must submit to random urine drug testing, to see whether people are taking the right medications and not mixing them with other drugs. The CDC recommends such testing for any patient younger than 65 with non-cancer pain who has been on opioids for more than six weeks.[66] The influential Federation of State Medical Boards also thinks they can be helpful in people at high risk for medication abuse.[67] A panel of experts convened to write opioid prescribing guidelines also recom-mends periodic urine testing, or some other monitoring information, for patients at high risk for abuse.[68]

But once again, we have to ask: Does urine testing yield clinically meaningful results? Is it overly stigmatizing? Who is it really protect-ing? Who really benefits, besides urine testing companies? And how reliable can it be when patients can buy "clean" urine on the Internet?[69]

There's another question, too: Is urine testing even constitutional? Randomly testing people simply because they seek treatment with opi-oids for chronic pain could, arguably, be considered a "suspicionless and warrantless search" that could violate both the Fourth and Fourteenth Amendments.[70] To be sure, it may make some patients feel secure to have urine tests that monitor medication levels or detect whether patients are mixing drugs inappropriately. But urine testing also may send a patient the message that the doctor does not trust him or her—an appropriate message for some people, but insulting and demeaning for others. (There's also some evidence that urine testing can be racially discriminatory, according to a Yale University study involving 1,612 patients.[71])

What is clear is that a sizable chunk of pain patients on opioids who take urine tests flunk. In a 2007 Harvard study, 45 percent of 470 patients had abnormal urine tests—a red flag for what's awkwardly called "aberrant drug-related behaviors," to be sure.[72] And that's not too surprising. Many people do not take their medications in the specific ways their doctors prescribe. A national survey of 76,000 urine tests for prescription drug medications by Quest Diagnostics, a testing company, showed that 63 percent of patients take their medications in ways inconsistent with their doctors' orders—including missing doses and combining medications.[73, 74, 75]

But even with something as seemingly objective as urine testing, it's impossible to come to definitive conclusions.[76] Some tests may also have built-in validity problems, in part because some drugs leave the body much more quickly than others.[77] This, of course, makes the timing of urine drug testing tricky. In other words, urine tests may only show a short snapshot in time and reveal nothing about longer term drug use or abuse.

It's also troubling that some studies that purport to show the effectiveness of urine testing are paid for by companies that make the urine tests. The profit motive, rather than public health, may be spurring the growing use of testing.[78] Indeed, some published studies claiming to show the value of urine drug testing are written by employees of or contractors from drug testing companies.[79, 80] A presentation on urine drug testing at the 2012 annual meeting of the American Academy of Pain Medicine, for instance, was sponsored by Ameritox, a drug test lab.[81, 82] But Ameritox has a troubled reputation. In 2011, Ameritox was forced to pay $16.3 million to the federal government to settle claims that it provided kickbacks to physicians for drug testing.[83, 84, 85] In June 2012, Ameritox and a competitor, Millennium, did battle in court over what Millennium alleged were false and deceptive advertising claims by Ameritox. (The court agreed, but did not assess monetary damages.[86, 87])

Urine drug testing also has cost considerations for pain patients. If office-based urine testing proves inconclusive, patients may have to pay out of pocket for additional, outside testing.[88]

Finally, for people in pain who find themselves subject to urine testing, there are some clear dos and don'ts. For example, *don't* eat a poppy seed bagel (or anything else with poppy seeds) before a urine test—the test might show morphine or its metabolites;[89, 90] and *do* be up front with your doctor—*before* any urine test—about all medications, legal and illegal, that you take, including dietary supplements. If you've been at a party where there was marijuana smoke, mention that, too, even if you didn't actually smoke yourself. Telling your doctor about everything you're taking is good for your *own* health and safety. And fessing up ahead of time preserves your credibility.

PRESCRIPTION DRUG MONITORING PROGRAMS (PMPs)

Among the most important strategies for combating opioid abuse and diversion are prescription monitoring programs (PMPs), also called prescription drug monitoring programs (PDMPs). In different forms, these state-based programs have been around for decades. Today, almost all states now either have PMPs in place or have enacted legislation to set up such programs.[91, 92, 93, 94, 95] Not surprisingly, the PMPs vary considerably state by state.[96]

In general, the goal of these state programs, which are funded in part by the federal Department of Justice and the Department of Health and Human Services, is to collect dispensing data in order to detect questionable patterns of drug use, such as "doctor shopping" or "pharmacy shopping," and thereby—in theory—reduce diversion of opioids.[97]

The data collected by PMPs are available, depending on specific state-by-state laws, to a *lot* of people—physicians and other practitioners; pharmacists; federal, state, and local law enforcement personnel; professional or occupational licensing authorities; and individuals whose receipt of prescriptions has been included in the PMP database.[98] This raises potential confidentiality concerns, although typically law enforcement personnel must show that they have probable cause—good reason—to be interested in the information. Just as troubling, there is no clear evidence that PMPs are either safe or effective—with safety, in this case, meaning doing no harm (such as reducing access to opioids by pain patients) and effectiveness meaning catching people who really are out to abuse or divert the drugs.

PMPs get dispensing data from pharmacies, then make them available to law enforcement agencies and prescribers. (How much access to this data law enforcement should have and under what circumstances are major points of contention.) The programs typically require pharmacies to put prescription data into a centralized, electronic database, including information that identifies the prescriber, dispenser, and patient, along with the drug, dosage, and amount dispensed.[99] In theory, PMPs could be the basis for a reasonably balanced opioid policy that would allow legitimate pain patients access to the opioids they need while restricting access to abusers, says June Dahl, a professor of neuroscience at the University of Wisconsin who is widely regarded as a leader in opioid policy research. "If we had effective PMPs," she told me, "we wouldn't have to be thinking about other federal mandates, which have great potential to adversely affect quality of care."[100]

But it's unclear how useful PMPs are.[101] A 2002 General Accounting Office review looked at PMPs in 15 states and found that PMPs did seem to reduce the time and effort needed by regulatory bodies to investigate drug diversion cases.[102] But the report also revealed a problem: States that border a state with a PMP often had an *increase* in the supply of prescription drugs, suggesting that patients went "doctor shopping" to get their drugs. In 2006, researchers for the federal Department of Justice reviewed the evidence on PMPs and concluded that when PMPs share their data readily with prescribing physicians and pharmacists, there is a 10 percent drop in prescription sales and a reduction in prescription drug abuse.[103] But this drop in prescriptions could mean more undertreatment of pain for legitimate patients. In a 2010 study, Boston-area pain specialist Nathaniel Katz focused on one state—Massachusetts—and tracked 11 years' worth of PMP data, from 1996 to 2006.[104] He found that it was only when people used four or more prescribers or got their drugs from four or more pharmacies that there were signs of questionable activity.

At best, PMPs address the problem of drug diversion stemming only from prescribing relationships, not the larger issue—getting drugs from family, friends, and unlocked medicine cabinets.[105] Moreover, many doctors don't even know about PMPs, which means that even well-intended state efforts are seriously underutilized. Prescription drug monitoring programs can also be cumbersome and expensive, as the state of California has discovered.[106]

One of the researchers concerned about the efficacy of PMPs is psychologist Robert Twillman, director of policy and advocacy at the American Academy of Pain Management, who thinks the programs do work, though that hasn't been scientifically shown yet.[107, 108] His findings are discouraging. He compared states with and without programs using data from a single year, 2003. In general, he found that in states with PMPs, there is a reduction in prescriptions for some opioids, but there's a concurrent *increase* in others such as Vicodin. While PMPs may trigger a shift in the pattern of prescribing, actual rates of abuse may not drop at all.[109] Moreover, even if a state with a PMP experiences a sudden drop in prescriptions, it's hard to know what that means. Does it mean less abuse and diversion? Or does it mean that doctors are getting even more scared of writing pain-reliever prescriptions?

In other words, while in theory PMPs should help control abuse and diversion, there's not much research to support that. The programs may indeed identify people who "doctor shop" and "pharmacy shop," but even doctor shopping and pharmacy shopping may simply indicate that pain patients are having trouble getting the help they need. PMPs may also create an unintended substitution effect, whereby doctors, fearful of getting ensnared in PMP red tape, write fewer prescriptions for some drugs and more for others that may not be as effective for chronic pain. Most important, PMPs may not accomplish a most basic goal—lowering the rates of overdose and death from opioids.

The most troubling—and controversial—assessment of PMPs came in 2011 from the government itself, specifically, the federal Centers for Disease Control and Prevention (CDC). It conducted the first major study assessing the effectiveness of PMPs, examining data from 1999 to 2005 across the United States. The study was flawed. PMP efforts in different states were set up so differently that comparisons were not easy. In some states, PMPs were just getting started. And federal funding to assist states in their PMP efforts kicked in only partway through the study.[110]

Nonetheless, the CDC study is provocative. It found that PMPs were not significantly associated with lower rates of drug overdose or opioid overdose mortality or lower rates of consumption of opioid drugs.[111] In fact, the effect of PMPs on overall consumption of opioids appears to be minimal. On the other hand, a 2012 study that looked at information from two drug abuse surveillance databases showed more encouraging results.[112] The analysis supports the idea that PMPs are associated with a mitigation of increasing opioid abuse and misuse over time in both the general population and in people seeking help at opioid treatment centers.

The potential downside of PMPs for pain patients remains a concern for pain patient advocates like Cindy Steinberg, the woman we met in Chapter 1 who has been in constant pain since office filing cabinets fell on her back nearly 20 years ago. Steinberg has devoted most of her life since the accident to the nonprofit Massachusetts Pain Initiative. She worries that with enhanced PMPs, prescribers may be targeted inappropriately for investigation.[113] And that pain patients who get prescriptions from more than one provider may be unnecessarily stigmatized and denied needed medication.

As I discovered in my own pain journey, legitimate pain patients often *do* see different specialists in the quest for better treatment, and many or all of these specialists may write prescriptions for pain medications. Instead of casting suspicion on all patients who get prescriptions from more than one provider, perhaps a fairer standard would be to raise red flags only on those who get pain medications from, say, more than four practitioners *and* visit more than four pharmacies.

RISK EVALUATION AND MITIGATION STRATEGIES (REMS)

Chances are, you've never heard of REMS, except in the context of rapid eye movement sleep. It's a bureaucratic term for a plan now required by the US Food and Drug Administration.

In 2007, the Food and Drug Administration Amendments Act gave the FDA the authority to require an opioid risk evaluation and mitigation strategy (REMS) from manufacturers, the idea being to reduce diversion, abuse, misuse, and overdose.[114, 115, 116] In April 2011, after considerable back-and-forth between the federal bureaucracy and industry, the FDA formally announced it would require REMs for extended-release and long-acting opioids,[117, 118, 119] and reiterated its position that opioid REMS would not be unduly burdensome on patient access.[120]

The REMS approach, finalized in July 2012, is a start—requiring that industry be more forthcoming about the risks of various drugs and that companies provide detailed educational materials about the drugs to providers. Under the program, manufacturers must pay for the development and implementation of the drug education materials by third-party providers.[121] It's not clear yet, however, what these educational materials would contain; they could contain language—for instance, suggested limits on daily doses of morphine—that could be detrimental to pain patients.[122] Moreover, do we really want the pharmaceutical industry to produce these educational materials? The industry has a vested interest in what might be called "creative risk/benefit messaging."[123]

The finalized REMS program applies to all extended-release (ER) and long-acting (LA) opioid analgesics, including, but not limited to, fentanyl, hydromorphone, morphine, oxycodone, and oxymorphone and is expected to affect more than 20 manufacturers.[124, 125] The impact could be huge. There were an estimated 22.9 million prescriptions for extended-release and long-acting opioids dispensed in 2011, according to industry tracking data cited by the FDA. More than 320,000 prescribers registered with the Drug Enforcement Administration wrote at least one prescription for these drugs in 2011.[126] Importantly, REMS do *not* make it mandatory that providers actually take the courses or use the educational materials in order to prescribe the extended-release or long-acting opioid drugs to patients. The Obama administration *does* want a mandatory training program on opioid prescribing that would be linked to DEA registration by providers, but such a program would require legislation that has not yet been approved.[127]

There's concern among patient advocates that REMS might limit access to opioids for pain patients by making doctors less likely to prescribe them, despite the FDA's insistence to the contrary.[128]

And the FDA's focus on long-acting medications could mean that doctors might switch to shorter-acting opioids like Percocet, Vicodin, and Tylenol #3, which can be less effective at pain relief and harder for patients to titrate.[129] (The oxycodone in Percocet and the hydrocodone in Vicodin, for instance, are effective pain relievers, but the doses are limited by the acetaminophen also contained in these medications.[130])

For what it's worth, industry seems amenable to the REMS program. "We embrace risk management," said Herbert Neuman, vice president of medical affairs at Covidien (which makes Exalgo). "The problems of overdose, abuse and death have to be worked on by everybody. Manufacturers have to be part of the solution as well."[131]

GUIDELINES

Government programs aside, there *are* ways to use opioids more safely. In fact, a number of guidelines exist for safe opioid prescribing. In general, they say that physicians should assess patients carefully for potential opioid abuse; assess and treat co-occurring mental health problems such as anxiety and depression; use published tables for converting dosages of one medication to another when doing opioid "rotations"; and try to avoid prescribing benzodiazepines with opioids (because both classes of drugs can depress breathing).[132]

In addition, guidelines often suggest that doctors start prescribing opioids slowly and advancing slowly, especially with methadone; assess patients for sleep apnea if they are on higher doses of opioids; tell patients to reduce opioid intake during upper respiratory infections or asthma episodes; and avoid prescribing long-acting opioids for short-term problems such as postsurgical pain.

Assessing a patient's risk for potential abuse is not as difficult as one might think. In a study of chronic pain patients by researchers from Boston's Brigham and Women's Hospital in 2004, Edward Michna and Robert Jamison showed that it's possible to predict opioid abuse by asking a few straightforward questions.[133] Patients who acknowledged a personal or family history of drug or alcohol abuse or a history of legal problems were more prone to the abuse of opioids, including a higher likelihood of lost or stolen prescriptions and the presence of illicit drugs in urine tests.

In 2009, the American Pain Society, the American Academy of Pain Medicine, and the Oregon Evidence-based Practice Center at Oregon Health and Science University published 25 specific recommendations for prescribing opioids, based on an intensive two-year collaboration among 21 experts who reviewed more than 8,000 published abstracts and studies.[134] The strongest predictor of possible drug misuse,[135] this evidence showed, is a personal or family history of alcohol and drug abuse. For patients who do have such a history, the guidelines advise telling patients to fill opioid prescriptions at only one pharmacy, to submit to random drug tests, to attend regular doctor's appointments, and to lock medications at home.

Similar recommendations have been promulgated by the Federation of State Medical Boards of the United States.[136] These guidelines have been endorsed by the American Academy of Pain Medicine, the Drug Enforcement Administration, the American Pain Society, and the National Association of State Controlled Substances Authorities. Many states have officially adopted all or part of these model guidelines. Still other guidelines have been proffered by a team of researchers from Harvard Medical School and the University of Illinois;[137] and other, similar, guidelines from Physicians for Responsible Opioid Prescribing (PROP).[138] Advice is also available from the educational group Opioids911-Safety.[139]

There are numerous recommendations for patients, too, most of which are common sense. Among the *dos* and *don'ts*:

> *Don't* take a pain medication that is not prescribed for you.
> *Don't* adjust your own doses.
> *Don't* mix opioids with alcohol.
> *Don't* take sleeping pills or antianxiety medications along with opioids without talking with your doctor first.
> *Do* be up front with your doctor about *all* medications and keep track of the schedule on which you take them.
> And, given the huge drug diversion problem in the US, *do* keep medications locked in a safe place and dispose of unused medications.

The state of Utah Department of Health inaugurated a plan incorporating these principles in 2007 and, by the end of 2010, had reduced overdose deaths dramatically.[140, 141]

But some people feel more drastic action is needed to control opioid abuse. Among them is San Francisco's Michael Katz, who in 2010 wrote that he has lost so much faith in opioids, at least for long-term use, that he recommends setting limits—a maximum dose—on them.[142] This is quite controversial.[143] And getting more so. On July 25, 2012, PROP, which opposes much of the current prescribing of long-term opioids, teamed up with Public Citizen's Health Research Group, an advocacy organization, to file a Citizen Petition to the FDA asking for labeling changes for most opioid analgesics.[144]

In the petition, the two groups voiced concern about the increase in opioid prescriptions, the fact that many pain patients continue to experience pain despite chronic opioid therapy, and the threat of addiction. The next day, several members of Congress endorsed the petition.[145] In addition to concerns about patient safety, the groups said their goal is also to keep drug companies from claiming that opioids are safe and effective long term for non-cancer patients.[146]

The groups note that the FDA-approved indication for nearly all instant-release opioid analgesics is "moderate to severe pain." For extended-release opioids, the indication is for "moderate to severe pain when a continuous, around-the-clock analgesic is needed for an extended period of time." The groups want the FDA to strike the term "moderate" from the indication for non-cancer pain. They also want drug labels to specify a maximum daily dose equivalent of 100 milligrams of morphine for non-cancer pain and a maximum duration of 90 days for continuous (daily) use for non-cancer pain.[147] The groups contend that these indications as currently written are overly broad and imply that the FDA thinks the drugs are safe and effective for long-term use, which the groups believe they are not.

What worries pain patient advocates is that if the FDA did change the labeling in this way, it would mean that only "severe" pain would be an approved indication. Granted, as I discussed in Chapter 7, there is less evidence than everybody would like on the efficacy of long-term opioids. *But absence of evidence does not imply evidence of absence.* There's also less evidence than everybody would like on the *risks* of long-term opioid use.

In any case, it seems unlikely that changing the labeling, limiting daily doses, and limiting opioid treatment to 90 days would fix much, especially since doctors can legally prescribe drugs "off label" and in higher doses than recommended on labels. (My severe neck pain, for instance, lasted about 240 days, not 90. I did not need opioids daily for this whole time, but what if I had?)

There does not appear to be any data to justify a 90-day limit on opioid prescriptions.[148] And limiting the daily dose to 100 milligrams also seems arbitrary. Some guidelines suggest a higher threshold, 120 milligrams a day, but even this limit is not absolute. If a patient is still in pain at this dose, the answer, ideally, is not automatically to stop the medication but to do a more careful assessment of the pain problem, and take it from there.

Bottom line? Yes, opioids have plusses and minuses. That's abundantly clear. But my take is that the PROP folks have hijacked the media and Congress on this one. Let's hear it for a more moderate approach.

CHAPTER 9

How the Immune System Cranks Up Pain

GLIAL CELLS

For decades, physicians trying to relieve pain have focused on opioid drugs like morphine. Their rationale made sense: Electrical pain signals travel along sensory nerve cells from the periphery—that's our fingers, toes, arms, legs—to a little structure in the spinal cord called the dorsal horn and from there up to the brain, where we actually *feel* the hurt. Opioid drugs fit into receptors on nerve cells all along the way, dampening pain signals, albeit not completely and not without serious side effects.

But in recent years, scientists have discovered that a very different kind of cell with no obvious connection to the traditional view of pain also plays a major role.[1] These are the *glial cells*, which live in the central nervous system, where they outnumber nerve cells nine to one. *Glia* comes from the Greek for "glue," so named because early neuroanatomists thought that glial cells were like glue or "bubble wrap" that just support the supposedly more important nerve cells. There are other, less lofty, translations of *glia*, too, including "slime," or even less respectfully, "snot." Glial cells are now thought to play key roles in a number of psychiatric illnesses such as schizophrenia and depression, perhaps Alzheimer's, as well as addiction, multiple sclerosis, brain cancer, aging, and sleep.[2, 3, 4, 5, 6, 7, 8] And now, pain. Yet they were completely overlooked by neuroscientists for decades.[9, 10]

"Like medieval astronomers who were shocked to learn that the earth is not the center of the universe, neuroscientists today are facing a similar revelation about neurons," wrote neuroscientist R. Douglas Fields in a 2011 article for *Scientific American Mind*.[11] For more than a century, scientists had been clinging to the *neuron doctrine*, the idea that all information in the nervous system is transmitted by electrical impulses over networks of neurons linked through synaptic connections.

But this bedrock theorem is deeply flawed, as Fields noted. New research proves that some information bypasses the neurons completely, flowing without electricity through networks of cells called glia. And *that* is completely upending the understanding of every aspect of brain function in health and disease.

It is now clear that neurons are not the only players that drive the establishment and maintenance of common clinical pain. This recognition is crucial because it offers a completely new treatment approach, as pain researcher Clifford Woolf of Children's Hospital in Boston put it, an approach that is sorely needed because current drugs don't work all that well against pain.[12]

In 2009, during a freak October snowstorm in Boulder, Colorado, I visited the glial cell research laboratory of Linda Watkins at the University of Colorado. Watkins is a vigorous woman in her late 50s, who, with her husband and colleague, Steve Maier, thinks nothing of biking 100 miles in a day. She runs 4 miles several times a week and lives in jeans, sneakers and fleece jackets. The four-footed joy of her life is her yellow Lab, Ike, whose toys—a green stuffed moose, bones, and water bowl—lie on the floor outside her office. Watkins seems both mom and mentor to her crew of "labbies," the young scientists who carry out the experiments she dreams up to test her theories. When the freak snowstorm dumped 17 inches of snow on Boulder, Watkins looked on with amusement as her labbies poured out into the hallway, shrugged into jackets and gloves, and had a massive snowball fight in the courtyard.

Their high spirits were contagious—one young woman rushed back in, giggling. "I forgot my mittens," she said as she dug into a box of surgical latex gloves, wiggled her fingers into them, and dashed back to the fray. Within a half hour, they all returned, rosy-cheeked, to their labs. Perched on a cluttered hallway table with her computer on her lap as her students worked nearby, Linda Watkins's face lit up and her eyes shone as she talked about the things she was discovering about glial cells, which come in three basic types—astrocytes, oligodendrocytes, and microglia.

Astrocytes, which look a bit like stars, carry nutrients and waste to and from blood vessels and mediate communication among neurons.[13] Although they come from nerve cell progenitors, they act like immune cells, pumping out pro-inflammatory substances called cytokines. One of the first clues about the role of glial cells in pain came in 1994 when researchers at the University of Iowa administered a poison to animals in whom pain had been induced. The poison was designed to selectively kill astrocytes. With their astrocytes knocked out, the animals exhibited far less chronic pain.[14] Oligodendrocytes also come from nerve cell progenitors; their job is to coat axons with myelin, a protective, fatty insulation that dramatically increases the speed at which pain signals travel along neurons. (In the peripheral nervous system, the task of coating nerves with myelin falls to a slightly different kind of glial cell called a Schwann cell.) The third type of glial cells is the microglia, which come from—and are—genuine immune cells. They fight infection, help repair damaged cells, and are crucial to brain functioning.[15]

Like many things in biology, glial cells have a Jekyll-and-Hyde personality—a good side and a dark side. A very dark side, as it turns out. Normally, glial cells are benign and quiescent. But if they become activated by pain signals from nerves, they send out chemical signals that *increase* pain. Sometimes, they even add insult to injury: They steal some of the very morphine a patient takes for pain relief and use it for evil, further revving up pain signals.[16] When the body senses that it is under attack—from things as diverse as physical trauma, chemotherapy, diabetes, direct nerve damage, inflammation, pain transmitters like substance P, and even bits of blood that leak out of blood vessels—chemical distress signals that Watkins calls " alarmins" land on an important receptor on the glial cell surface called TLR-4. (TLR-4 stands for toll-like receptor 4.)[17]

Once that landing occurs, glial cells swing into action, pumping out a swarm of chemicals, most importantly, the cytokines IL-1 (interleukin 1), IL-6 (interleukin 6), and TNF (tumor necrosis factor). These cytokines are also both good guys and bad guys. IL-6, for instance, is a great immune stimulant. When a person gets an infection, IL-6 signals the brain to produce fever, which raises body temperature, which in turn helps kill bacteria. IL-1 is a good actor, too: It helps white blood cells flock to the site of an infection to fight bacteria. But these pro-inflammatory cytokines, particularly Il-1, are devils as well as angels. In addition to their helpful immune-boosting role, they act as *neuroexcitatory molecules*, that is, molecules that excite nerve cells and thus boost pain.

When triggered by an activated TLR-4 receptor, pro-inflammatory cytokines float around in the spinal cord until they land on nerves carrying pain signals up to the brain, explained Watkins. This TLR-4 stimulation amplifies the original pain signal, keeping the pain pathway in a constant state of activity. As a result, nerve cells wind up firing faster and faster, generating ever more pain signals headed for the brain. In part through this mechanism, what started out as short-term, acute pain turns into long-term, chronic pain.[18] The good news, noted Watkins, is that more than 200 animal studies show that preventing glial activation can reduce pain.[19] In people with fibromyalgia, too, researchers have shown that stopping microglial cells from pumping out cytokines (with low-dose naltrexone, a drug normally used to block opioids) can reduce pain.[20, 21]

One of the first questions Watkins asked as she began delving into TLR-4 receptors was this: If activation of TLR-4 cranks up production of IL-1 and ultimately, more pain, could drugs that block IL-1 also block pain? The answer was yes, but there was a downside. If a drug blocks only IL-1, other cytokines take over.[22] Which made Watkins wonder if a different way of blocking Il-1 might work better. Perhaps, she thought, she could use a cytokine called IL-10 to block its cousin Il-1. Indeed, it turns out that Il-10 can block not just IL-1, but TNF and IL-6 as well. By reducing all three, IL-10 can slow down the revved-up chronic pain cascade.

In an ideal world, doctors could get more IL-10 into the spinal cord by simply giving a drug containing IL-10, thereby reducing pain. But IL-10 drugs do not cross the blood-brain barrier, the network of blood vessels around the brain and spinal cord that has evolved to keep potentially dangerous substances out. But what if there were another way to get IL-10 where it is needed, around the spinal cord? Watkins decided to try another idea: gene therapy—injecting a gene that makes high quantities of IL-10 into the intrathecal space around the spinal cord.

To be sure, the gene therapy approach is controversial, and has had a bad name ever since 18-year-old Jesse Gelsinger died in an early gene therapy trial at the University of Pennsylvania in 1999. (In that trial, scientists used a virus to carry the needed gene into Gelsinger's body; Watkins's approach does not use a virus, a decided advantage.) And pharmaceutical companies may look askance at gene therapy.

"If you can't put it in a pill and take it twice a day, they aren't interested," says a glial scientist, sighing.[23] Nonetheless, the approach does have promise. In a series of experiments, Watkins showed that, administered this way, IL-10 can indeed shut down IL-1 in animals and make neuropathic pain disappear—for at least three months at a time.[24, 25, 26] (In 2011, researchers from the University of Michigan found that a different kind of gene therapy reduced pain in a small, human study.[27])

Watkins is convinced there may be other ways to boost IL-10 as well, including with a drug that closely mimics a chemical, adenosine, that we all make naturally in our bodies. To explore this approach, Watkins started with rats in which nerve pain had been triggered by a poke on the paw with a tiny mechanical hair. It typically takes 8 to 10 grams of force to elicit the normal pain reaction—the rat lifts its paw away from the stimulus.

Once it's clear that a rat has a normal response to pain, the rat is put under anesthesia and given surgery on one leg to constrict the sciatic nerve. This causes a partial nerve injury similar to the sciatica that leads to chronic pain in people. After the operation is over, chronic neuropathic pain develops in the rats over the next 10 days, then stays stable for about three months.

What happens next in the rats is much like what happens in people with chronic, neuropathic pain. The animal—or person—becomes far more sensitive than before, even to very mild pain stimuli. Now, when the rat's paw is stimulated by the mechanical hair, it lifts its leg sooner and sooner, and after much less forceful poking—clear signs of hyper-reactivity to pain stimuli. In technical language, this is called *allodynia*. Mere touch has become exquisite pain. Stanford University pediatric anesthesiologist Elliott Krane demonstrates this vividly in a TED talk, showing how, in people, the slightest touch on the skin with a feather feels like the burning agony from a blow torch.[28] Once Watkins is sure that her rats have allodynia, she injects the space around their spinal cords with either an adenosine-like drug called ATL313 or a placebo.

It's almost like magic. The rats that get the adenosine-like drug quickly go back to normal in terms of responsiveness to pain stimuli. In other words, their hypersensitivity to pain—their allodynia—is gone. The other rats—the ones that got placebo—remain hypersensitive. The beneficial effect seems to last for at least four weeks.[29]

And there's still more to the unfolding TLR-4 story. TLR-4 receptors also seem to play a role in the body's processing of the opioid, morphine. Morphine has an attraction to opioid receptors on nerve cells, as we've seen. But it also has an affinity for TLR-4 receptors on glial cells. And when it lands on theses receptors, it *increases* pain rather than decreasing it. This unfortunate phenomenon may help explain opioid-induced hyperalgesia, an increase in pain caused by the very opioids patients hope will make the pain go away.

But there's a silver lining in all this complexity. The very fact that morphine goes to two different receptors—the ones on nerve cells and the ones on glial cells—suggests that, in theory, scientists could tinker with things to keep morphine's good, pain-reducing effects on nerve cells and block its bad effects on glial cells. Which is precisely what Watkins is now trying to do.[30] In experiments with rats, she has found that blocking glial cells means that rats do not become *tolerant* to morphine. (Tolerance occurs when a drug becomes less and less effective over time.) Blocking TLR-4 receptors may also be a way to reduce drug *dependence* and the withdrawal symptoms that occur when opioids are discontinued abruptly.

"With our little rat addicts," said Watkins, "if we make them go 'cold turkey,' they get withdrawal symptoms." But if she gives them glial inhibition—by blocking their TLR-4 receptors—they get very little withdrawal.[31] So far, there's only one anti-glial drug in human trials that appears to reduce these morphine complications: Ibudilast (also known as AV-411 and MN-166), which is on the market in Japan for asthma.[32, 33, 34] Studies in rats show that the drug, now being developed by MediciNova, crosses the blood-brain barrier, can be given orally, reduces glial activation, and helps combat neuropathic pain.[35] It appears to reduce the risk of developing tolerance to opioids as well. It's currently being tested as a treatment for addiction and medication overuse in headache pain.[36]

Across the country from Linda Watkins, another glial cell researcher, Joyce De Leo, a pharmacologist at Dartmouth Medical School, is also pursuing glial cell biology in search of better pain treatments. In 2005, Joyce De Leo and her team were actually the first to discover the role of TLR-4 in pain.[37, 38] Her team looked at rats given experimental spinal cord injuries. Untreated rats showed the classic revving up of pain signals. But "knockout" rats (those that had been genetically altered so that they lacked TLR-4 receptors) showed much less hypersensitivity. So did mice with spinal cord injuries that were given a form of DNA that blocked the gene that makes TLR-4. But De Leo was more interested in a potential pain blocker called propentofylline, a caffeine-like substance that protects nerve cells from the damage in strokes.[39] She has shown that propentofylline can block both microglial and astrocyte activation—and reduce pain.[40, 41] She has shown that an antibiotic called minocycline, which prevents microglial activation, can reduce chronic pain in rats.[42, 43, 44] (A different drug, fluorocitrate, can do the same thing.[45, 46]) And she has shown that propentofylline can help with morphine tolerance in rats.[47]

A few years ago, things were looking great. Hopes for propentofylline were soaring. Armed by the encouraging animal studies and backed by Cambridge, Massachusetts-based Solace Pharmaceuticals, De Leo set out on a big proof-of-concept trial of propentofylline—in human patients, not rats. She selected people suffering from a stubborn pain syndrome, postherpetic neuralgia, which often follows shingles, a painful condition caused by the chickenpox virus. The drug, under its Solace name, SLC022, was hot. And unlike Watkins's intrathecal injections, this was a pill, just what Big Pharma wanted. In 2009, Solace trumpeted the $12 million trial on its website, noting that the study design was based on a large body of preclinical and clinical data.[48] The study was meticulously designed. It was double-blind, placebo-controlled, with 185 people per arm. This meant that some patients got the drug, some a dummy pill, and neither patients nor doctors knew until the code was broken who got what. The trial took place at multiple medical centers, another way of reducing researcher bias. Patients got the pills three times a day. Tests showed that, as hoped, propentofylline did reach the central nervous system.

Then things fell apart. The drug just didn't work, said De Leo with frustration and disappointment in her voice. This happens in science. Perhaps postherpetic neuralgia was the wrong pain condition to study.

Perhaps scientists simply need better ways to tell whether glial cells are being activated. And, of course, drugs that work beautifully in rats sometimes don't work at all in humans, and nobody knows why.[49]

Whatever the explanation, the study results were tough to swallow, raising the question of whether glial cells will live up to their promise as good targets for human pain therapy.[50] Pharmaceutical companies, which are already cutting back on neuroscience drugs because the brain and central nervous system are so complex and expensive to study, might get further discouraged.[51]

Still, the bad news "doesn't mean I will lose my enthusiasm totally," De Leo told me.[52] And other pain researchers remain excited about targeting glial cells. In addition to the TLR-4 receptors, scientists are studying other receptors, including one called P2X4. When nerve cells are damaged, microglia go ballistic, ramping up spinal cord pain.[53, 54] But when the P2X4 receptor is blocked, pain is blocked, too, Japanese researchers led by Kazuhide Inoue of Kyushu University have shown.[55] Inoue, a neuropharmacologist, said he remains very optimistic about targeting glial cells for pain.[56] Microglial cells also have receptors for chemicals called *fractalkines*, which are also pumped out by damaged nerve cells. When rats in chronic pain are given a drug that blocks fractalkine receptors, the animals are freed from their chronic pain.

All this work makes for an astonishing transition in medical science, according to neuroscientist R. Douglas Fields of the National Institutes of Health. "It's as if a door has been cracked open into a room filled with an entirely new stock of drugs to cure chronic pain."[57]

OTHER WAYS THE IMMUNE SYSTEM INCREASES PAIN

It's not just glial cells that have captured pain researchers' imaginations. T cells, the so-called managers of the immune system, are now believed to play a key role, too, explains Michael Costigan, a neurologist and pain researcher at Children's Hospital in Boston. Microglial cells are part of the *innate* immune system, an evolutionarily older part of the immune system that finds and attacks invaders like viruses and bacteria by engulfing and eating them.

"Essentially, they are the first responders, executioners and trash collectors, all rolled into one," Costigan said.[58] By contrast, T cells, which orchestrate the entire immune response, and B cells, which make antibodies, are part of the *adaptive* immune system, a more sophisticated and recent evolutionary development. In fact, the adaptive immune system is downright clever. Cells in the adaptive system shuffle their genes to produce many different cells, each of which has the unique ability to identify and lock onto a particular protein on the outer shell of a particular invader. The body is constantly producing millions of these cells.

Astonishingly, it's a random process—at first. By sheer chance, one immune cell will glom onto the "right" protein on a particular invader. Then things become nonrandom. That special immune cell then cranks up its cell division, making lots and lots of cells that also fit perfectly onto that particular invader. Meanwhile, T cells signal other cells to gobble up what's left of the invading germs. And, importantly, the winning T-cell line that has emerged doesn't "forget" its achievement. The highly specific T cells now stick around, "remembering" their successful battle, ready to attack if that invader ever enters the body again. All of which, scientists now think, plays into the problem of pain as well.

T cells are not normally found in a healthy central nervous system, as microglia are. In fact, the central nervous system is supposed to be an immunologically privileged site—no T cells allowed. But in some autoimmune diseases such as multiple sclerosis, T cells *do* find their way into the central nervous system. Once there, they make a big mistake. They "see" the myelin sheath surrounding nerve cells as foreign ("nonself")—that is, they see it as an invader, and proceed to attack it; without the myelin sheath, the nerves then can't function normally. Costigan and others now think that something similar may happen with chronic pain, specifically, that T cells somehow do gain entry to the spinal cord and other parts of the nervous system and work with microglia to ramp up pain signals.

Costigan's team demonstrated this dramatically in 2009. Like Linda Watkins, Costigan created a peripheral nerve injury in rats, in his case, in both adult and newborn rats. After the injury, the adult rats showed ongoing neuropathic pain, but the babies did not. (In humans, too, while babies feel acute pain, they do not develop the long-term, neuropathic pain that is a disease in itself.) Why? Costigan suspected that T cells might be the culprits, ramping up pain in adults, whose adaptive immune systems had had enough time for T cells to mature, but not in newborns. In newborns, he thought, T cells might simply not be present, and thus could not have entered the nervous system. Sure enough, when Costigan looked at spinal cord tissue, he found that T cells had infiltrated the dorsal horn in the spinal cords of adult rats—and not in the newborns.[59] Boosting this theory is the fact that a particular strain of mice that do not have T cells also do not develop neuropathic pain.[60]

That strongly suggests, Costigan says, that T cells—and the genes that control them—are involved in neuropathic pain. Once again, this suggests that neuropathic pain may be as much an immune problem as a nervous system problem. And that suggests that damping down T cells, just like damping down microglia, may be yet another way to combat neuropathic pain.

And there's yet another important way in which the immune system may be involved in some types of chronic pain. Researchers at the Mayo Clinic in Rochester, Minnesota, have recently found that in some people with chronic pain, antibodies to a potassium channel may contribute to—and may possibly even be one cause of—the chronic pain.[61, 62] In other words, in some people with apparently normal nervous systems, targeting these antibodies could open yet another new avenue for pain treatment.[63]

EINSTEIN'S BRAIN: A GLIAL SYMPHONY

Glial cells are becoming so important in neuroscience research today that, to hammer home this point, I can't resist telling this story, originally reported in the 2000 book *Driving Mr. Albert*.[64]

In 1955, when the brilliant physicist Albert Einstein died, a pathologist named Thomas Harvey performed the autopsy of his brain, holding in his hands the three pounds of convoluted tissue that changed our view of physics forever. After finishing his task, Harvey irreverently took Einstein's brain home, where he kept it floating in a plastic container for the next 40 years, as neuroscientist R. Douglas Fields wonderfully retold the story in a 2004 article in *Scientific American* and again in a 2009 book, *The Other Brain*.[65, 66]

Every now and then, Harvey would dole out small brain slices to scientists and pseudoscientists around the world who probed the tissue for clues to Einstein's genius. But when Harvey reached his 80s, he placed what was left of the brain in the trunk of his Buick Skylark and embarked on a road trip across the country to return it to Einstein's granddaughter. Four pieces of the famous brain wound up in the hands of a distinguished neuroanatomist at the University of California at Berkeley, Marian C. Diamond, who found nothing unusual about the number or size of its neurons.

What she did find, in the association cortex, which is responsible for high-level cognition, was a surprisingly large number of glial cells. In fact, this "excess" of glial cells seemed to be the only difference between an average brain and Einstein's. Perhaps, Fields speculated, glial cells might be the cellular basis of genius. And perhaps they could be the next key to unraveling the mysteries of pain.

CHAPTER 10

Marijuana

The Weed America Loves to Hate

THE BATTLE TO STUDY CANNABIS

Beth McCauley, a 57-year-old Los Angeles business executive, had a vicious case of trigeminal neuralgia, a facial pain condition so excruciatingly painful it's often called "the suicide disease." "It feels like my entire face is on a greasy griddle at 350 degrees, with someone pushing my face down on it," McCauley told me. She tried Buddha-like acceptance of her fate, which helped somewhat. Biofeedback, which also helped. And a pain medication that helped until its side effects made her cut her dose drastically.[1] Finally, in desperation, she tried marijuana, or, more correctly, cannabis, which comes from the plant *Cannabis sativa.*

"It was the most amazing thing," she said. Now when she gets breakthrough pain, she takes a puff or two of a joint. "The pain stays there, but it moves about a foot and a half off my face. All of a sudden, I can just breathe," said McCauley, who has formed a company that tests the purity of cannabis. She can completely forget about the pain and go about her business, with relief coming in less than a minute. "I don't even think about my face anymore," she told me. "I can keep going. It changed my life."

Cannabis has changed Marcy Duda's life, too. Duda, 50, a skinny, blond Massachusetts grandmother of two, told me marijuana is the only thing that touches her migraines, which she describes as "hot, hot ice picks" in the left side of her head.[2] Duda has had migraines her whole life. But they got much worse a decade or so ago after she had two operations to remove aneurysms, weak areas in the blood vessels in her brain that could have ruptured—fatally—at any moment. She survived the surgeries but was left with chronic pain all down her left side, as if her body were cut in half. Doctors gave her drugs, but nothing really worked. Then she tried cannabis, which she smokes—researchers prefer the term "inhales"—through a vaporizer. Her experience is much like McCauley's. "It doesn't miraculously wipe the headaches away," Duda said, "but it's better than any other drug." And unlike drugs that must pass through the digestive system, she has found, inhaled marijuana gives her instant relief.

Beth McCauley and Marcy Duda are among the countless Americans—nobody knows the actual number—who use marijuana for a variety of medical problems, including pain. But lost in the headlines about unscrupulous marijuana smugglers and teenage abusers is what scientific research says about how marijuana works in the body.

In this chapter, we'll explore what that evidence does—or does not—show about medical marijuana's safety and effectiveness. We'll see how marijuana interacts with pain circuits in the brain. How effectively it may combat pain. How serious the side effects are, and for whom.

And of course, what the risks of dependence and addiction are. Whether marijuana creates tolerance (the need to keep increasing doses to get the same effect). And whether the government-approved, single-ingredient pills are as effective as inhaling the real stuff with all the components nature concocted. (We will not get into the distracting issue of dangerous *synthetic cannabinoids* such as "Spice," "K2," and "Aroma," which should not be confused with medical marijuana.[3, 4, 5, 6]) At the end of the chapter, we will, of course, address the legal and political issues surrounding marijuana, and offer one solution.[7]

But first, a startling contrast. In the United States, the federal government still seems to see marijuana, even medical marijuana, as dangerous and seductive.[8] In spite of significant evidence that marijuana is remarkably safe. Put bluntly, people do not die from marijuana. There are simply no deaths—zero—attributable to marijuana, according to the government's own statistics, from the federal Centers for Disease Control and Prevention, as well as from other studies.[9, 10] In stark contrast, government figures show that 443,000 American adults die every year from cigarette smoking, and more than 80,000 die annually from excessive alcohol use.[11, 12] Even nonsteroidal anti-inflammatory drugs (NSAIDs) like ibuprofen are more dangerous than marijuana—they kill an estimated 7,000 to 10,000 American adults a year.[13]

The main reason marijuana is so nonlethal is that, unlike opioids, it does not cause respiratory depression. This means it is unlikely to cause a person to stop breathing. With marijuana, overdosing is extremely rare and is usually accompanied by the use of other drugs, such as alcohol, as McGill University researchers noted in a 2005 review.[14] In fact, they add, a lethal dose of tetrahydrocannabinol (THC) has never been reported. Two other large studies support this, showing no increase in the death rate attributable to cannabis.[15] Even the National Institute on Drug Abuse acknowledges the nonlethality of cannabis.

"Marijuana does not kill directly," acknowledged Steven Gust, special assistant to the director of National Institute on Drug Abuse (NIDA), though it can contribute to risky behavior, such as driving while stoned and drunk.[16] This safety profile has held true for decades, as even an administrative law judge for the Drug Enforcement Administration noted in 1988 in an official finding of fact: "There is no record in the extensive medical literature describing a proven, documented cannabis-induced fatality." (By contrast, the judge noted, aspirin causes hundreds of deaths a year.)[17]

So what *is* this plant that is causing such controversy? Cannabis (and scientists prefer this term to *marijuana*) is a psychoactive plant with significant healing properties that has been around for millennia. It is believed to contain hundreds of different chemicals. Usually smoked as a cigarette, it's the most commonly used illegal substance in America, according to NIDA.[18] In 2010, 17.4 million Americans were current users of marijuana, up from 14.4 million in 2007.[19]

But cannabis is also one of the most potent natural herbal medicines in the world, a staple of traditional Chinese medicine. Indeed, flowers from the female cannabis plant were found in the 2,700-year-old tomb of a medicine man in Northern China. From China, the medicinal use of marijuana spread to India. There, a British surgeon "discovered" its healing properties and introduced it into Western medicine in the 1840s. (There's even a story—false, as it turns out—that Queen Victoria used cannabis for menstrual cramps.[20, 21, 22])

Among other uses, cannabis was used as a treatment for migraines in many ancient cultures, not just the Chinese and Indian, but Egyptian, Assyrian, Greek, and Roman as well.[23], [24] By the early 1900s, it wasn't just ancient cultures that appreciated cannabis. Americans were catching on, too, including pharmaceutical companies, which saw the promise of marijuana and began creating their own preparations, according to cannabis researcher Donald Abrams, an AIDS and cancer specialist at the University of California, San Francisco.[25] This placid state of affairs continued until 1937, when a prominent Prohibitionist, Harry J. Anslinger, who later became the head of the Federal Narcotics Bureau, got Congress to pass the Marijuana Tax Act. He tried to describe marijuana "in so repulsive and terrible terms that people wouldn't even be tempted to try it," noted the late Yale University drug historian David Musto.[26]

Even back in Anslinger's day, there was no evidence that cannabis was demonic. In fact, the American Medical Association opposed the Marijuana Tax Act out of fear that the act would impede future research. (Which it did.) In 1942, the La Guardia Commission in New York likewise concluded that marijuana, despite allegations to the contrary, would not lead to crime or mental illness. Nonetheless, that same year, amid growing anti-pot fervor, cannabis was removed from the US Pharmacopeia, the nonprofit, nongovernmental public health organization that sets standards for medicines and food.[27]

Then, in 1970, Congress enacted the Controlled Substance Act, which classified marijuana, like heroin, as a Schedule I drug, the "worst" category. A substance in this category is deemed to have a high potential for abuse and no accepted medical use. The result is what *Time* magazine in 2010 called a "flawless bureaucratic catch-22.... Pot is listed as Schedule I because science hasn't found an accepted medical use for it, but science can't find a medical use for it because it's listed as Schedule I."[28] (Actually, even the government may not be so sure marijuana is medically useless. In October 2003, the Department of Health and Human Services took out a patent on cannabinoids for potential use as antioxidants and neuroprotectants.[29])

Until the 1970 act, laws in all states that prohibited marijuana allowed exceptions for using marijuana as a medicine, according to Michael Cutler, a Massachusetts lawyer who works on reforming marijuana laws.[30] On the plus side, the 1970 law also called for a study on marijuana, which was duly performed by a national group, the Shafer Commission.[31] In 1972, the commission recommended a medical exemption for marijuana, as well as decriminalization. But once again, Congress was not buying. It rejected this idea, and antidrug sentiment continued to grow.[32] In 1986, President Reagan signed the Anti-Drug Abuse Act, which ordered mandatory sentences without parole for those convicted of possession or sale of all illegal drugs, including stiff sentences for cannabis.[33]

* * *

Today, in the Orwellian world of the federal bureaucracy, it is extremely difficult for American scientists to obtain legal marijuana to study, although a handful of California researchers have managed to do it. For research on *any* controlled substance provided by the government, three things have to happen. The researcher must get investigational new drug (IND) approval from the Federal Drug Administration (FDA). The researcher must also get the appropriate registration from the Drug Enforcement Administration (DEA). And the protocol for the proposed study must be deemed to have scientific merit by one of three processes—a grant review from the National Institutes of Health, an ad hoc review by NIDA, or, in the case of marijuana, a Public Health Service (PHS) committee review for studies that are funded by non-government sources.[34]

In 1999, the Public Health Service established a special process for evaluating proposed studies of marijuana that would involve use of government-provided marijuana. Not surprisingly, advocates of research on marijuana see this as the government singling out marijuana as forbidden territory for study.[35, 36, 37, 38] As a practical matter, what all this means is that in order to conduct a clinical study of cannabis, a scientist has to pass muster with the FDA, the DEA, *and* the PHS, at which point NIDA then may give the scientist federally grown marijuana to study.

And therein lies a problem. NIDA's stated goal is to study marijuana to look for evidence of *harm*, not to find potential benefits. It is "not NIDA's mission to study the medicinal use of marijuana or to advocate for the establishment of facilities to support this research," NIDA director Nora Volkow told the *Boston Globe* in 2006.[39] And, as Steven Gust, told me, "NIDA is in the business of studying, for the most part, the detrimental effects of drugs."[40] But the real catch is that the only legal source of marijuana is that grown by the government itself on a single, 12-acre farm run by the National Center for Natural Products Research (NCNPR) at the University of Mississippi.[41, 42] That farm is overseen by NIDA.

"We are the farmer," as NIDA's Gust put it. It is misleading, he says, to view NIDA as the obstacle or gatekeeper for research on marijuana: "If a study has been approved by the DEA, the FDA and the PHS, if all those agencies say yes, once those three boxes are checked, we will send the marijuana."[43]

But that's not how would-be marijuana researchers see it. They see NIDA as having a de facto monopoly on all the carefully cultivated, standardized strains of cannabis that they would like to study. (Scientists could, of course, study black market marijuana, but not only would this be illegal, it would be bad science: Strains of marijuana sold on the street vary widely in potency and constituents.)

The government justifies this de facto monopoly in part on the basis of an international treaty called the Single Convention on Narcotic Drugs of 1961, which the government interprets as saying the United States may have only one source of cannabis.[44] Others dispute this interpretation, among them, Mary Ellen Bittner, a DEA administrative law judge. In a finding in 2007, she recommended ending the government's monopoly on medical marijuana research.[45]

A number of legitimate researchers have been stymied by the government's reluctance to part with its marijuana. In the mid-1990s, Donald Abrams, the California AIDS researcher mentioned earlier, got FDA approval to study cannabis's potential benefits for AIDS/HIV patients. With the FDA's approval in hand, he then petitioned NIDA for the federally grown cannabis he needed for the study. He was turned down. Abrams was frustrated.

"I must tell you that dealing with your Institute has been the worst experience of my career," Abrams wrote to NIDA. He eventually reworded his proposal to appeal to what NIDA wanted—that is, to look for harms. This time, he was approved, and he got $1 million to boot.[46, 47] To be sure, some professional medical associations—most notably, the American Society of Addiction Medicine—approve of this restricted state of affairs.[48] But other medical groups lament the obstacles facing scientists trying to grow marijuana in order to study it, among them the American College of Physicians and the American Medical Association.[49, 50]

Among the most frustrated scientists is Lyle Craker. Craker is a friendly, white-haired crop physiologist and professor of plant and soil sciences at the University of Massachusetts. In 2001, he applied to the DEA for a license to cultivate cannabis for use in clinical trials by medical doctors. The research was to be privately funded, so he wasn't even looking for federal money. He is still waiting for the DEA's answer, despite an administrative judge's ruling that it is in the public interest for Craker to be granted a license.

Craker is hardly a wild-eyed pothead. "He's the Rosa Parks of medical marijuana," Rick Doblin told me. Doblin holds a PhD in public policy from Harvard's Kennedy School of Government and founded an advocacy group called MAPS in 1986.[51, 52] "Craker is "perfect. He doesn't smoke, he's not an advocate for legalization. He's a senior faculty member. He can't be intimidated. He's simply saying there should be more research."

Craker is a patient man. But three years after he filed his initial application for a license and got no response from the DEA, he sued. His suit was supported by the American Civil Liberties Union (ACLU), the late US Senator Edward Kennedy, and numerous medical, patient, and advocacy groups.

In a sense, Craker's initial lawsuit was partially successful. The Court of Appeals in the District of Columbia ordered the administration to stop stalling and respond.[53] The DEA did respond—by rejecting Craker's petition. It argued that the Single Convention treaty requires the government to maintain only one source of marijuana and that allowing Craker to run a facility at UMass would violate government policy. Judge Bittner disagreed.[54] In a final ruling in February 2007, she recommended that Craker be allowed to grow research cannabis. Finally, thought Craker.

But it turned out that the ultimate decision wasn't hers to make. It was DEA acting administrator Michele Leonhart's. In January 2009, just as President George W. Bush was leaving office and six days before President Barack Obama was to be inaugurated, Leonhart, a Bush appointee, rejected Bittner's recommendations and ruled against Craker. To the surprise of many people who had believed Obama's pro-medical marijuana campaign statements in 2008, Obama went on to reappoint Leonhart, who was confirmed as head of the DEA in 2010.

During his presidential campaign, Obama had told the editorial page editor for the *Mail Tribune*, a southern Oregon newspaper, that he took a "practical" view of medical marijuana, adding that "there is really no difference" between a doctor prescribing medical marijuana as a treatment for glaucoma or as a cancer treatment "and a doctor prescribing morphine or anything else." Obama went on to say in that interview that he would not "punish doctors" for prescribing cannabis in an appropriate way, even though "that may require some changes in federal law."[55, 56]

His administration did keep that promise—for a while. When asked during a press conference on February 25, 2009, if recent raids on medical marijuana providers in California represented American policy going forward, his attorney general, Eric Holder, said, "No. What the president said during the campaign, you'll be surprised to know, will be consistent with what we'll be doing in law enforcement." In October 2009, David Ogden, a deputy attorney general, also seemed to hew to the Obama campaign rhetoric. Ogden wrote a memo saying that while the Department of Justice remains committed to prosecuting significant traffickers of illegal drugs, including marijuana, the government should not focus federal resources on individuals who are in clear compliance with state laws on medical marijuana.[57] Ogden added that it would not be an efficient use of limited federal resources to prosecute people with cancer or other serious illnesses who use marijuana as part of a recommended treatment regimen.

But something snapped in Washington. On June 29, 2011, a different deputy attorney general, James M. Cole, changed the administration's tune.[58, 59] In *his* memo, Cole noted a big increase in large-scale, commercial cultivation and sale of medical marijuana. From now on, the Cole memo said, people in the marijuana cultivation business "are in violation of the Controlled Substances Act, regardless of state law."[60, 61] Today, more than a decade after he first applied for a license to cultivate marijuana, Craker's case is still tied up in court. In May 2012, Craker's legal team once again presented their case against the DEA, in federal court.[62] So far, there has been no resolution.[63]

Craker is not the only cannabis researcher to run afoul of the government's obsessive fear of marijuana. Ethan Russo is a neurologist who treated migraine patients for a quarter of a century in Missoula, Montana. He now lives on an island off Seattle. The author of several historical reviews of cannabis, Russo tried for more than 15 years to study herbal cannabis for migraine. His first proposed study was turned down at NIDA in 1997. He tried again in 1998. Same result. "I thought it was a good protocol, but politics entered into this, I'm afraid," he told me.[64] His hopes rose briefly in 1999, when the prestigious Institute of Medicine acknowledged the promise of medicinal marijuana.[65] Suddenly, the FDA did accept his application and approved his study.

But then he bumped into that old catch-22. He couldn't proceed until he got an additional review from the Public Health Service. His migraine study was rejected. Although Russo arguably knows more about the biology of cannabis than any other scientist on the planet, he gave up fighting the government.[66] He now consults for a UK company called GW Pharmaceuticals that makes Sativex, an oral-mucosal spray made from extracts of two standardized cannabis strains that are mixed to give fixed doses of THC and cannibidiol (CBD). (Sativex is approved in several countries, but not in the United States, although it is now in an FDA-approved trial for cancer pain.)

To be sure, there have been a few scientists who have scored government marijuana to study. They are a team of researchers led by Igor Grant, Thomas Coates, and J. H. Atkinson, physicians who run the Center for Medicinal Cannabis Research at the University of California, San Diego. In 2001, they received $8.1 million from the state of California for cannabis research—and somehow got NIDA to part with enough government-grown marijuana from Mississippi to sponsor 14 studies, including the first clinical trials of inhaled marijuana in more than two decades.[67, 68] It wasn't easy.

Many scientists "are just not going to go through this kind of effort," Atkinson acknowledged. But the California team's persistence did pay off in research showing that cannabis is indeed a promising therapy, especially since its mechanisms of action are different from those of standard treatments.[69] That's the good news. The bad is that the center has now spent all its money. It is still a resource for other scientists, but it won't fund any new research projects. Meanwhile, as Craker, Russo, and the California scientists were fighting to study cannabis, an entirely separate effort has also being going on, this one spearheaded by Jon Gettman.

As leader of the Coalition for Rescheduling Cannabis (CRC), Gettman filed a petition in 1995 and again in 2002 to get marijuana taken out of Schedule I, arguing that there *is* enough evidence of its medical usefulness that the government should not claim it has none.[70, 71] He suggested that marijuana be regulated as a Schedule III, IV, or V (over-the-counter) substance or simply be regulated like alcohol or tobacco. In June 2011, the Global Commission on Drug Policy, an august, nonpartisan group, also recommended the rescheduling of certain drugs—cannabis, coca leaf, and MDMA—because the current scheduling has "obvious anomalies."[72]

Remarkably, Gettman's petition cited 87 healthcare or state government entities supporting medical marijuana use, including the American Academy of Family Physicians, the American Public Health Association, the National Association of [state] Attorneys General, the National Institute of Medicine, and many others. After years of government inaction, Gettman went to court to compel the DEA to respond to his petition. On July 8, 2011, nine years after the second petition, the DEA finally did rule—it denied Gettman's petition.[73, 74]

Although Gettman's coalition had argued that cannabis is *less* likely to lead to dependence than other Schedule I or II drugs, that argument didn't fly. The DEA insisted that long-term, regular use of marijuana "can lead to physical dependence and withdrawal following discontinuation as well as psychic addiction or dependence." The government also reiterated its standard line, saying that it would not reschedule marijuana because it "has a high potential for abuse, has no accepted medical use in the United States, and lacks an acceptable level of safety for use even under medical supervision." Strikingly, while referencing studies on potential health *risks* of marijuana, the DEA made no mention of other studies showing medical efficacy. It also failed to note its own role in blocking studies that the FDA had already approved.[75, 76]

Advocates for medical marijuana howled. "The federal government is making no bones about its aggressive policy to undermine medical marijuana," complained Americans for Safe Access, one of the groups supporting the Gettman petition.[77]

It's been known since 1964 that the primary psychoactive ingredient in marijuana is THC, or cannibidiol, a substance first isolated by Raphael Mechoulam, an Israeli chemist.[78] But it was not until decades later that scientists stumbled upon something even more interesting.

All human beings, and indeed other mammals, birds, fish and even reptiles, are born with the ability to make both marijuana-like chemicals called cannabinoids and the cannabinoid receptors into which they fit. Cannabinoid receptors can be triggered not only by these endogenous cannabinoids, but also by externally obtained cannabinoids like THC and CBD from the marijuana plant itself and by synthetic cannabinoids made in the lab. In fact, to scientists' surprise, cannabinoid receptors turn out to be all over the place, among the most abundant receptors in our bodies.[79]

Why on earth would our nervous systems be so full of cannabinoid receptors? So that our caveman ancestors might someday stumble upon a marijuana plant and smoke it to get high? Probably not. More likely, evolution favored us with all these cannabinoid receptors for a more practical reason, like dampening pain. And perhaps to give us that "runner's high," which is fueled, it turns out, not just by endorphins but by endogenous cannabinoids as well.[80, 81]

Two of the most important endogenous cannabinoids are anandamide and 2-arachidonyl-glycerol, or 2-AG, lipids that have a wide range of biological functions, including pain processing.[82] Basically, they make us "relax, eat, sleep, forget and protect."[83, 84]

When people are deficient in endocannabinoids, they may be more susceptible to certain pain conditions, including migraine, fibromyalgia, and irritable bowel syndrome.[85, 86] Italian researchers, for instance, have shown that cannabinoid levels are too low in migraine sufferers. Certain mutations in the receptor for anandamide can also raise the risk of migraine.[87] On the other hand, *boosting* levels of endocannabinoids— in part by blocking substances that break them down—is a promising a new approach to reducing pain.[88] In fact, some pain drugs that we already use, such as NSAIDs, or nonsteroidal anti-inflammatory drugs, seem to work in part by stopping this breakdown of endocannabinoids.[89]

The two most important cannabinoid *receptors* are CB1 and CB2. The CB1 receptors reside mostly in the central nervous system and on peripheral nerves, while CB2 receptors are mostly in immune cells, including microglia and, to a lesser extent, in the central nervous system.[90, 91] These receptors are clearly vital to survival. Mice genetically engineered to lack CB1 receptors show increased anxiety and susceptibility to depression.[92] They don't respond normally to reward stimuli.[93] And they eat less and lose weight.[94] CB1 receptors also seem to play a role in the placebo response.[95]

THC triggers its high when it lands on CB1 receptors.[96] The other cannabinoid, CBD, doesn't bind strongly to *either* CB1 or CB2 receptors, though it does seem to partially block the binding of THC to CB1.[97] When CB2 receptors are activated, the main effect is reduced inflammation and activity in spinal cord pain relay centers, as well as protection of nerves from oxidative damage.[98, 99, 100]

The holy grail of marijuana pain research is to unravel the mysteries of the two cannabinoid receptors and the two major cannabinoids from plants, THC and CBD. In theory, teasing apart this biochemistry will allow the creation of fine-tuned marijuana strains that *decrease* the psychoactive effects of marijuana—the high—and *increase* pain-relieving effects.

There's a catch in this theory, though. It may be that a little of the psychoactive effect from smoking marijuana is what helps pain patients like Marcy Duda and Beth McCauley dissociate emotionally from their pain, even though the physical pain is still there. A 2013 study from Oxford University showed that cannabis does indeed make pain less unpleasant, at least in healthy volunteers studied in a pain lab.[101] Using fMRI brain scanning, the researchers found that while THC did not reduce the intensity of pain, it did reduce the emotional impact. In other words, the CB1 effect from the plant itself may be unwanted in the eyes of people opposed to marijuana, but its very "mood-altering effect may be an important part of the overall therapeutic response" note McGill University researchers Mark Ware and Vivianna Tawfik.[102]

And of course, it's the high from THC that recreational marijuana users and abusers seek. In recent years, precisely because it does not trigger a high, CBD has actually been bred *out* of marijuana strains sold illegally.[103] With any cannabis on the black market in North America, "the CBD just isn't there. The black market cannabis is virtually all high-THC strains," Ethan Russo told me.[104]

Back in the early 1970s, there was a perfect balance of THC and CBD in natural cannabis plants from Afghanistan. This balance produced a modulatory effect. The CBD blocked the intoxication, rapid heartbeat, and sedation of THC alone, but also boosted the good effects—pain control and reduced inflammation.[105] Drug companies have been trying to come up with man-made equivalents. Several have tested CB2-only drugs, but so far, the results have been disappointing.[106, 107, 108, 109] As for the two synthetic cannabis medications on the US market, the jury is out. Both drugs act on both CB1 and CB2 receptors, and Marinol, which contains THC, can produce a high if the dose is sufficient. So far, both Marinol (dronabinol) and Cesamet (nabilone) are approved only for anorexia and nausea, though they can be used "off label" for pain, as well as for improving sleep.[110]

In truth, nothing man-made appears to be as effective—or as quick— for pain relief as smoking or inhaling the cannabis plant itself.[111, 112] Cesamet is perceived to produce more undesirable side effects, to take a long time to work, and to be more expensive than smoked cannabis.[113] Marinol has shown efficacy as an add-on to opioid therapy in some people with chronic pain.[114] But it can be hard for people to find the right dose because of individual variations in how their digestive systems absorb the drug.[115]

There's a downside to smoking the real plant itself, though. Even one puff of high-potency cannabis may overshoot what you need for pain control.[116] That's because smoked cannabis has a *narrow therapeutic index*—a small gap between symptom control and side effects. The overshoot problem typically occurs, however, chiefly with people who have not used marijuana much; experienced users become quite good at getting their doses right. By contrast, the marijuana extract Sativex, which contains both THC and CBD, seems to have a wider therapeutic index. This suggests that people may be able to spray just enough into their mouths to control pain without producing unwanted side effects. Sativex is used in Canada, Great Britain, Spain, and Germany for neuropathic pain, cancer pain, and multiple sclerosis, though its effectiveness for multiple sclerosis is questionable.[117, 118, 119, 120, 121] It also appears mildly effective in people with rheumatoid arthritis pain, according to company-sponsored trials.[122] It is not approved in the United States, but a 2012 international, randomized, double-blind, placebo-controlled trial for poorly controlled pain in 263 people with advanced cancer was promising, showing both efficacy and safety at low and medium doses.[123]

THE MEDICAL BENEFITS OF MARIJUANA

Since the focus of this book is chronic pain, we'll concentrate here on marijuana as a pain reliever, not on its other medical effects, such as reducing nausea and anorexia. But just for the record, it's worth noting that there have been two major reviews in recent years of more than 100 randomized, double-blind, placebo-controlled clinical trials involving more than 6,100 patients with a variety of medical conditions.[124, 125]

These and other studies show that marijuana is effective at combating nausea, vomiting, appetite loss, glaucoma, irritable bowel disease, muscle spasticity in multiple sclerosis, muscle spasms, Tourette's syndrome, epilepsy, and symptoms of amyotrophic lateral sclerosis (ALS, or Lou Gehrig's disease).[126, 127, 128, 129, 130] There may be another benefit as well. In animals, at least, there's preliminary evidence that marijuana can block the growth of tumors, according to a 2003 review by Spanish researchers.[131] Specifically, cannabinoids seem to fight tumors by blocking inflammation, cell proliferation, and cell survival, other research shows.[132, 133] It may also be possible to block cancers that start in immune cells by targeting CB2 receptors on those cells, though this is very preliminary.[134]

But pain is the point here. And, to put it bluntly, marijuana works. Not dazzlingly, but about as well as opioids. That is, it can reduce chronic pain by more than 30 percent.[135, 136] And with fewer serious side effects. To be sure, some researchers think it's too soon to declare marijuana and synthetic cannabinoids a first-line treatment for pain, arguing that other drugs should be tried first.[137] But that may be too cautious a view.

Overall, marijuana and its prescription cousins show a significant analgesic effect compared to placebo in people with all sorts of chronic, non-cancer pain, according to a 2011 review of 15 high-quality studies.[138] And one of the huge advantages may be that marijuana can allow people in severe pain to take *lower* doses of opioids. While doctors often shy away from prescribing opioids to patients who also use marijuana, this may be backward: There's evidence that marijuana can make opioids *more* effective and allow patients to take *less* of them.[139, 140, 141] In general, marijuana seems to work best, ironically enough, for people with the most intractable pain. It is less effective for acute pain, such as pain after surgery.[142, 143] And it has only mixed efficacy against acute pain intentionally induced in the lab.[144]

Some conditions in particular—neuropathic pain, fibromyalgia, and pain from multiple sclerosis—seem amenable to the pain-reducing effects of cannabis and its synthetic cousins. There is less research on other problems, such as migraine and cancer pain, in part because of the US government's restrictive access policies. With neuropathic pain, which affects 1 to 2 percent of the population, cannabis is quite a promising treatment, according to a report from the San Diego–based Center for Medicinal Cannabis Research.[145] Research from the Canadian Consortium for the Investigation of Cannabinoids has come to the same conclusion.[146] And, as Beth McCauley and Marcy Duda discovered on their own, most of the reduction in pain comes from the first marijuana cigarette, with subsequent doses not adding significantly to the effect.[147] In other words, you don't have to get stoned out of your mind to get pain relief.

In fact, a steady drumbeat of studies has confirmed the effectiveness of cannabis for neuropathic pain relief. In a 2008 UC Davis study, 38 patients rated their neuropathic pain after inhaling cannabis or placebo: Smoking cannabis clearly reduced their daily pain.[148] In 2009, other researchers followed 28 patients who puffed away—under direct observation in a hospital. Again, cannabis yielded significant pain relief, as well as improvements in mood and daily functioning.[149]

In 2010, a different study set researchers buzzing at the annual meeting of the International Association for the Study of Pain. The study was done by Mark Ware, a McGill University anesthesiologist with a big smile and a passion for scientific rigor. Ware looked at 21 neuropathic pain patients and found that one puff through a pipe three times a day for five days yielded significant pain relief, as well as better sleep. And patients smoking marijuana with the highest concentrations of THC got the most benefit.[150, 151]

As a Canadian researcher, Ware isn't caught up in cannabis politics the way American scientists are. Scientists "should study herbal cannabis the same as any other substance," he told me one day in his Montreal office overlooking the St. Lawrence River. "We should establish its safety profile, its efficacy, etc. If it's as good as everyone says it is, it could be considered as rational medical therapy."[152]

People with fibromyalgia seem to be helped by marijuana or the synthetics, too. A 2008 randomized, double-blind, placebo-controlled Canadian study in 40 fibromyalgia patients found that the patients getting Cesamet got pain relief but also complained of side effects such as drowsiness, dry mouth, vertigo, confusion, and dissociation.[153] A 2011 Spanish study compared 28 fibromyalgia patients who inhaled cannabis or consumed it orally to 28 nonusers. The cannabis users had less pain and stiffness, were more relaxed, and had increased feelings of well-being. They also scored higher on a questionnaire for mental health.[154]

For multiple sclerosis (MS) pain, the prescription Sativex spray seems to work, reducing pain and sleep problems more than placebo.[155] As for migraines, American scientists, as we've seen, have had trouble getting legal marijuana from the federal government to study. In theory, though, marijuana should work for migraines because it can activate CB1 receptors.[156, 157, 158]

THE RISKS OF MARIJUANA

Remember those syllogisms they used to teach in college logic classes? "John is a human. All humans have legs. Therefore John has legs." My version goes like this: Marijuana, like alcohol, caffeine, and opioids, is a drug. All drugs have risks. Therefore marijuana has risks.

That said, the evidence shows that marijuana has a remarkably safe profile. And this is in spite of the fact that the US government has lopsidedly supported studies of risks rather than benefits. But because anti-marijuana politics has focused so much on the risks, we'll address them one by one, and see what the research shows.

One of the most often alleged risks of marijuana is that it is a "gateway" drug that leads to other illegal drug use. This is only partly true. Because it is the most widely used illicit drug, marijuana is predictably the first illicit drug most people encounter, acknowledged a 1999 review by the Institute of Medicine, an arm of the National Academy of Sciences.[159] "Not surprisingly," the report said, "most users of other illicit drugs have used marijuana first." But here's the catch. Most drug users *begin* their drug using with the legal drugs alcohol and nicotine. Because underage smoking and alcohol use typically precede marijuana use, the report said, marijuana is not the most common, and is rarely the first, "gateway" to illicit drug use.

Assessing the medical risks of marijuana is tricky, in part because most research has been done in young, recreational users. In general, adolescents and young adults who use cannabis recreationally tend to be heavier users, while older people who use cannabis medicinally tend to use smaller doses for symptom relief.[160] When researchers look at medicinal use, they don't find much harm. In a review of 23 randomized controlled trials and eight observational studies of medicinal use, McGill University researchers Tongtong Wang and Mark Ware found that the overall risk of adverse events for short-term (two-week) use of cannabinoids and cannabis extracts was minor.[161] The most common problem was dizziness. But by and large, the rates of serious adverse events did not differ between people taking medicinal cannabis and controls. And, as would be predicted from the biology of marijuana itself, the risks that do exist are lower when people take formulations that include both THC and CBD rather than THC alone.[162] So, let's take a look at the medical risks one by one—dependence and addiction, cancer, schizophrenia and other forms of psychosis, other psychiatric problems, cognitive problems, respiratory damage and cardiac issues.

Dependence and Addiction

Dependence is a physical adaptation that leads to withdrawal symptoms if a drug is stopped, especially if it's stopped abruptly. Addiction is different—it's a neurobiological condition characterized by impaired control over drug use, compulsive use, continued use despite harm, and craving. But many people, including doctors, researchers, and federal agencies, confuse the two terms. With marijuana, there are reports of withdrawal symptoms in both adults and adolescents, especially among heavy users.[163] But even when mild physiological withdrawal does occur in heavy users, the symptoms are not as impairing as those caused by alcohol.[164] NIDA insists, though, that marijuana users run the risk of both dependence and addiction.[165, 166, 167]

And that's slightly true. But the research shows that cannabis has a *lower* rate of dependence/addiction than alcohol, cocaine, heroin, or tobacco, although the risk increases with dose.[168] Among users of tobacco, for instance, 32 percent become addicted, Susan Weiss, acting director of the office of science policy and communications at NIDA, told me. For heroin, it's 23 percent, for cocaine, 17 percent, for alcohol, 15 percent—and for marijuana, 9 percent.[169, 170]

Cancer

Historically, one of the big fears about smoking marijuana was that it might raise the risk of cancer. This does not appear to be the case. A 2009 study by researchers at the University of Leicester in England did find that cannabis smoke can damage DNA, raising the theoretical possibility that the damaged DNA could produce cancer.[171]

But the bulk of the evidence points the other way. In fact, as we noted earlier, a 2003 review by Spanish researchers suggested that marijuana may actually block the growth of tumors, at least in animals.[172] In human studies, it appears that once the effect of smoking *tobacco* is accounted for, there's no extra risk from smoking marijuana, as a landmark 2006 California study showed. In this research, scientists from France, the University of Michigan, the Albert Einstein College of Medicine, UCLA, and other medical centers pooled their efforts to study 1,212 people with lung and oral cancers and 1,040 people without.[173]

The team asked all the participants about marijuana habits, using a standardized questionnaire. When the researchers controlled for tobacco smoking, there was no positive association of the cancers and marijuana. The researchers had hypothesized that long-term heavy use of marijuana would increase the risk of lung and head and neck cancers. But after controlling for cigarette smoking, they found no evidence of that.[174]

In 2009, many of the same researchers looked more specifically at head and neck cancers. They pooled data from other studies involving more than 4,000 people with these cancers and more than 5,000 people without and asked them about marijuana use.[175] Once again, there was no elevated risk of the cancers from marijuana. Even NIDA, on its website, acknowledges that studies have not found an increased risk of lung cancer in marijuana smokers.[176]

Schizophrenia and Other Psychoses

Another concern is whether marijuana raises the risk of psychosis, especially schizophrenia. This is not a big concern for older people who use marijuana medically, but it may be for adolescent and young adult recreational users whose brains are still developing and who are at the age when schizophrenia is most likely to develop. In 2002, British researchers analyzed data on more than 50,000 people (97 percent of all males aged 18–20) who had been drafted in 1969–1970 into the Swedish army.[177] The study, published in the *British Medical Journal*, found that cannabis use was linked to a higher risk of schizophrenia, and the more the men smoked, the higher the risk. The link could not be explained away by the use of other drugs or personality traits. In that same issue of the journal, other British researchers studying 759 New Zealanders also found that early adolescent use of cannabis was a risk factor for schizophrenia, with use at age 15 carrying more risk than use after age 18.[178]

That same year (2002), yet another team, this time a group of Dutch, British, and French researchers, came to similar conclusions.[179] These researchers looked at more than 4,000 psychosis-free people and 59 others who been diagnosed with a psychotic disorder. They tracked all the subjects' marijuana use for three years. They found that smoking marijuana increased the risk both of a person becoming newly psychotic and of faring poorly if the person already had a diagnosis of psychosis. In 2004, a different Dutch team reviewed five other studies and found that cannabis use seems to raise the risk of schizophrenia, especially in vulnerable people.[180] In 2007, a meta-analysis of data pooled from 35 other studies further strengthened the link. If a person smokes cannabis during his or her youth, this analysis found, there's a significantly increased risk of psychosis later in life.[181]

Other studies hammer this home. In 2010, Australian researchers found that teenagers who started using cannabis early, around age 15, and kept smoking for six years until they were 20 had more than twice the normal risk of psychosis.[182] In 2011, Australian researchers who analyzed pooled data from 83 studies concluded that cannabis users who develop psychosis do so at an earlier age (by about two years) than nonusers.[183] You might think, then, that it's an open-and-shut case for the link between adolescent marijuana use and schizophrenia. But it's not that simple. If marijuana use really does increase the risk of schizophrenia, this should show up in large populations as marijuana use has increased over the years.

It doesn't.

In 2009, United Kingdom researchers from Keele University looked at the medical records of almost 600,000 people, more than 2 percent of the entire UK population aged 16 to 44. They studied the years from 1996 to 2005, when there was a substantial rise in cannabis use. They found no evidence of increasing schizophrenia or psychoses in this time period.[184] If there is an increased risk, then, perhaps it occurs in people genetically susceptible to psychosis.[185] But that raises the question of what a biochemical link between cannabis and schizophrenia might be, and the data on that are inconclusive.[186, 187]

Bottom line? There is only equivocal evidence for the hypothesis that cannabis can cause schizophrenia.[188] Young, recreational users should probably be cautious, McGill University researchers concluded, but older people using marijuana medically probably need not worry.[189]

Other Psychiatric Problems

Research on potential links between cannabis and anxiety or depression is inconclusive. In 2002, Australian researchers reported that teenage girls who inhaled marijuana at least once a week were twice as likely as less frequent users to experience depression or anxiety over the next seven years.[190] But other research shows that, while anxiety, paranoia, and disorientation do occur in new cannabis users, these problems are uncommon in regular users. Indeed, a systematic review of the data does not find a strong association between chronic cannabis use in young people and psychosocial harm.[191]

Cognitive Problems

Cognitive problems attributed to marijuana have also been a concern, but again, the jury is still out. In 2002, researchers from Harvard's

McLean Hospital studied 122 long-term, heavy cannabis users and 87 people who had minimal cannabis exposure, and subjected them all to a number of cognitive tests. As hypothesized, the people who started using cannabis earlier in adolescence did do more poorly on cognitive tests. But it's not clear how to interpret this. The heavy cannabis users may have been on a bad track to begin with. As the authors put it delicately in this and a subsequent study, these people may already have "eschewed academics and diverged from the mainstream culture."[192, 193] In 2008, Australian researchers used magnetic imaging (MRIs) to scan the brains of 15 men in their late 30s who had inhaled more than five joints a day for an average of almost 20 years. The men had not used other drugs or had any neurological problems. They were compared to 16 similar men who had not used cannabis. The brains of the marijuana group showed reduced volume in two areas key to emotional and cognitive functioning, the amygdala and the hippocampus, suggesting possible damage.[194]

In 2009, a different group of Australian and Irish researchers used fMRI scans and also documented changes. They found that several brain regions, particularly the anterior cingulate cortex and right insula, were underactive in chronic cannabis users.[195] This is troubling, to be sure, as was a 2010 study from McLean Hospital in which researchers looked at 33 chronic marijuana users and 26 nonusers and put them all through neurocognitive tests and brain scans to assess the ability to plan and do abstract thinking.[196] The McLean team found that age of initial heavy use of marijuana was crucial. People who started before age 16 made twice as many mistakes on the tests, a pattern that got worse the more the teenagers smoked. Even when told they had made errors, the marijuana users kept making mistakes and had more trouble following rules and maintaining focus. In 2012, researchers from Duke University's Center for Child and Family Policy analyzed data on 1,037 people from birth to age 38 and found that those who were diagnosed with marijuana dependency as teenagers and who continued to use it had cognitive declines.[197]

Pretty worrisome stuff, to be sure. But other data suggest that once a person stops using marijuana, some cognitive changes like memory bounce back to normal.[198, 199] And when San Diego researchers pooled data from a dozen studies on 704 cannabis users and 484 nonusers, they found that while chronic marijuana users sometimes showed a decreased ability to remember new information, other cognitive functions weren't affected at all.[200]

Respiratory Problems

Since the main way marijuana is taken in to the body is by inhalation, one of the persistent concerns has been whether smoked cannabis causes respiratory damage. In many ways, smoking is not an ideal "drug-delivery system" because of respiratory risk. (The flip side of this is that inhalation of any drug—whether marijuana or inhaled analgesia—is great if the goal is to get the drug to the brain quickly.) The challenge for researchers has been to tease apart the potential respiratory damage from smoking marijuana from that due to smoking tobacco because the same people often do both. In 2007, New Zealand researchers did just that. They recruited 339 people from four different groups—those who smoked only cannabis, those who smoked only tobacco, those who smoked both, and those who smoked neither.[201] They found that smoking one marijuana joint had similar adverse effects—in terms of airflow obstruction—as 2.5 to 5 cigarettes, although inhaled marijuana was not linked to chronic obstructive pulmonary disease (COPD), as cigarettes are.[202]

In a 2012 American study of more than 5,000 men and women in four cities, researchers found that occasional and low cumulative marijuana use was not associated with adverse effects on pulmonary function.[203] In a more high-tech study, Canadian researchers used smoking machines to compare the ingredients in smoke from both tobacco and marijuana.[204] They found that ammonia was 20 times more prevalent in marijuana smoke, as were other substances, but different potentially harmful ingredients were less prevalent. In yet another study, a different Canadian team, McGill's Mark Ware and Vivianna Tawfik, scoured 79 research papers on adverse effects of cannabis published from 1966 through 2004. Long-term, heavy cannabis smokers did get more bronchitis, they found. And inhaled marijuana did contain many of the same constituents as tobacco smoke, as well as higher concentrations of polyaromatic hydrocarbons, which are known carcinogens.[205]

But—and here's the surprise—the researchers couldn't find any lung damage in long-term users, nor any link between smoking pot and the cancers typically associated with tobacco smoking. Moreover, whatever respiratory risk there may be from smoking marijuana can be at least partially offset by vaporizing (inhaling marijuana smoke through a gadget that delivers just the vapor). This allows the active ingredient of marijuana, THC, to get into the bloodstream without toxic carbon monoxide, a constituent of both marijuana and tobacco smoke. Vaporizing heats the cannabis to between 180 and 200 degrees Celsius. This releases the cannabinoids on the surface of cannabis flowers and leaves, but avoids the combustion (which happens at 230 degrees Celsius or higher) that yields smoke toxins. In a pivotal 2007 study, California scientist Donald Abrams asked 18 healthy subjects to inhale standardized marijuana for six days and measured the carbon monoxide (CO) in their expirations. When the subjects used vaporizers, he found little if any increase in CO.[206] Researchers from the State University of New York at Albany confirmed the benefits of vaporizing in a 2010 study.[207]

Cardiac Risks

Overall, the cardiac risk from marijuana appears small. Marijuana can increase heart rate and blood pressure and can increase the risk of heart attack in the first hour after smoking, which suggests that people with uncontrolled hypertension or active heart disease should be cautious about marijuana use. Marijuana also lowers the resistance in blood vessel walls, meaning that if a person stands up suddenly, there can be a sudden drop in blood pressure. There have also been a few reports of minor strokes (transient ischemic attacks) right after marijuana use. But by and large, there appears to be no link between marijuana use and hospitalization or death from cardiovascular disease.[208, 209, 210]

* * *

After analyzing all these potential risks, the conclusion is inescapable. It's a dumb idea to drive if you're high on marijuana.[211] And it's probably prudent for anyone at risk of schizophrenia, especially teenagers and young adults, to steer clear of it.

But aside from that, marijuana is a valuable option for pain control. "To reject the therapeutic potential of cannabis and cannabinoids on the grounds of toxicity and potential abuse is to throw the baby out with the bathwater," as Mark Ware, the McGill anesthesiologist and marijuana researcher put it.[212]

Marijuana is simply not the dangerous drug that the federal government claims it is. In fact, it meets the standard criteria for any good drug—it is both safe and effective.

THE LEGAL BATTLES TODAY—AND ONE SOLUTION

Frankly, I didn't start out researching this chapter as a proponent of the legalization of marijuana. I don't even like the stuff. But I have slowly become an advocate, which puts me in some rather unexpected company—like that of evangelical leader Pat Robertson. "I really believe we should treat marijuana the way we treat beverage alcohol," Robertson told the *New York Times* in March 2012. "I've never used marijuana and I don't intend to, but it's just one of those things that I think: this war on drugs just hasn't succeeded."[213]

More and more Americans agree.[214, 215] A Gallup survey in October 2011 showed that a record-high 50 percent of Americans now say the use of marijuana should be legalized, up from 46 percent last year.[216] This attitude has been growing steadily since Gallup first asked the question in 1969, when only 12 percent of Americans favored legalization. Among the supporters is California's lieutenant governor, Gavin Newsom.[217]

Even the presidents of key Latin American countries—Costa Rica, Guatemala, El Salvador, Colombia, and Mexico—now say they want to discuss the option of legalizing drugs because of the violence associated with the failing drug war.[218, 219] In fact, the momentum for legalization in Latin America seems to grow almost daily. In 2012, Uruguay's president Jose Mujica called for the regulated and controlled legalization of marijuana. Across Latin America, leaders appalled by the spread of drug-related violence are mulling policies that would once have been inconceivable, the *New York Times* reported in July 2012.[220] Indeed, the *Times* noted, if Uruguay completely legalizes marijuana, it would go beyond the Netherlands and Portugal, which have had lenient marijuana policies for years. No other country has seriously considered creating a completely legal state-managed monopoly for marijuana or any other substance prohibited by the 1961 United Nations Single Convention on Narcotic Drugs. Even Sanjay Gupta, CNN's chief medical correspondent, has publicly renounced his opposition to marijuana (http://www.cnn.com/2013/08/08/health/gupta-changed-mind-marijuana), arguing the government is wrong to say marijuana has no medical use and has high abuse potential.

In the United States, *medical* marijuana is currently legal, albeit still controversial, in the District of Columbia and in 18 states, with the biggest use—and biggest ongoing battles—in California and Colorado.[221] As of the 2012 election, marijuana is also legal for recreational use in Colorado and Washington.[222]

Some people oppose this trend, among them Kansas physician Eric Voth of the Institute on Globe Drug Policy, who derides what he calls the "medical excuse movement." Ballot initiatives and legislative initiatives are "not the way we bring medicines to market. We bring them to market through the FDA," he told PBS in August 2011.[223]

Gil Kerlikowske, the White House "drug czar," has sounded a similar theme. Responding to a petition to legalize marijuana, he insisted that marijuana use is "not a benign drug."[224] (Of course, neither is tobacco or alcohol, both of which are legal.)

The groundswell for outright legalization is clearly growing. In the summer of 2011, congressmen Barney Frank (D-MA) and Ron Paul (R-TX) filed one bipartisan bill to end prohibition of marijuana at the federal level and another to remove marijuana from Schedule I or II in the federal categorization of controlled substances.[225] Initially, the bills went nowhere. But by early 2012, several more bills had been filed in Congress. The bills would have the federal government regulate marijuana the way it regulates alcohol, and oversight of marijuana would be removed from the Drug Enforcement Administration and given to a newly renamed Bureau of Alcohol, Tobacco, Marijuana, and Firearms.[226]

Even Obama, who has acknowledged using marijuana as a teenager, has begun changing his tune. After the 2012 election, he told ABC-TV's Barbara Walters that prosecuting recreational users in states that have made marijuana legal should not be a "top priority."[227] Obama called the marijuana issue "a tough problem, because Congress has not yet changed the law. . . . How do you reconcile a federal law that still says marijuana is a federal offense and state laws that say it's legal?"

Suppose we *did* make marijuana legal? What might happen? Among other things, it would make economic sense. Harvard University economist Jeffrey A. Miron calculates that legalizing marijuana could save $7.7 billion per year in enforcement of marijuana prohibition, most of which would accrue to budget-strapped states, but some to the federal government as well. Beyond that, taxing legal marijuana would yield $2.4 billion, Miron calculates, if it were taxed like all other goods. And a whopping $6.2 billion if it were taxed comparably to alcohol and tobacco.[228]

Maine now allows qualified patients—with a doctor's approval—to buy marijuana from small growers and nonprofit centers, a move that has created jobs and turned underground businesses into taxpaying operations, according to a 2012 *Boston Globe* analysis.[229] The growers collect a 5 percent sales tax and pay tax on their own income as well.

Frankly, in an ideal world, I would like to see marijuana not just legalized and taxed, but treated as a dietary supplement. This would make it subject to postmarketing surveillance by the US Food and Drug Administration. Recategorizing marijuana as a dietary supplement wouldn't be easy.[230, 231, 232] But if it were a supplement, and if a given product were linked with harm when used as directed on the label, producers could be forced to withdraw that brand from the market. Wouldn't it be nice to be able to go into any health food store and buy a packet of marijuana with an accurate, informative label showing how much psychoactive THC and how much nonpsychoactive CBD that product contained? Right now, there is no way for consumers to know whether what they're buying is pure and produced by licensed, reliable growers. There's no easy way to know whether your marijuana was grown, dried, and packaged safely, without molds such as aspergillus, pesticides, formaldehyde, or other toxins. Consumers have a right to know such things, and manufacturers, a duty to inform.

To me, the argument for legalization boils down to this. Marijuana is not the "gateway" drug for illicit drug use that opponents of legalization say it is. Underage drinking and smoking are the real culprits. Marijuana is quite safe—far safer, mortality data show, than NSAIDs, acetaminophen, alcohol, and cigarettes, not to mention illegal drugs like heroin and cocaine. Marijuana is a reasonably effective pain reliever, on a par with opioids. Moreover, when used with opioids, it can reduce the amount of opioids needed to control pain.

Beyond those arguments, though, there's a practical one: The war against marijuana has failed. Why not bow to scientific, social and economic reality? If we made marijuana legal, we could focus law enforcement efforts on real criminals. Not on responsible adults and people in pain.

No one has put this better than Gustin L. Reichbach, a pancreatic cancer patient and justice of the State Supreme Court in Brooklyn. In May, 2012, Reichbach wrote an op-ed piece in the *New York Times*. He noted that he did not "foresee that, after having dedicated myself for 40 years to a life of the law, including more than two decades as a New York State judge, my quest for ameliorative and palliative care would lead me to marijuana."

Despite ongoing mainstream treatment, "nausea and pain are constant companions," the judge wrote. "Every drug prescribed to treat one problem leads to one or more drugs to offset its side effects. Pain medication leads to loss of appetite and constipation. Anti-nausea medication raises glucose levels, a serious problem for me with my pancreas so compromised. Sleep, which might bring respite from the miseries of the day, becomes increasingly elusive."

To his surprise, Reichbach found that "inhaled marijuana is the only medicine that gives me some relief from nausea, stimulates my appetite and makes it easier to fall asleep. The oral synthetic substitute, Marinol, prescribed by my doctors, was useless.... I find a few puffs of marijuana before dinner gives me ammunition in the battle to eat. A few puffs more at bedtime permits desperately needed sleep."

"This is not a law and order issue; it is a medical and a human rights issue," the judge went on. "Because criminalizing an effective medical technique affects the fair administration of justice, I feel obliged to speak out as both a judge and a cancer patient suffering with a fatal disease." He concluded his piece poignantly: "Medical science has not yet found a cure, but it is barbaric to deny us access to one substance that has proved to ameliorate our suffering."[233]

Judge Reichbach died two months later.[234]

CHAPTER 11
Beyond Opioids, Part I

Western Medicine

In this chapter on non-opioid pain treatments in Western medicine—and in the next on complementary and alternative approaches, as well as in the chapter after that on exercise—we focus mostly on low back and neck pain for one simple reason: Low back and neck pain are the biggest causes of chronic non-cancer pain in America. Indeed, more than 28 percent of all people with chronic pain have pain in their lower back and another 15 percent have it in their neck.[1] This includes both *axial* pain, which is pain that doesn't radiate down an arm or leg, and *radicular* pain, which does.[2]

Chronic low back pain, the fifth most common reason for doctor visits, is big business. In recent years, there have been "dozens of highly promoted new interventions, thousands of studies, millions of lost work days and billions of dollars spent," according to a provocative 2008 editorial in *The Spine Journal*.[3] Sadly, though, there's been very little convincing evidence that any one of the treatments we'll talk about here is all that effective, although overall, noninvasive treatments are generally safer and should be tried before more drastic or invasive approaches.[4]

Even multidisciplinary rehabilitation, which incorporates several of the best things Western medicine has to offer, yields only moderate benefits. More often than not, treatments for chronic low back pain "do not result in complete resolution of pain or functional limitations," according to a high-powered team of researchers from the Oregon Health and Science University, the University of Washington, Stanford

University, Harvard Medical School and other prestigious institutions.[5] There's no way to give this a truly positive spin. But there is some cause for hope among the estimated 200 treatment options for low back pain. Obviously, we can't evaluate all those options here. But we can take a look at the most important ones.

ELECTRICAL STIMULATION: FROM ELECTRIC EELS TO SPINAL CORD STIMULATION

Electrical stimulation is actually "just a fancy way of rubbing," says University of Washington neurosurgeon John Loeser. "Activating non-pain systems—with nerves that respond to temperature, pressure or vibration—inhibits the pain system."[6] Indeed, animals, including people, have instinctively used electrical stimulation to ease pain for millennia. Dogs lick or rub a hurt paw to make it feel better. Mothers the world over rub little kids' stubbed toes and bumped knees. This rubbing action fits with the theory proposed in 1965 by Ronald Melzack and Patrick Wall—the *gate control theory*.[7] Nerves carrying painful signals from the periphery and those carrying sensations of touch and vibration all converge in a structure in the spinal cord called the dorsal horn. If non-pain nerves can be stimulated, this can swamp incoming signals from pain nerves, and pain signals to the brain can be reduced, at least somewhat.

Electrical stimulation is a way of using the language of nerves to jam the signals, according to anesthesiologist Scott Fishman of the University of California, Davis: "We can add a signal that changes the signal from 'here comes pain' to 'here comes gentle vibration or gentle tapping.' "[8] Or, put another way, "Nerve stimulation induces white noise or gibberish so that the brain doesn't recognize the incoming signal as pain," as Stephen Parazin, chief of spine surgery at New England Baptist Hospital in Boston, describes it.[9] The brain doesn't understand gibberish so "it ignores it."

The earliest trial of this concept took place in ancient Greece, where a healer named Scribonius Largus reportedly put electric eels (torpedo fish) on the skin of people in pain and, so the story goes, even had people put their aching limbs in a pool of water full of eels.[10] Whether this actually worked is unclear, but Largus may have been on the right track. The modern equivalent of Largus's trick—without the "ick" factor—are little devices called transcutaneous electrical nerve stimulation (TENS). These devices send mild electric currents noninvasively through the skin.

The evidence for the effectiveness of TENS is mixed at best. A 2007 meta-analysis of pooled data from 38 studies did show that TENS was effective for musculoskeletal pain.[11] But a slew of other studies found no clinically significant benefit.[12, 13, 14, 15, 16] In March 2012, Medicare announced it would withdraw most coverage of TENS treatments.[17] But TENS does have one major advantage: "It's dirt cheap," says Loeser. "And no risk."[18] And it's possible that some of the studies that found that TENS didn't work didn't use high enough intensity stimulation.

Slightly more invasive than TENS is an approach called peripheral nerve field stimulation (PNFS). This involves stimulating peripheral nerves by putting electrodes through a needle under the skin. After implanting the electrode, surgeons withdraw the needle; the electrode is hooked up to a power pack implanted under the skin. This approach helps with some types of superficial pain, and the risks are low. But a distinct downside is that the electrodes sometimes migrate away from where they were inserted. A more invasive technique is peripheral nerve stimulation (PNS), though some pain specialists question how applicable either PNS or PNFS is for low back pain. Sometimes done through a needle, PNS is more often done through an open surgical incision, through which an electrode is placed directly on a nerve. (As with PNFS, the electrode is hooked up to a battery pack implanted under the skin.) Typically, a temporary electrode is implanted for a week to see whether it reduces the patient's pain; if it does, a permanent one is then implanted. Ideally, instead of pain, the patient feels just a mild, tingling sensation.[19]

This technique is useful for painful limbs. But it's not financially profitable: Demand for the procedure is so low that manufacturers are reluctant to tinker with electrode design. So surgeons have had to jury-rig electrodes for the spinal cord to make them fit peripheral nerves, a tricky task. The procedure can provide short-term relief, but it's not clear how good the long-term results are.[20] And these electrodes can migrate, too, especially if they are inserted in areas—like limbs—that move a lot.

The big gun in all this is spinal cord stimulation (SCS). Once again, an electrode is implanted either through a needle or an open operation called a laminectomy. This time, the electrode is placed in the epidural space right around the spinal cord. This is a permanent implant, and the procedure carries the risk of local complications such as infection, bleeding, and electrode migration; on the plus side, surgeons usually insert a temporary implant first to see whether the patient will truly benefit. Sadly, at least in the United States, the main reason people get spinal cord stimulation is because they have what's known as *failed back syndrome"*—that is, they have already had back surgery for pain and ended up worse than when they started. Sometimes failed back syndrome occurs because back surgery was the wrong approach in the first place. Other times, back surgery was appropriate but didn't work. Indeed, as many as 20 percent of back operations in this country don't help, leading to failed back syndrome.

Not surprisingly, there has been growing concern over the years that surgeons are doing far too many back surgeries.[21, 22] Even surgeons themselves are worried they are too quick to cut: A 2010 study found that surgeons today are actually less likely than family physicians or patients to view surgery as a preferred treatment for pain.[23] Spinal cord stimulation has only been shown to work in certain cases of failed back syndrome—those in which the surgeries were technically well done, but still left the patient with pain.[24] The good news about spinal cord stimulation is that it does reduce pain for some people with failed back syndrome, at least for 24 months, according to a 2008 study.[25] Two 2009 reviews also came to positive conclusions for spinal cord stimulation.[26, 27, 28]

There's one last type of electrical stimulation for pain control, and it's the most invasive: deep brain stimulation (DBS). It's been used for 50 years for various purposes, but it's still not clear how well it works for chronic pain relief. The research is encouraging, though, with the best results occurring when electrodes are placed in brain regions called the periventricular/periacqueductal gray and the sensory thalamus/internal capsule.[29] All in all, however, electrical stimulation is still something of a crapshoot. "Those who get pain relief love it," acknowledges Loeser. "Those who don't are angry."[30]

TRANSCRANIAL MAGNETIC STIMULATION—NOT JUST FOR DEPRESSION ANYMORE

Transcranial magnetic stimulation is a noninvasive procedure in which plastic-covered coils of wire are placed on the skull to induce electrical currents that activate specific brain regions.[31] It can be used both to help diagnose certain chronic pain conditions and, increasingly, to treat them.

With TMS, the physician or researcher passes a strong electrical current very quickly through a coil of wire, according to neurologist Alvaro Pascual-Leone of Beth Israel Deaconess Medical Center in Boston, a pioneer in TMS. This creates a magnetic field that rises up fast and decays fast—in other words, a field that changes very quickly.

The magnetic field goes through the skin, scalp, and skull, and when it reaches the brain, it induces a secondary current that can influence the activity of the affected brain regions. (While the brain is essentially an electrical organ and therefore a great conductor of electricity, the bone and skin of the skull are not, which means the current from the TMS device passes through the skull without change.) In a sense, the term *transcranial magnetic stimulation* is a misnomer. There is a magnetic field involved, but it's just a kind of bridge that induces electrical currents that act in the brain. Technically, TMS should be renamed "electrical stimulation via electromagnetic induction," but that's quite a mouthful.

In the brain, the electrical stimulation from TMS can decrease the excitability of specific regions involved with pain. And because the skin and skull bone don't respond to the magnetic field, strong currents can be applied without causing pain. (This is in stark contrast to electroconvulsive shock therapy, ECT, which uses direct electrical currents—no magnetic fields involved—to treat severe depression. Unlike TMS, ECT does cause intense pain, which is why ECT is administered under general anesthesia.)

So far, most research on therapeutic applications of TMS has focused on depression. But a number of labs in the United States and elsewhere are now studying its potential for pain relief: One study involves a handheld device that a patient could place on his or her head to abort a migraine in progress. Other research, too, suggests that TMS might be useful to relieve chronic pain.

One small French study in 2001 suggested that TMS can provide short-term pain relief in some patients.[32] A 2004 study similarly showed that TMS can temporarily reduce chronic pain, as did a 2009 study.[33, 34] More important than any single study, a 2009 meta-analysis that pooled data from five other studies showed that TMS works better for pain originating in the central nervous system than for pain in the peripheral nervous system.[35]

More recently, a 2010 study of people with migraines showed TMS reduced pain two hours after treatment.[36] A 2010 randomized study in Barcelona involving 39 people with neuropathic pain following spinal cord injury showed that TMS, combined with walking visual illusion, significantly reduces pain.[37] (In the illusion group, patients watched a movie of legs walking. It was projected under their own head and trunk and reflected in a mirror so that they could imagine that they were walking.) And a small French–Brazilian study in 2011 showed that repeated TMS treatments significantly reduced pain intensity in people with fibromyalgia for up to 25 weeks.[38] But it remains to be seen how long these pain-relieving effects might last.[39] More research is needed, especially since a 2010 Cochrane Collaboration review found that, at least at low frequencies, TMS was *not* effective for chronic pain.[40] (For more on the use of magnets for pain and the highly controversial area of pulsed electromagnetic fields therapy, see Chapter 12.)

INJECTIONS—NERVE BLOCKS, STEROIDS, BOTOX: WHAT WORKS AND WHAT DOESN'T

I have never been so grateful for anything as for the four steroid injections I had in my neck several years ago at New England Baptist Hospital in Boston. The pain from my inflamed nerve roots, bone spurs, and spondylolisthesis (vertebrae slipping over each other) was off the charts. I could barely walk because the slightest motion-induced jiggling of my head sent my pain skyrocketing. My irritated nerves were firing so constantly that the muscles in my left shoulder went into uncontrollable spasms, pulling my head over at a bizarre angle toward my left shoulder. I was so desperate I would have consented to injections of almost anything.

Thankfully, for me, the steroids worked, probably by damping down the inflammation around my nerves. (Or was it our old friend, the placebo effect?) But they don't work for everyone. Epidural steroid injections, that is, injections into the space around the spinal cord, have been used for more than 50 years for low back pain—and often for neck pain as well. In fact, for low back pain, epidural steroid injections are the most common intervention in pain clinics throughout the world.

But their effectiveness is very much open to question. Of around 35 controlled studies evaluating such injections, only a bit more than half show any benefit, lamented Steven P. Cohen, a Johns Hopkins anesthesiologist and director of pain research at Walter Reed Army Medical Center, in a 2011 editorial in the *British Medical Journal*.[41] And even in the trials that did show a benefit, the benefit was short-lived—8 to 12 weeks.

The occasion of Cohen's editorial was a fascinating study by Norwegian researchers who divided 461 chronic low back pain patients into three groups.[42] One group got "sham" (fake) injections under the skin in the back. The second group got real injections into the epidural space—but instead of medicine, the injections contained only saline (salt water). The third group got genuine steroid injections. (The addition of a control group getting saline injections was clever because some researchers had thought even plain saltwater might reduce pain by washing away pro-inflammatory molecules called cytokines, a major cause of pain.) The surprise was that, at the end of the study, there were no differences among the groups in disability, pain, or quality-of-life scores. Not exactly a slam-dunk endorsement for steroids. And not exactly breaking news, either.

In the 1990s, studies in the *New England Journal of Medicine* had already questioned the value of steroid injections.[43, 44] To be sure, steroid injections may work better, some data suggest, when combined with local anesthetics, a 2005 study showed.[45] But overall, the emerging picture has been grim. In 2007, Dutch researchers reviewed 30 studies of low back pain and concluded that steroid injections did not help.[46] It was much the same story in 2008 and 2010, according to reports from three different teams of researchers.[47, 48, 49] Similarly, a Cochrane Collaboration review of 18 randomized controlled trials on low back pain was forced to conclude that there is simply no strong evidence for or against the use of any type of injection therapy.[50]

In a more recent blow to epidural steroids, Cohen's team studied 84 people with low back pain and sciatica in 2012 and found the steroids may provide some pain relief, but that relief is only modest and short term, and may involve nothing more than normal healing.[51] In a 2013 study, other researchers found that epidural steroids not only didn't help, but were actually linked with less long-term benefit in people with spinal stenosis.[52]

And it's not just *epidural* steroids that can't be counted on to relieve spinal pain. Steroid injections into *facet joints* don't work so well, either.[53] (Facet joints are the bony protrusions that stick out from vertebrae and help stabilize the spine.)

Steroid injections can also carry risks, as a 2012 outbreak of fungal meningitis showed. More than 100 people with low back pain came down with meningitis after being injected with contaminated steroid injections, prompting criticism, once again, that such injections are among the most overused procedures in the United States.[54]

But it's not just steroids that doctors are injecting into the backs of chronic pain patients. Cohen's lab at Johns Hopkins, for instance, is testing injections of drugs that directly block cytokines, those pro-inflammatory molecules that ramp up pain. Doctors also inject ordinary local anesthetics such as lidocaine and bupivacaine, the same medications that dentists use before drilling teeth. Called nerve blocks, these injected anesthetics can be used both diagnostically, to stop pain temporarily in a particular area so doctors can determine exactly which nerves are probably causing the pain, and therapeutically, to temporarily control pain.[55] Increasingly, doctors now use continuous peripheral nerve blocks, in which a particular nerve is blocked for longer periods with the anesthetic supplied by a portable pump.[56]

In addition to injections of steroids and local anesthetics, some pain patients are helped by injections of Botox, or botulinum toxin, though it's expensive and the effects don't last long. I had Botox injections myself in the trapezius muscle in my shoulder and neck, and it did seem to help. Botox is increasingly being used to treat chronic migraine, too.[57]

Finally, there are *trigger-point injections*, which target hyper-irritable spots in taut bands of muscle, and prolotherapy. The latter involves injections of irritating substances into ligaments to trigger a controlled, acute inflammation that supposedly can lead to stronger ligaments and reduced pain—after an initial period of intense pain. But neither of these therapies seems to work very well. A Cochrane Collaboration review of five studies on prolotherapy came out negative.[58] So did another review in 2008 and another in 2009.[59, 60] A 2011 review by Ohio State University researchers found prolotherapy "promising," but noted that much more research is needed.[61]

As for injections of saline, local anesthetics, or other substances into "trigger points," no luck there, either. There's virtually no evidence of efficacy.[62] My own experience confirmed this. I had trigger-point injections, and they did nothing, except trigger more pain.

So far, we've been talking about injections for necks and backs, but injections of various sorts are also frequently offered for other pain problems, including knee pain from osteoarthritis. But once again, the evidence for efficacy is mixed and, often, distinctly less than convincing.

In 2012, for instance, Cleveland Clinic researchers looked at published studies on knee injections and concluded that steroid injections for rheumatoid arthritis and osteoarthritis were linked to significant improvements in pain and function, with the benefit sometimes lasting as long as a year.[63] And, they said, injections of a lubricating substance called hyaluronic acid may have even longer-lasting effects.

But Swiss researchers also reporting in 2012 said that they had pooled data from 89 other studies involving 12,667 adults with knee osteoarthritis and found that the methodological quality of these studies was so poor overall that it was difficult to draw conclusions.[64] That said, there was some evidence that injections of hyaluronic acid reduced knee pain moderately. On the other hand, there was also evidence that in some people, the injections actually increased knee pain. And a 2013 study showed that steroid injections did not seem to help with tennis elbow.[65]

Overall, many injections seem to carry small benefits and can be quite expensive.[66, 67, 68, 69]

NERVE KILLING: DOES IT WORK?

Since pain nerves cause so many problems, why not just get rid of them? After all, there's no shortage of ways to do this—injections of alcohol or phenol (carbolic acid), scalpels, lasers, radio-frequency waves, you name it. All these methods work murderously well for *denervation*, the technical name for nerve-killing.[70] The trouble is, cutting nerves is not very helpful for chronic pain. Wiping out nerves can sometimes relieve chronic pain, but it also can make things a whole lot worse. If a doctor cuts a peripheral nerve, for instance, the result is often a neuroma, an overgrowth of nerve tissue, which itself can become a source of pain, although there is an important exception to this. Cutting branches of the trigeminal nerve in the face can reduce the pain of tic douloureux, a painful, stabbing pain—at least until the nerve regrows.[71]

But the big problem is that peripheral nerves are multitaskers—that is, they are multifunctional. This means that if doctors cut a nerve, this can deprive the patient of all sorts of necessary incoming sensory stimulation, not just pain. Moreover, cutting doesn't work for all types of pain.

If the pain is neuropathic—that is, caused by damage to the nerve itself—cutting nerves can make things worse. "Cutting a nerve always injures that nerve," Steven Cohen of Johns Hopkins told me.[72] And when nerves grow back, they are sometimes more damaged than before. On the other hand, cutting nerves *may* help with non-neuropathic pain, including the pain from arthritis. Arthritis often causes pain in the facet joints along the spine. In this scenario, the tiny peripheral nerves feeding the facet joints can be cut safely. In fact, cutting these tiny nerves has become the gold standard for treating facet joint pain.[73]

It's also possible to cut nerves in the spinal cord (the central nervous system). This technique, called *cordotomy*, has been used—with some success—for nearly 100 years, especially in advanced cancer patients who don't have long to live. Traditionally, cordotomies have been done under direct vision with a small scalpel, so the surgeon can see what he or she is doing. When it works, the operation reduces pain from the spot where the spinal nerve was destroyed to about three levels (vertebrae) down the spinal cord.[74] But it's far from a free lunch. There are obvious risks to cutting spinal nerves: paralysis and phantom limb pain.[75, 76]

Increasingly, cordotomies are being done with radio-frequency energy. In this method, a needle containing an electrode is inserted through the skin (under X-ray guidance) toward the spot where the nerve is believed to be, and then radio-frequency current is turned on, killing the nerve. Radio-frequency energy produces a kind of controlled burn—the heat is generated from the friction of electrons vibrating rapidly. Radio-frequency ablation is a more accurate way to kill nerves than simply dousing nerves with alcohol or other chemicals, which can ooze all over, hitting neighboring nerves as well as target nerves. But the trouble is, even with radio-frequency ablation, doctors can't see what they're doing.

They can use X-rays to find the patient's bony structures, and they can use their general knowledge of anatomy to make an educated guess as to where the target nerves *probably* are in relation to the bones. But the nerves themselves do not show up on X-rays. To get around this invisibility problem, many doctors first inject a nerve block. If the numbing medication yields pain relief, doctors know they are in the right place and can go ahead and kill nerves with radio-frequency waves. In some cases, it may not be necessary to do this preliminary step—and skipping it could save money, as a 2010 study suggested.[77] But this study also revealed a depressing truth in the pain world: Radio-frequency nerve-killing doesn't work in everyone. More than half of the patients in the study did not get lasting pain relief from radio-frequency ablation.

In some situations, like pain in the sacroiliac joint in the lower back, radio-frequency ablation may provide a reasonable option, according to a 2010 review of 10 studies.[78] But another 2010 review came to a different conclusion—that radio-frequency ablation doesn't help with pain in the lower back.[79] Sound familiar? Once again, there is a paucity of really good, randomized trials; some of the trials that do exist have so many methodological problems that the results are hard to interpret.[80]

Where does that leave the nerve-killing option for back pain? Nowhere near where we'd like to be. The jury is still out, or at least, underwhelmed. As a 2009 review put it, "Few nonsurgical interventional therapies for low back pain have been shown to be effective in randomized, placebo-controlled trials."[81]

SURGERY—DON'T LEAP!

Okay, then. What *about* surgery? There's no question that back surgery is still more popular than it should be, in part because patients in chronic pain are so desperate but also, as one back surgeon privately confessed to me, because of the surgical mindset: "I am a surgeon.

I have a hammer. Therefore you are a nail." Not to mention, of course, that back surgery is a veritable gold mine, with surgeons getting paid boatloads of money to operate. Some estimates say the average cost of such surgery is $70,000 per patient.[82] Indeed, in recent years, there have been billions of dollars spent worldwide on surgery for low back pain and thousands of research articles, as Stanford University researchers discovered when they combed through the literature.[83]

Every cool new surgical device or fancy gizmo seems to spur new twists on old techniques for eager back surgeons. For spinal fusion surgery in particular (in which two adjacent vertebrae are grafted together to reduce pain and increase stability), rates of surgery soared dramatically in the 1980s and even more so in the 1990s, Dartmouth Medical School researchers found when they probed the issue.[84] It's truly mind-boggling: Between 1992 and 2003, Medicare spending for lumbar surgery more than doubled, *even though*, as the Dartmouth team noted, the explosion of fusion surgery far outpaced any evidence that it worked.

Part of the problem is that it's not all that easy to figure out who should and who should not be a candidate for surgery. X-rays and MRI scans are not nearly as informative as one might think: In fact, there's surprisingly little correlation between what scans show and the back pain a person feels. "I have patients with MRIs so hideous I want to throw up, and they say they're in no pain," says Stephen Parazin, the chief of spine surgery at New England Baptist Hospital in Boston. "Then, 20 minutes later, I see an MRI so beautiful it would make angels weep and the person is all curled up in the fetal position because it hurts so much. You just can't always equate images on an MRI with back pain."[85]

Surgery is not even recommended for certain types of neck and back pain. In the case of my neck pain, for instance, the pain stemmed from irritated nerve roots—called radiculopathies—which means the pain originates inside the nerve itself. "We treat radiculopathies conservatively," Parazin explained. "You basically do supportive things like acupuncture, physical therapy, chiropractic that will make you feel better and buy you time until Mother Nature takes care of it."

Even for people with back pain not caused by radiculopathies but with pain that *is* appropriate for back surgery, the results are disappointing. In a clinical trial conducted between March 2000 and November

2004, a different team of Dartmouth researchers randomized 501 back pain patients from 13 spine clinics in 11 states to surgery or nonoperative care.[86] All had been deemed good candidates for surgery on the basis of persistent pain and scans that showed herniated spinal discs. (Discs are the soft, cushioning material that acts as a shock absorber between vertebrae. If there is a tear in the outer ring of a disc, the soft, central part of the disc called the nucleus pulposus bulges out, releasing inflammatory chemicals that can cause severe pain. A bulging disc can also press directly on small nerves or the spinal cord itself, which also causes pain.)

The goal of the study, published in 2006, was to see which worked better—surgery or nonsurgical care—up to two years later. The first surprise was that things didn't work out as planned. Half of the patients who had been randomly assigned to get surgery opted out for one reason or another. And almost a third of those who were *not* supposed to get surgery did. Even more surprising was that over the course of two years, there was substantial improvement in pain and disability symptoms in *both* groups. The people who got surgery did a little bit better, but the differences were small and not statistically significant, although the surgery patients did feel better faster.

In a 2009 review of 161 randomized trials, a different team of researchers—this time from the Oregon Health and Science University—concluded that outcomes are so iffy that it's incumbent upon doctors to tell potential back surgery patients the truth: that there is only a small to moderate average benefit from surgery.[87] "The majority of such patients who undergo surgery do not experience an optimal outcome," that is, having minimal or no pain, reduction of pain medications, and a return to high-level functioning, the Oregon team said.

To be sure, the Oregon team was talking specifically about fusion surgery, not other types of back surgery such as discectomy (the removal of a herniated disc), according to Roger Chou, the lead author.[88] The evidence is better for discectomy and decompression for spinal stenosis than for fusion in people with nonspecific, nonradicular low back pain.

And surgery is a good solution for some things, including trauma and deformity, in which the biggest need is to restore stability to the back.[89, 90, 91] Still and all, given the less than stellar outcomes, it's curious that surgery for back pain ever became so widespread.

Thirty years ago, spinal fusion seemed to be the perfect fix for people whose discs were degenerating from arthritis. "It was the gold standard for 'black disc disease,'" Stephen Parazin told me.[92] *Black discs* were so named because they contained so little water that the discs looked black on certain MRI scans. And the surgery worked—sometimes. On average, about two-thirds of people usually got better. But they had to be in body casts for six weeks and weren't really functional for six months. Worse yet, the pain—and degeneration—often shifted to the discs above and below the ones that had been fused.

So surgeons starting putting screws and rods into degenerating backs to stabilize the fusion, and this kind of worked, too, at least reducing the need for body casts and lengthy recuperations. But again, many of the people still wound up in pain. So surgeons tried taking out the bad discs and putting in artificial discs. Again, this helped some people, but failed to help many others, making it unclear whether it's any better than standard fusion surgery.[93]

Overall, fusion in the lower back "appears to offer limited relative benefits," as one 2008 review put it. Artificial discs rate the same tepid assessment.[94] Basically, spinal fusion should be a last, not first, resort for back pain stemming from degenerated discs.[95]

That said, there is a new surgical technique that may hold more promise. It's called *decompression* or *disc nucleoplasty*. In this procedure, surgeons, using thin needles inserted through the skin, drill tiny holes inside a damaged disc to relieve pain. A 2008 review concluded that nucleoplasty is simple and relatively safe, involves minimal tissue damage, and has fewer downsides than fusion.[96] But it's too soon to get too excited about it yet. So far, there have been no randomized trials comparing nucleoplasty to fusion, so any firm conclusions are premature.[97]

CHEMOTHERAPY PAIN

We haven't focused much on cancer pain in this book because, compared to chronic, non-cancer pain, doctors generally do better with it. They are less likely to dismiss the pain as all in the patient's head. Friends and family members are more likely to believe cancer patients' pain. And there is much less political controversy about using the big guns of pain control—opioids—to control it.

But there is one facet of cancer pain that hasn't attracted the attention it deserves, and that is chronic pain that comes not from the spreading cancer itself, but from the very treatments, specifically chemotherapy, used to treat it. (Interestingly, radiation is not a big cause of cancer-related pain because it does not directly damage pain nerves. It does damage the blood supply *to* nerves, which indirectly damages nerves. But a drug given before radiation, Amifostine, can protect blood vessels, thus minimizing damage to nerves.[98])

To be sure, in most cancer patients, chemotherapy does not lead to peripheral neuropathy—damage to pain nerves. But some chemotherapy patients—nobody is quite sure what percent—do get peripheral neuropathy. Of these, about 20 percent have numbness and often pain, which can be severe. In fact, painful peripheral neuropathy is the most common reason for stopping chemotherapy, according to Gary Bennett, a neuroscientist at McGill University in Montreal. Doctors could give *more* and potentially more effective chemotherapy if it were not for peripheral neuropathy. Doctors can't give maximally effective doses of chemotherapy to kill tumors because they are limited to maximally tolerable doses, Bennett told me, the limit being peripheral neuropathy.[99]

Many different chemotherapy drugs can trigger neuropathy, including Paclitaxel, Cisplatin, vinca alkaloids such as vincristine and vinblastine, and so-called proteosome inhibitors such as Velcade.[100] These drugs are believed to cause pain by poisoning mitochondria—tiny powerhouses that produce energy in every cell—in the axons of nerve cells. (Axons are long projections from nerve cell bodies that carry pain signals from one nerve cell to the next.) "The mitochondria inside neurons get sick with chemotherapy—they get all swollen and part of the inner membrane collapses," explained Bennett.

If chemotherapy actually *killed* all sensory nerve fibers, patients would feel no pain in response to a stimulus. The reason they do feel pain from chemotherapy is that nerve cells still function to some extent, but with a severe energy deficit because of the injured mitochondria. Instead of dying outright, in other words, the axons degenerate. And degenerating axons spontaneously discharge, or fire, causing pain. The good news is that there are two drugs that can protect mitochondria against damage from chemotherapy—at least according to research in animals. One is a dietary supplement called acetyl-l-carnitine (ALCAR). But in order to protect nerves, it has to be taken *with* chemotherapy, not afterward.[101] The other is Olesoxime, a drug made by the French company Trophos. It is currently under study for various neurological problems.[102]

There may be another way to guard against chemotherapy-induced pain as well—cannabidiol, a component of marijuana, as Temple University researchers have recently shown.[103] (For more on marijuana and pain, see Chapter 10.)

EMERGING PAIN DRUGS

Resolvins

Scientists are now studying a number of new pharmacological approaches to pain control. Among the most interesting are those based on substances made naturally in the body called *resolvins*.

In response to invaders like viruses and bacteria, the body mounts an aggressive, acute inflammatory response. It also mounts a strong inflammatory response to injuries that occur *without* infection, including surgical operations like knee surgery. During such operations, surgeons clamp off arteries to control bleeding. But the minute the clamp on the artery comes off, an aggressive inflammatory response begins. White blood cells rush in to the area to mop up tissue damage. The cells flock to the lungs, too, where they can cause serious congestion, according to Charles Serhan, who studies inflammation and its role in pain at Boston's Brigham and Women's Hospital.[104]

In the past, nobody thought too much of this. Scientists figured that as soon as the inflammatory response—with its hallmark chemicals, including prostaglandins and leukotrienes—was over, all this frantic chemical activity would dwindle away on its own. But Serhan told me he "had one of those Eureka moments 10 years ago." He realized that instead of a passive slowing down of inflammatory activity, there is an *active* shutoff—a resolution of the acute response that is orchestrated by anti-inflammatory chemicals he dubbed *resolvins*.

Resolvins, which are made in the body from two common fatty acids, actively shut down the inflammatory response, returning the body to normal. The intriguing part, for pain researchers, is that resolvins don't just turn off the inflammatory response but also bind to receptors in the dorsal root ganglion. Once there, they damp down pain. The implications are obvious: Boosting resolvins might help damp down pain. So far, there have been no resolvin-type drugs on the market, but one is in clinical trials.

Adenosine

Adenosine is another promising pharmacological strategy. Adenosine, which has a widespread calming influence on the body and damps down the pain system, is made in the body from the ubiquitous energy molecules adenosine triphosphate (ATP) and its cousin adenosine monophosphate (AMP). Recently, researchers from the University of Rochester stirred considerable excitement by showing that acupuncture may reduce pain by triggering release of adenosine.[105]

And there may be other ways of boosting adenosine as well, says Mark Zylka, a pain researcher and associate professor of cell and molecular physiology at the University of North Carolina.[106] Doctors could simply give pain patients adenosine as a drug. There are two adenosine drugs already on the market—an anticancer drug called deoxycoformycin (Pentostatin), which keeps adenosine levels up by inhibiting an enzyme that destroys it, and Adenocard, which is used to slow abnormal heart rhythms. But these drugs are far from ideal for pain patients—slowing heart rhythm is not necessarily something pain patients need. And the adenosine in the current formulations has a short half-life, meaning the body destroys it quickly.

So Zylka is trying to find other ways to boost adenosine for pain control. One way, his team has found, is by administering an enzyme called prostatic acid phosphatase (PAP) that is made naturally in the body. (Technically, this type of enzyme is called an *ectonucleotidase*.)[107, 108, 109, 110] PAP creates adenosine in the body by chopping off a piece of a precursor molecule, AMP, leaving pure adenosine. Like the "energizer bunny," PAP can keep chopping away for extended periods of time.

In studies so far, Zylka has injected PAP directly into the intrathecal space around the spinal cord in mice given experimental injuries to produce pain. The animals got fairly long term pain relief—three days.

But Zylka has shown that if PAP is injected *before* the injury, pain relief can last as long as nine days. The PAP-induced pain relief is also powerful—eight times more effective than opioids, with no side effects, Zylka has found. His team is also studying ways to use a similar enzyme called NT5E to achieve long-lasting pain relief.[111] In a 2012 study in mice, Zylka's team injected PAP directly into a well-known acupuncture point behind the knee (the Weizhong acupuncture point) and found that pain relief lasted six days, far longer than the hour-long relief obtained by acupuncture alone. He calls the technique "PAPupuncuture."[112]

AC1

Another promising drug target is an enzyme called AC1, a chemical messenger made inside nerve cells that enhances transmission of pain signals. A compound that could block this enzyme is the dream of University of Toronto neuroscientist Min Zhuo, who has been studying AC1 in animals for 10 years.[113, 114] In animal tests so far, the anti-AC1 drug seems to work in a part of the brain called the anterior cingulate cortex (ACC).[115] Whether given by injection or orally, the drug seems to block chronic pain without side effects. More important, unlike opioids, which block sensitivity to both acute and chronic pain, the anti-AC1 drug blocks only chronic pain. This is important because, while chronic pain has no protective value, acute pain does.

Monoclonal Antibody Technology

Another innovative pharmacological approach is to use monoclonal antibody technology to fight chronic pain. Monoclonal antibodies are specialized molecules made in the lab that are designed to attach to tiny markers (proteins). In the case of pain, the goal has been to make monoclonal antibodies that attach to and block nerve growth factor (NGF), a chemical made in the body that, as its name implies, stimulates nerves to grow.[116, 117, 118] The drug company Pfizer has already spent years testing its monoclonal, called tanezumab, for knee and hip pain from osteoarthritis.[119, 120] It works. In two studies presented in May 2011, tanezumab showed promise in reducing the pain of this type of arthritis.[121]

Another encouraging study was one published in 2010 in the *New England Journal of Medicine*.[122] In this study, researchers looked at 450 people with knee arthritis who were taking various doses of the drug, and found it reduced pain a remarkable 45 to 62 percent, far more than the 30 percent or so achievable with opioids.

But there was bad news, too. A number of patients wound up requiring joint replacement surgery, and it's not clear why. The speculation is that perhaps the drug reduced not just chronic pain but acute pain as well and that as a result of blunting all pain *too* much, patients overdid it, indulging so much in their newfound ability to exercise that they may have damaged their knees and hips to the point where they needed surgery.[123, 124] It's also possible that the problem was caused by taking tanezumab along with nonsteroidal anti-inflammatory drugs (NSAIDs).[125] At the request of the US Food and Drug Administration, Pfizer (like other companies testing similar products) suspended its studies of tanezumab for arthritis, back pain, and diabetic neuropathy in the summer of 2010.[126] In the fall of 2012, Pfizer was allowed to resume its studies.[127]

Protein Kinase C-Epsilon (PKC-Epsilon)

In yet another potential approach, researchers from the University of California, San Francisco, are studying an enzyme called protein kinase C-epsilon (PKC-epsilon), that appears to be involved in the transition from acute to chronic pain.[128] Blocking this enzyme could potentially lower the risk that temporary pain becomes persistent. But this remains to be seen.

TYO27

In May 2012, at a meeting of the Pain Consortium at the National Institutes of Health, Victor Hruby of the University of Arizona, Tucson, offered yet another potential approach, this one involving a peptide dubbed TYO27 that acts on two different sites at the same time, with potentially effective analgesia but less risk of addiction.[129, 130] At that same conference, University of Michigan scientist David Fink reported that it's possible to use a changed form of the herpes simplex virus

(HSV, the virus that hides in nerve cells) as a vector to carry certain genes to nerves in the dorsal root ganglion to combat pain.[131, 132, 133]

PAIN RELIEVERS BY ANY OTHER NAME

Fortunately, it's not just drugs specifically designed to combat chronic pain that fight pain. Drugs originally designed for other purposes can also help, and many are already on the market. In some cases, pain relief has been added as an official FDA-approved "indication" for these non-pain drugs; in others, the drugs are not specifically approved for pain, but can be used legally off-label to treat pain.

The most fascinating of these drugs is an anti-epileptic drug called gabapentin (sold as Neurontin, Fanatrex, Gabarone, Gralise, and Horizant), and its close cousin, pregabalin (Lyrica), which is often pre-scribed for people with fibromyalgia. (Both gabapentin and pregabalin are FDA-approved for pain.)[134, 135]

The gabapentin story began in the mid-1990s, recalls McGill University's Gary Bennett.[136] He was testing an anti-epileptic drug called felbamate in rats to see whether it worked against experimentally induced pain. He thought it would because felbamate works on many different biochemical pathways, including some for pain.[137] Bennett discovered that it did work—like a charm. "We were getting excellent results in terms of pain," Bennett told me, the old excitement still audi-ble in his voice. "We were just beginning to write up our results when the FDA sent out a letter saying felbamate was killing people." The FDA had discovered that the drug could cause aplastic anemia, a potentially fatal disease, in adults. The FDA banished it from the market, except for babies with rare form of epilepsy who would die without it. "We were heartbroken," recalled Bennett. "You obviously can't give that danger-ous a drug to a pain patient."

But no sooner had the felbamate news sunk in than Bennett received a phone call from a physician in Ohio. The doctor had been treating a handful of patients suffering from both epilepsy and complex regional pain syndrome, a chronic pain condition that can affect the entire body but often affects just one arm or leg. Three of the physician's patients surprised him by saying that when they started taking Neurontin for epilepsy, their pain also disappeared. Bennett was thrilled by this news, and soon word spread. Doctors all over the country began giving pain patients Neurontin—with promising results. By 1998, researchers had confirmed that the drug worked for painful neuropathy.[138] A number of other studies since have confirmed the efficacy of anti-epileptics for pain, including a 2010 Cochrane Collaboration review of Lyrica in 19 studies involving 7,003 patients.[139]

And it's not just anti-epileptics that can relieve pain. Other drugs, especially some antidepressants, can, too, though the evidence is some-what mixed.[140] Antidepressants called serotonin and norepinephrine reuptake inhibitors (SNRIs) such as duloxetine (Cymbalta), venla-faxine (Effexor), and milnacipran (Savella) often help with chronic pain.[141, 142, 143, 144] (For a more complete discussion of antidepressants and pain, see Chapter 6.) Antidepressants called tricyclics including nortriptyline (Pamelor and Aventyl), amitriptyline (Elavil, Endep, and Vanatrip), and desipramine (Norpramin and Pertofrane) can also reduce pain somewhat.[145, 146, 147]

Antipsychotics drugs such as olanzapine (Zyprexa) may also help with pain. And, for severe muscle spasms, Carisoprodol (Soma), cyclo-benzaprine (Flexeril), and diazepam (Valium) may help.[148, 149, 150, 151]

OVER-THE-COUNTER PAIN RELIEVERS: HOW SAFE? HOW EFFECTIVE?

NSAIDs

Last, but decidedly not least, there are the nonsteroidal anti-inflam-matory drugs (NSAIDs) and acetaminophen, sold over the counter. These drugs can be very effective for moderate pain and are an appro-priate first step for treating many types of pain.

But there's a huge irony here. While many people are highly fearful of opioids, they are often *not fearful enough* of acetaminophen and NSAIDs. For all their much-publicized risks, opioids do *not* cause specific organ toxicity such as damage to the liver, kidneys, brain, or other organs.[152] Acetaminophen and NSAIDs can.[153] The big culprit is acetamino-phen, which is the active ingredient in Tylenol. But acetaminophen is not just in Tylenol, and that's part of the problem. Acetaminophen is everywhere—mixed in with cold and cough medications as well as with opioid drugs, though you have to read the fine print to figure this out. Vicodin, Lortab, Percocet, Tylox, and Darvocet, for instance, are all combinations of opioids and acetaminophen.

In 2008, approximately 25 billion doses of acetaminophen were sold in the United States, according to the Food and Drug Administration. While acetaminophen is reasonably safe used by itself, because it's in so many other medicines and because it has such a narrow *therapeutic index*—the dose at which it helps is very close to the dose at which it harms—it's potentially dangerous.

In fact, acetaminophen is a leading cause of acute liver failure. There are roughly 30,000 hospitalizations a year linked to acetaminophen overdose, according to government figures.[154] It's especially dangerous in combination with alcohol, which is why the FDA now says flatly, "Do not drink alcohol when taking medicines that contain acetaminophen." In January 2011, the FDA issued a safety announcement asking drug manufacturers to limit the amount of acetaminophen in combined products to 325 milligrams per dose. It also demanded that labels carry a "boxed warning" to highlight acetaminophen's potential for severe liver damage.[155]

NSAIDs, the most famous of which is ibuprofen, the main ingredient in Motrin and Advil, are hardly risk-free, either. NSAIDs can cause severe and potentially fatal bleeding in the stomach and intestines, among other problems.[156] Since April 2005, the FDA has required boxed warnings on NSAID labels. In its 2009 guidelines, the American College of Gastroenterology noted that gastrointestinal bleeding and perforation send 100,000 people to the hospital every year and cause 7,000 to 10,000 deaths, particularly in people at high risk.[157]

Unfortunately, as the American Geriatric Society noted in *its* 2009 guidelines, age is one of those risk factors.[158] The risk of a serious NSAID-associated gastrointestinal bleed for people aged 16 to 44 is 5 in 10,000, with the risk of death being 1 in 10,000; for people 75 and over, the risk of a serious bleed is 91 in 10,000, and the risk of death from the bleed, 15 in 10,000.[159] The implication of this is sobering: Some older people in pain cannot take these drugs and must turn to opioids for lack of better options. (It's worth noting, however, that since 2009, the geriatric society has received $344,000 in funding from opioid manufacturers, according to records the group provided to the *Milwaukee Journal Sentinel*, which published a report on the issue in May 2012.[160])

NSAIDs have also been linked to a small but potentially important increased risk of atrial fibrillation (an abnormal heart rhythm that can increase the risk of stroke) in a huge Danish study in 2011 involving more than 32,000 patients with the arrhythmia.[161] Other studies have also raised concern about cardiac risks with NSAIDs. In 2010, for instance, a large Danish study showed that a number of NSAIDs can raise the risk of cardiovascular problems, with rofecoxib (Vioxx) and diclofenac (Voltaren, Cambia) among the more dangerous, and naproxen (Aleve) among the least.[162]

In 2011, Swiss researchers from the University of Bern did a complex analysis of pooled data from 31 trials involving 116,429 patients who had taken a variety of different NSAIDs.[163] Once again, Vioxx was associated with the highest risk of heart attack; ibuprofen was linked to the highest risk of stroke, and naproxen appeared to be the least harmful. "Although uncertainty remains," the authors concluded, "little evidence exists to suggest that any of the investigated drugs are safe in cardiovascular terms." Also in 2011, Canadian researchers did their own review of NSAID use in 2.7 million people—the largest study to date—and came to similar conclusions, namely that naproxen (Aleve) and low-dose ibuprofen are the least likely to raise cardiovascular risk whereas diclofenac (Voltaren, Cambia) carried more risk.[164] In 2013, British researchers reported on a meta-analysis of 639 randomized studies involving more than 300,000 patients that showed NSAIDs raise by about one third the risk of major vascular events such as nonfatal heart attacks, strokes, and death.[165]

Topical Treatments

In addition to NSAIDs and acetaminophen, oral drugs that act systemically, there are a number of local—topical—treatments that can help with minor pain. In general, topical treatments have a huge advantage over oral pills. With swallowed pills, the chemical ingredients pass through the stomach, enter the bloodstream, and then pass through the liver, where they are processed in such a way that the concentration of active medication is reduced by as much as a half. This means that half the drug is wasted before it can begin to fight pain.[166]

When medications are absorbed through the skin, by contrast, much lower doses may be needed because the drugs do not pass through the liver. (Special drug stores called compounding pharmacies can custom-make many pain-relieving topical formulations.)

The simplest topicals, of course, are ice, to reduce inflammation, and heat, to relieve muscle soreness. Beyond that, there are over-the-counter products that can be rubbed or sprayed onto the skin, including "counter-irritants" containing menthol (such as Bengay) that create a mild burning or cooling sensation that can distract you from the pain, and irritants like Zostrix and Icy Hot Arthritis Therapy that contain capsaicin, the main ingredient in hot chili peppers.[167]

Capsaicin, the substance used in pepper sprays for riot control, is particularly interesting.[168, 169, 170] When absorbed through the skin via ointments or a high-dose dermal patch, capsaicin can reduce pain. A 2009 review by the Agency for Healthcare Research and Quality, part of the US Department of Health and Human Services, confirmed that capsaicin can relieve pain.[171] A 2011 review also found capsaicin gel effective for relief of osteoarthritis.[172]

In addition to the irritants and counter-irritant topicals, there are a number of creams and patches containing the anesthetic lidocaine.[173] These, too, can be somewhat effective for minor pain. On the other hand, salicylate skin creams such as Aspercreme or Bengay Arthritis do not seem to help with osteoarthritis pain.[174]

DEVICES: IMPLANTABLE PUMPS FOR PAIN RELIEF

Finally, there are increasingly good ways to deliver long-term pain relief by infusing drugs directly into the area around the spinal cord—the intrathecal space. The big advantage to this is that, since the drugs go right to the area of pain, much lower doses of medication can be very effective. Medication is typically delivered with a *pain pump*, albeit an expensive and invasive approach. The growing use of intrathecal drug delivery has "dramatically reduced" the need for other surgical procedures for pain, University of Washington neurosurgeon John Loeser told me.[175]

To be sure, it takes a three- to four-hour operation to implant the pump—about the size of a hockey puck—under the skin in the abdomen, and to run a catheter from the pump to the intrathecal space in the lower back so that the drug can be pumped directly to this area.[176] The pump can be programmed to deliver the drug at desired times and can be refilled by inserting a needle through the skin of the abdomen into the pump's reservoir. Some pumps even have rechargeable batteries. For people with cancer pain and neuropathic pain, there is strong evidence for the short-term improvement of pain with intrathecal pumps.[177] The evidence is moderate for long-term management of persistent non-cancer, non-neuropathic pain.

Historically, the drug infused through a pump has been morphine. But other pain relievers can be administered this way as well, including local anesthetics, Clonidine, an antihypertensive drug also used for neuropathic pain, and zinconotide (Prialt), a nonopioid derived from the toxin of a cone snail.[178] Prialt is promising, but tricky. It was approved in 2004 by the US Food and Drug Administration for severe and chronic pain. But it is a potentially dangerous drug with many side effects and can't be used in people who have a history of psychosis.

NERVE TRANSPLANTATION

In a dramatic new approach, pain researchers Allan Basbaum and Joao Braz of the University of California, San Francisco showed in May 2012 that it is possible to transplant fetal nerve cells that produce the inhibitory neurotransmitter GABA into mice with neuropathic pain and thereby reduce that pain. (Strikingly, this does not affect other types of pain, such as inflammatory pain.)[179]

The Basbaum-Braz team knew that in neuropathic pain—that is, pain caused by damage to nerves themselves—there is often a loss of neurons that make gamma aminobutyric acid (GABA). GABA damps down excitatory neurons, including those that transmit pain signals. Without this inhibitory activity, pain nerves keep firing, creating the torture of neuropathic pain. The goal of the study was to see whether missing GABA-producing neurons could be replaced.

The team harvested immature precursors of GABA-producing neurons from the brains of fetal mice and injected them into the spinal cords of adult mice with laboratory-induced neuropathic pain. In a series of steps, the team showed not only that the transplanted neurons survived in the recipient mice but that they grew into mature, functioning neurons that hooked themselves up to the local spinal circuits of the mice. Within a month or so, the neuropathic pain in the animals' paws was significantly reduced. If the technique can be shown to work in humans, it would represent a major advance. There are drugs on the market that can boost GABA, but these also lead to sedation, an unwanted side effect. The transplantation approach appears to sidestep this problem.

Taken together, the treatments discussed in this chapter are options to consider. None work as well as patients—or doctors—would like. And, of course, some work in some people but not others. But even if they work only partially, they are worth exploring and worth combining. If any given approach works 10 percent of the time, using several approaches may result in a 50 percent reduction in pain. Definitely worth a try. While the treatments discussed in this chapter are all in the realm of traditional, Western medicine, there are many other options from the world of complementary and alternative medicine. They are not perfect, either. But, as you'll see in the next chapter, they, too, are worth exploring.

CHAPTER 12

Beyond Opioids, Part II

Complementary and Alternative Medicine

OVERVIEW: AMERICANS AS TRUE BELIEVERS

Complementary and alternative medicine (CAM) is wildly popular among Americans, with chronic pain the chief reason people turn to this form of care.[1, 2, 3] A whopping 83 million of us, including me, used some of these ancient-to-New-Age techniques in 2007, the latest year for which data are available. That's 38.3 percent of adults (plus 11.8 percent of children).[4] Collectively, we forked out $33.9 billion that year on complementary treatments—out of pocket![5] (By the way, I will use the term *complementary medicine* from here on, not *alternative*, because most people, appropriately, use these techniques in addition to, not instead of, Western medicine.[6])

Such is the growing popularity of complementary treatments— herbal remedies, breathing and meditation techniques, chiropractic, massage, acupuncture, and the like—that the government had virtually no choice but to set up, in 1998, a separate structure with the National Institutes of Health called the National Center for Complementary and Alternative Medicine (NCCAM).[7] The center's goal is to scientifically evaluate, using Western standards of research methodology, the CAM practices for which Americans so clearly clamor.

Critics of NCCAM question whether the millions of dollars that NCCAM and the rest of the National Institutes of Health have spent on CAM from 1999 to 2009 are justified. Eugenie Mielczarek, an emeritus physics professor at George Mason University and Brian D. Engler, a retired US Navy commander, spent a year analyzing total NIH spending on complementary and alternative medicine and concluded that there were simply "no discoveries in alternative medicine that justify the existence of the center [NCCAM]." [8]

"Did Americans really need to spend millions of dollars to learn that 'distance healing' cannot cure brain cancer or HIV/AIDS?" they ask in a scathing article in the January–February, 2012 issue of the *Skeptical Inquirer*. Did we need to spend $2 million, they ask, to see whether magnetic mattress pads helped with fibromyalgia? (They didn't.)

Even to a more sympathetic eye, the results from taxpayer-funded research on CAM have been disappointing. Indeed, there is only "limited evidence of clinical efficacy" for complementary medicine overall, as a 2008 government report admitted.[9] In a sense, this is not surprising, since, "by definition, CAM techniques are not part of conventional medicine [precisely] because there is insufficient proof that they are safe and effective," the report noted.

When researchers combed through the National Library of Medicine journal database (PubMed), for instance, they found 40 systematic reviews of acupuncture, massage therapy, naturopathy (which emphasizes a holistic approach to healing), or yoga published between 2002 and 2007. Of all these reviews, only 10 (25 percent) found sufficient evidence that a given therapy was effective for a given problem. Similarly, when *Consumer Reports* surveyed 45,601 subscribers online and asked how well complementary medicine worked for them, subscribers reported that the results were "far less helpful than prescription medicine" for most of the conditions studied.[10]

Yet we keep turning to complementary medicine, no matter how skimpy or poor quality the evidence is.[11] Indeed, there is no correlation at all between how popular a CAM technique is and whether it is backed by vigorous study. In fact, CAM techniques that are *less* often used by the public, like biofeedback, hypnotherapy, and acupuncture, may actually be among the more effective, at least in the eyes of mainstream physicians.[12]

Part of the explanation for this irrational state of affairs, I suspect, is our old friend the placebo effect, which helps 30 to 60 percent of patients feel better despite conditions ranging from arthritis to depression.[13]

(See Chapter 6 for more on placebos.) The sheer belief that something—anything—will make us feel better often does. I suspect we also turn to complementary providers out of a spiritual hunger for a more holistic, emotional, even mystical approach to health and illness, as well as out of a craving for a deeper bond with a provider. An hour spent with a kindly soul who believes that our pain is real and who offers empathy and unrushed attention goes a long way toward healing. (Mainstream physicians could and often want to offer this, too, but probably won't unless we alter the reimbursement system to pay doctors more for spending spend time talking with patients and less for dispensing pills, injections, and other interventions. Unfortunately, changing the entire insurance reimbursement system is outside the scope of this book.)

In this chapter, as in the previous chapter, we'll focus mainly on chronic back and neck pain, since these are the main reasons people turn to complementary medicine. We can't evaluate all the complementary practices on the market today, but we can hit the highlights, starting with acupuncture, whose popularity has increased significantly since 2002.[14]

ACUPUNCTURE: MORE THAN JUST A PLACEBO

I have to confess that I love acupuncture, the ancient Chinese practice of inserting thin needles into one or more of 360 specific points in the skin that lie along 12 putative "meridians" through which a postulated kind of energy called Qi (pronounced "chee") flows. I've been using it for decades for general stress reduction and minor aches and pains. I have to also confess, however, that acupuncture didn't help a bit with my severe neck pain—in fact, it made it worse.

In Chinese theory, the beneficial effects of acupuncture come from releasing blocked Qi, partly by triggering what acupuncturists describe as a dull, aching sensation called De Qi.[15, 16] (Neuroscientists at Massachusetts General Hospital in Boston are trying to measure De Qi with a special scale, the MGH Acupuncture Sensation Scale.[17]) What all this needling is doing, in Western terms, has been the subject of considerable research—and controversy, although recent evidence strongly supports the efficacy of acupuncture.[18, 19, 20, 21, 22]

On the downside, despite multiple attempts, nobody has ever been able to find the acupuncture meridians along which Qi is supposed to flow. And some studies have been flat-out wrong. In the late 1990s, researchers using brain scans reported that acupuncture on the foot seemed to increase activity in the visual cortex of the brain—just what Chinese theory would have predicted.[23] Everybody got excited. But nobody was able to replicate the study and it eventually had to be retracted.[24, 25, 26]

In some ways, acupuncture lies in the crosshairs of a culture war—true believers versus the skeptics. Among the most prominent doubters are Edzard Ernst, a British physician and professor of complementary medicine at the University of Exeter, and his colleague, science journalist Simon Singh. They contend that there is no significant evidence that acupuncture works apart from the placebo effect.[27, 28] They do acknowledge that there are somewhat positive research results on acupuncture for pelvic and back pain during pregnancy, some types of low back pain, headaches, postsurgical nausea and vomiting, chemotherapy-induced nausea and vomiting, neck disorders, and bedwetting.[29]

But for chronic pain overall? There is "little truly convincing evidence that acupuncture is effective," Ernst proclaimed in 2011 after a review of 57 studies.[30] (He confirmed this finding in 2012.[31]) The exception, interestingly, was neck pain, for which Ernst did find evidence of effectiveness. (Except, sadly, for me).

In terms of published results on acupuncture, it's hard to sort things out because there's a large publication bias at work. Over the years, a gullible mainstream press has hyped stories on acupuncture, lauding studies that purport to show a benefit. In part, that's because the lay press takes its cues from the scientific and medical journals, which are more likely to publish positive studies. Negative or inconclusive results may never see the light of day. When researchers, such as those from the Cochrane Collaboration, an international group that analyzes research results, take the time to look systematically at multiple studies at once, the data on acupuncture's effectiveness become less clear.

Methodologically, one of the big problems in trying to assess acupuncture is figuring out what kind of control groups to use: Do you just compare acupuncture to no acupuncture? That could miss a lot of subtleties, including whatever benefits might accrue from the calming ritual of acupuncture procedures. A better way, researchers now think, is to compare real acupuncture—sticking needles into known acupuncture points—to "sham" or fake acupuncture. Sham acupuncture can be done in various ways—sticking a toothpick on the skin in real acupuncture points but not penetrating the skin, sticking needles into the skin but on points other than acupuncture points, even using fake, nonpenetrating needles on real points. (With fake needles, the needle slides up inside the shaft so it looks as if it's inserted.)

Some researchers also use lasers for sham acupuncture. Unlike fake acupuncture with a toothpick, which slightly stimulates the skin and hence the nervous system, cool laser acupuncture creates no apparent sensation, thus making it a potentially better control, says biomedical engineer and acupuncturist Vitaly Napadow at Massachusetts General Hospital.[32] In still another twist, some researchers compare real electroacupuncture—in which small electric currents are passed through the needles—with a sham procedure in which researchers insert the needles and turn on an electrical stimulating machine, with all the bells and whistles going, but they don't actually connect the wires.

By rights, if Chinese theory is correct, real acupuncture should work better than sham. And sometimes it does. With postsurgical pain, a 2008 systematic review of 15 randomized, clinical trials found that real acupuncture resulted in less need for supplementary opioids than sham procedures and that patients getting real acupuncture reported significantly less pain.[33] For osteoarthritis of the knee, too, there's evidence that real acupuncture, but not sham, may improve pain and function.[34, 35] That's true for low back pain as well, according to Peter Wayne, an evolutionary biologist turned research director at the Osher Center for Integrative Medicine at Harvard Medical School.[36, 37] And myofascial pain of the jaw.[38]

But in other cases, strange things happen when researchers compare real to sham acupuncture. The most perplexing—and the most challenging to traditional Chinese theory—is that while acupuncture often *is* superior to usual care for pain relief, sham acupuncture is nearly as effective.[39, 40] In one intriguing 2009 study at the Center for Health Studies in Seattle, researchers gathered 638 adults with chronic low back pain and randomly assigned them to customized acupuncture, standard acupuncture, sham acupuncture, or no acupuncture (usual care).[41] The acupuncture groups were treated twice weekly for three weeks, then once weekly for four weeks. Eight weeks later, everybody felt much better—*except* the folks getting no acupuncture. A year later, all the acupuncture groups were still doing better, at least in terms of improved back *function*, though some of the initial improvement in pain *symptoms* was gone.

A number of German trials have done much the same thing, dividing patients into several groups—those getting real acupuncture, those getting sham acupuncture, and those getting no acupuncture. Once again, real acupuncture significantly reduced pain in about half of patients, but sham acupuncture did, too. So what does it mean if fake acupuncture is as good as the real thing? Does it mean that any old kind of skin stimulation helps? That it's the placebo effect doing the magic? That some unknown mechanism is at work? Ernst and Singh think it's the placebo effect. "The fact that real and sham acupuncture are roughly as effective as each other implies that real acupuncture merely exploits the placebo effect," they write. "But does this matter as long as patients are deriving benefit? ... In other words, does it matter that the treatment is fake, as long as the benefit is real?"[42] A valid question.

Still, it would certainly be more satisfying if there were proof of plausible, physiological reasons for acupuncture's putative benefits. If there were such explanations, what might they be? It's possible, for instance, that acupuncture triggers potentially beneficial changes in blood flow and immune function.[43] But there are other, potentially more interesting, hypotheses as well.

In a series of now-classic experiments, Chinese researchers hooked together the circulatory systems of two animals, but performed acupuncture on only one. Both animals showed evidence of less pain, leading, with time, to the hypothesis that this might be due to increased endorphins circulating from one animal to the other. (Endorphins are the endogenous opioids that the body makes in response to pain.[44])

Getting to this hypothesis was not a linear process. Western neuroscientists were decidedly skeptical of the early Chinese acupuncture experiments, one of those skeptics, Bruce Pomeranz, now a retired neuroscience professor from the University of Toronto, told me.[45] In the early 1970s, Pomeranz, a young MD–PhD with degrees from Harvard University in physiology and medicine from McGill University, had been hired to work with legendary pain researcher Patrick Wall, then at MIT. Wall had heard of the Chinese acupuncture work, went over to China to check it out, and concluded that if acupuncture did relieve pain, it was probably a placebo effect, remembered Pomeranz.

"I was out to disprove it. We set up our experiments reluctantly. We had no grants for it. We did these experiments in the wee hours of the morning." said Pomeranz who returned to his native Canada in the mid-1970s. Dutifully, Pomeranz began measuring pain signals from single cells in animals' brains while they were acupunctured. It was puzzling, he said.

"If we gave pain in the toe, then acupunctured the hand or paw, to our shock and amazement, it blocked the pain message, at the level of the spinal cord. I was shook up, actually." His young Chinese assistant would call and tell him to go into the lab at 3 a.m.

"I went in, to make sure he wasn't kidding me," he told me. "We didn't even publish. We figured most journals wouldn't even accept it, it was so way out there." They kept gathering data to make sure it was not a mistake.

With his exciting, but puzzling acupuncture research in the back of his mind, Pomeranz went off to Amsterdam for a conference on how morphine blocked pain. One scientist at the conference announced he had found something he called an endorphin.

"Here I am at this conference," Pomeranz said, the memory of the moment energizing his words. "It was the most exciting thing, like discovering insulin. I thought maybe *we* were dealing with endorphins in the acupuncture work. I took the next plane home."

It all began to make sense. Opioid pain relievers typically took about 20 minutes to kick in and block pain. So did acupuncture. That might be what happened, Pomeranz reasoned, if acupuncture triggered endorphins. And if acupuncture *did* stimulate endorphins, Pomeranz figured, there was one sure way to tell: with naloxone, a drug that blocks the effects of opioids. If naloxone blocked the effect of acupuncture, it would strongly suggest that acupuncture did indeed work through endogenous opioids—the endorphins. "Lo and behold," Pomeranz said. It did. "Suddenly, we had a possible mechanism. It was publishable." Ultimately, Pomeranz would publish more than 50 papers on the subject.

Pomeranz's work kicked off a flurry of other experiments, with a number of studies suggesting that acupuncture works by boosting endorphins.[46, 47, 48] By 1997, even the National Institutes of Health acknowledged the endorphin theory.[49] More evidence along these lines came in a 2009 study by researchers at the University of Michigan. They found, on brain scans, that real acupuncture, but not sham, increased specific opioid receptors called mu-receptors in parts of the brain governing pain. Today, researchers think acupuncture may relieve pain by releasing other chemicals as well. In 2010, researchers showed that, at least in mice, acupuncture stimulates adenosine, a powerful, endogenous pain reliever.[50]

But of all the research on acupuncture, perhaps the most encouraging are the studies involving brain scans—functional magnetic imaging (fMRI), positron emission technology (PET), and other methods. These techniques can show in real time what happens during acupuncture, especially in brain regions involved in pain processing. In 2006, Massachusetts General Hospital researcher Napadow documented with fMRI scans that people with wrist pain from carpal tunnel syndrome—pressure on the nerve that supplies sensation to the hand—have abnormal changes in their brains.[51, 52] He then showed that acupuncture can not only reduce their pain and numbness, but can change patients' brains back to a more normal pattern, probably, he told me, thanks to neuroplasticity (changeability) in the brain's primary somatosensory cortex. Napadow has also found that chronic pain patients respond more dramatically to acupuncture than healthy people—that is, their brains show a greater increase in activity in the hypothalamus and a greater decrease in activity in the amygdala, which governs fear.[53, 54] He has also shown that acupuncture can change the normal (resting) degree of connectedness among the various brain regions involved with pain.[55, 56, 57]

Perhaps most provocatively, Boston researchers in 2009 showed that people getting real acupuncture, but not sham, had changes in nerve pathways *descending* from the brain, a sign that acupuncture may also work by dampening pain from the top down, more evidence, perhaps, that acupuncture activates more than just the placebo effect.[58] Intriguing, isn't it? So intriguing that even the US Navy now uses acupuncture for people with traumatic brain injury.[59] Indeed, a positive bottom line is now emerging.

A 2007 review deemed the scientific evidence for acupuncture only "fair," at least for low back pain.[60] But despite that tepid endorsement, both the American College of Physicians and the American Pain Society now include acupuncture in their guidelines for low back pain. More recently, the North American Spine Society concluded that acupuncture has some value, at least as an add-on to other treatments.[61, 62] Similarly, in the United Kingdom, the National Health Service has decided to offer acupuncture for people with low back pain.[63, 64] Two Cochrane reviews, in 2010 and 2011, also came to mildly positive conclusions. In 2010, the Cochrane review found acupuncture somewhat effective for neck pain.[65] In 2011, a separate review of 35 randomized studies found that real acupuncture (but not sham) yielded at least short-term relief for low back pain.[66]

Most recently, and most provocatively, in 2012, researchers from the Sloan-Kettering Cancer Center in New York reviewed data on nearly 18,000 patients from previously published randomized controls. For chronic back and neck pain, osteoarthritis, chronic headache, and shoulder pain, they found, real acupuncture was superior to both sham acupuncture and no acupuncture. A clear indication that, as they put it, acupuncture "is more than a placebo."[67]

Ah, music to my ears. For the record, there's one last point. Acupuncture is not totally without risks. Serious adverse effects are rare, but there have been isolated cases of pneumothorax, or collapsed lungs.[68, 69] Since 2000, by one researcher's count, there have been five acupuncture-related deaths in published reports.[70] But that's out of presumably millions and millions of treatments—rare indeed.

MASSAGE: POPULAR AND EFFECTIVE

Like acupuncture, massage therapy is booming in America. It's now a multibillion-dollar-a-year industry, backed by fair to strong evidence that, in the hands of trained massage therapists, it is reasonably effective for low back pain.[71, 72, 73, 74, 75, 76] For acute pain, unfortunately, there's no good evidence that massage helps much.[77] But for chronic pain, the kind that lasts for weeks or months, massage works fairly well. And, again, I have to confess my personal bias: I love massage for unkinking painful, tight muscles.

In 2003, a review of three randomized controlled trials found that massage therapy was effective for chronic back pain.[78] In 2007, researchers looked at eight trials of massage therapy and found that it was just as effective as exercise and even a little better than general relaxation techniques or acupuncture.[79] In 2010, a review of 13 studies similarly concluded that massage can be beneficial for low back pain, especially when combined with exercise.[80]

What's less clear is whether the specific type of massage matters. In 2011, researchers from the Group Health Research Institute and the University of Washington in Seattle reported on a study of 401 adults that attempted to sort this out.[81] The team compared Swedish massage, which aims to promote relaxation through long strokes, kneading, and deep circular movements, with "structural" massage, intended to correct soft-tissue abnormalities. (Structural massage requires more training and is more often reimbursed by health insurers.) Both massage groups had one session a week for 10 weeks. There was also a control group of patients getting usual care. By the end of the 10-week study, both massage groups showed significant improvements in disability and the "bothersomeness" of pain. They functioned better, spent fewer days in bed and used less anti-inflammatory medication.

In fact, one-third of those who got massage said their back pain was either gone or much better by the end of the study, compared with only 4 percent of those in the no-massage group. The benefits often lasted up to six months. Surprisingly, though, there was no difference *between* the two massage groups, which raises obvious questions. Is it massage per se that helps or is the benefit, once again, a placebo effect? Or could it be just the comfort of being touched? Or being in a relaxing environment?

On the other hand, other researchers *have* found evidence that Swedish massage may do something special—perhaps by triggering the release of beneficial hormones. In a 2010 study at Cedars-Sinai Medical Center in Los Angeles, researchers assigned 53 healthy adults to get one session of Swedish massage for 45 minutes or a 45-minute session of light touch with the back of a hand.[82] (Light touch here was virtually a placebo; unfortunately, this study did not compare Swedish massage to other types of vigorous massage.) Blood samples were taken before and after the sessions to determine levels of certain hormones and white blood cells. Curiously, there was no difference between the groups in levels of the stress hormone cortisol, as one might expect with general stress reduction. But those who got the Swedish massage did show significant decreases in a blood pressure regulating hormone (arginine-vasopressin), and significant decreases in certain pro-inflammatory chemicals called cytokines. In another study that compared massage to light touch, researchers at 15 US hospices studied 380 patients with advanced cancer and randomly assigned them to massage or light-touch therapy for six 30-minute sessions over a two-week period.[83] Both groups experienced immediate improvements in pain and mood, although the benefits were greater for the massage group.

Bottom line? Massage can help with pain. Consumers clearly love it—in fact, overall, consumers rate massage therapy (along with yoga and Pilates) as equal to prescription medication for low back pain.[84]

ENERGY HEALING: VOODOO MEDICINE OR REAL TREATMENT?

Now we come to the murky world of "biofield therapies." These include Therapeutic Touch, Reiki, and an array of other spiritual and touch techniques. Frankly, most of these are too "woo-woo" for the skeptical science writer in me. But these practices are out there, and some pain patients I respect swear by them, so I feel duty-bound to take a closer look. As a whole, these therapies postulate that it's possible to use a subtle, natural energy to stimulate the body's healing processes, something akin to the biblical "laying on of hands."[85] The idea that there's some kind of "vital energy" in and around us is thousands of years old and is prevalent in many cultures. The Indians call it "prana," the Chinese, Qi or Ch'i, and the Japanese, Qi. Practitioners of Johrei, a Japanese healing ritual, call it "divine light" energy.[86] In the West, we may simply call it "spiritual energy." There are many extravagant claims for these therapies—and hardly any data. But there are some hints.

In 2008, a Cochrane Collaboration review of 24 studies of Healing Touch, Therapeutic Touch, and Reiki found that, although there were not enough data to reach firm conclusions, touch therapies might help with pain reduction.[87] In 2009, researchers Shamini Jain, from the UCLA Division of Cancer Prevention and Control Research, and Paul J. Mills, from the department of psychiatry at UC San Diego, reviewed 13 studies of various biofield therapies. They found strong evidence for reducing pain intensity, though they acknowledged the positive effects may be indistinguishable from a general relaxation effect.[88]

On the negative side, the British skeptics Simon Singh and Edzard Ernst, authors of the provocative 2008 book *Trick or Treatment*, take a predictably dim view of spiritual healing in general. "The concept of healing 'energy' is utterly implausible," they write, noting that some initially encouraging studies later turned out to be fraudulent.[89] At best, they conclude, spiritual healing "may offer comfort; at worst, it can result in charlatans taking money from patients with serious conditions who require urgent conventional medicine."

Let's look at some specifics.

Alexander Technique

This movement therapy teaches patients to change their posture and body position in hopes of improving overall functioning of the body and to treat conditions such as low back pain and symptoms of Parkinson's disease.[90] (For the record, the Alexander technique does not rate a mention on NCCAM's list of "Health Topics A–Z."[91])

With a gentle, hands-on approach, the Alexander therapist guides the patient to relearn postures and body movement, which, proponents say, might help with respiratory problems, Parkinson's disease, and chronic back pain.[92] In 2002, researchers at a clinic in central London compared the Alexander technique to massage or no treatment in 93 people with Parkinson's disease. The Alexander technique did yield more improvement in symptoms than no treatment at all, but not much more than massage.[93] In 2008, other British researchers found that the Alexander technique was effective for low back pain.[94] In 2011, still other researchers found the technique changed muscle tension near the spine and hips and reduced stiffness.[95] Translation? The Alexander technique might help with pain—if you can commit to dozens of sessions and have the money to pay for them.

Craniosacral Therapy

This involves gentle manipulation of the skull and sacrum, supposedly to facilitate movement of cerebrospinal fluid. It *might* be better than no treatment for some tension headaches, NCCAM says.[96] But, again, solid data are scarce. I'm inclined to believe the British skeptics, Ernst and Singh, who conclude that there is "no convincing evidence to demonstrate that craniosacral therapy is effective for any condition." [97]

Feldenkrais Method

This approach aims to teach people how to be more flexible mentally and physically by moving and holding their bodies differently.[98] The practitioner often uses light touch to teach the patient to become more aware of how the body moves through space. Once again, there's almost no supporting research. It's conceivable that through this "somatic re-education," the brain might rewire itself in a positive way, which would fit with neuroplasticity theory. But the Feldenkrais method does not rate a mention on NCCAM's "Health Topics A–Z list."[99]

Healing Touch

This involves a practitioner placing his or her hand on or just above the patient's body, supposedly to engage the patient's own healing energy. According to a Harvard Health Publications newsletter in 2005, one study found that patients had shorter hospital stays if they received healing touch before or after open-heart surgery.[100] But this technique, too, doesn't make it to NCCAM's "Health Topics A–Z" list.[101]

Reiki

Developed in the 1920s in Japan, this approach uses "palm healing" to channel "the healing energy of the universe" to the patient for the "highest good of the patient," explains Pamela Pettinati, a retired Boston surgeon, Reiki "master" and practitioner of other forms of energy healing.[102]

Reiki can involve actual touch, or just placement of the hand near the body of the patient. Reiki does rate a mention on the NCCAM website, and 2007 government data suggest that 1.2 million Americans have used this or similar techniques.[103, 104] Basically, anybody can do it (and you can do it on yourself), though many practitioners take first-, second-, and third-degree training. On the downside, there is no governmental regulation of Reiki practitioners. And, once again, the evidence is skimpy. In 2008, a systematic review of nine randomized clinical trials of Reiki failed to find any evidence of efficacy for any condition studied.[105] A 2009 review by Canadian and Dutch researchers similarly found that studies on Reiki have been so few and so shoddily done as to be useless for assessing effectiveness.[106]

Rubenfeld Synergy

This technique, also known as *somatic therapy*, is a form of "body psychotherapy," in which the therapist puts his or her hands lightly on the patient's body, and "listens" to what the patient's body is communicating. Rubenfeld therapy does not rate a mention on the NCCAM website.[107] And a word of warning: Rubenfeld practitioners do not have to be trained psychotherapists, which means they may not have the skills to deal with whatever emotional issues emerge during sessions. That said, those who practice it believe it has value. "By putting your hands on different places on the patient's body, you receive information that the body is communicating and you can help guide the patient to listen to him or herself," says Joanne Gaffney, a nurse and psychotherapist in Provincetown, Massachusetts, who is trained in the technique.[108]

As for research on Rubenfeld, there is one tidbit. In 2002, Pettinati, the Boston surgeon, did a study on 100 nuns, all retired Sisters of Notre Dame de Namur.[109] These women, whose average age was 78, lived in two retirement communities and had various types of chronic pain. Pettinati divided them randomly into five groups—a control group, which got no touch therapy; and four groups that employed different types of CAM therapy: Reiki; Focusing, which involves no touch and asks the patient to focus on different bodily sensations and discuss them with the therapist; Zero Balancing, which involves touching the patient on various body points to release "stuck energy"; and Rubenfeld

Synergy. The patients were not given details of which type of therapy was being used on them. Pettinati was both investigator and therapist for all the techniques, a potential cause of bias. For what it's worth, she found that Rubenfeld Synergy was the most effective for reducing chronic pain.

Therapeutic Touch

This approach, which has been popular among nurses for years, involves the practitioner placing a hand on or near the patient, the goal being to stimulate the patient's "energy field" to enhance healing. But once again, caveat emptor. There's a now-famous experiment designed by a nine-year old girl, Emily Rosa, and published in 1998 in the *Journal of the American Medical Association*. In the study, 21 practitioners of Therapeutic Touch placed their hands on a table underneath a towel strategically hung in front of them so they couldn't see what was going on. An investigator on the other side of the towel then held a hand over one of the practitioner's hands. The idea was to see whether Therapeutic Touch practitioners could detect energy changes and figure out which of their own hands the investigator's hand hovered over.[110] The Therapeutic Touch practitioners flunked badly, guessing right only 44 percent of the time. They would have done better with simple coin flips. Enough said. Even staunch proponents of energy therapies like Pettinati admit that these techniques are more about faith than science. "The data," she says, "simply are not there."[111] On the other hand, for believers, a little faith can go a long way.

SPINAL MANIPULATION: CHIROPRACTORS SWEAR BY IT—SHOULD YOU?

Spinal manipulation—mostly performed by chiropractors, but also by osteopathic physicians and physical therapists—is a method of applying controlled force to a joint and moving it beyond the normal range of motion in an effort to restore health.[112, 113] It is among the most popular—and, historically, one of the most controversial—of complementary medicine approaches.

The American Medical Association once deemed chiropractic an "unscientific cult" and boycotted it until it lost an antitrust case in the 1980s.[114] Now, the AMA takes a softer view, letting physicians refer patients to chiropractors if they deem it advisable.[115] Chiropractors once held to some pretty bizarre teachings, including the belief that spinal problems—including *subluxations*, or misaligned vertebrae—underlie most diseases.[116] Luckily, things have changed considerably. Some chiropractors still identify as "straights," those who cling to the idea that subluxations are the cause of all disease, but most now see themselves as "mixers," those who are more open to mainstream medical views.[117] In addition to having different philosophies, chiropractors differ in that they use a wide range of techniques, from high-velocity dynamic thrusts to gentle, low-force manipulations. (High-velocity thrusts with the chiropractor's hands are usually termed *manipulation*, while manual force on a joint without a thrust is often called *mobilization*.)

Historical controversies aside, there's no question that consumers love chiropractic. In a 2009 *Consumer Reports* survey of subscribers with back pain, chiropractic was rated as *the* most popular treatment (59 percent satisfaction), followed closely by physical therapy and acupuncture, with care from primary care physicians ranking lowest.[118] Even some people with complicated neuromuscular problems such as amyotrophic lateral sclerosis find chiropractic the most effective form of pain relief.[119] Chiropractic's popularity is helped by the fact that it's relatively cheap, about $60 a visit, and is sometimes covered by insurance.[120, 121] Recent guidelines include it as one treatment option for low back pain.[122, 123, 124]

But scientifically, the research is mixed. Some data show that spinal manipulation along with strengthening exercise works as well for low back pain as prescription NSAID drugs plus exercise.[125, 126] In fact, a 2005 Australian study showed that spinal manipulation actually worked *better* for back and neck pain than acupuncture or medications such as NSAIDs or acetaminophen.[127] Other data show that to *maintain* improvements in pain reduction, though, spinal manipulation must often be continued long term.[128] Chiropractors, among them Scott Haldeman, who is also a neurologist at the University of California, Irvine, firmly believe that spinal manipulation is equal to or better than *any* other kind of treatment except exercise for neck and back pain.[129]

But that's a complicated comparison. Other researchers, among them, Roger Chou, an associate professor of medicine at Oregon Health & Science University, find that "studies comparing spinal manipulation directly to exercise don't show much difference."[130]

In a 2006 UCLA study, for instance, researchers randomized 601 people with low back pain to spinal manipulation or standard medical care. People getting chiropractic (or physical therapy) were more likely to *perceive* improvement in symptoms. But overall, there were no *clinically meaningful* differences.[131] A 2003 meta-analysis of results from 26 randomized controlled trials of spinal manipulation for back pain came to similar conclusions. Spinal manipulation, the researchers said, does have benefits, but they are small.[132] A 2004 British randomized trial compared exercises classes, spinal manipulation alone, manipulation followed by exercise, and regular care in 1,334 people with back pain. After three months, the researchers did find that manipulation was the best treatment—*if* it was combined with exercise.[133] In a 2007 study, Brazilian and Australian researchers randomly assigned 240 people with low back pain to general exercise, special exercises to strengthen the trunk, or spinal manipulation. It didn't settle the debate. By six and 12 months later, the groups were equivalent.[134]

In 2011, Australian researchers looked at 12 studies of chiropractic in low back pain patients and concluded that there was simply not enough evidence for or against chiropractic, compared to other interventions.[135] A 2012 British review analyzed 22 studies of various pain conditions and concluded that the data fail to show that spinal manipulation is an effective intervention for pain management.[136] A 2012 Swiss study of people with acute or chronic low back pain suggested that chiropractic treatment can help, but the study was flawed because there was no control group and because back pain often gets better on its own over time.[137, 138] And a 2012 Dutch review found much the same thing, at least for acute back pain.[139]

With neck pain, as opposed to low back pain, it's a bit more complicated. A 2002 Australian study of 183 people with neck pain found manipulation was more effective than exercise therapy or standard care.[140] A 2007 Canadian review also found that spinal manipulation helped with neck pain.[141] So did a 2012 randomized study of 272 adults with neck pain.[142] But, as often happens in complementary and alternative medicine, some studies are of such poor methodological quality that it's hard to trust the results.[143]

There is also a small, but lingering safety question about chiropractic for neck pain. Edzard Ernst, the British skeptic, dug around in the medical literature and found 26 reported deaths after chiropractic for neck pain. Presumably, the deaths occurred because abrupt twisting of the neck can dissect (tear) the vertebral artery, potentially triggering a stroke.[144]

Other researchers have also tried to calculate the risk from neck chiropractic, generally finding it's tiny, but not zero. In 2001, a team led by neurologist-chiropractor Scott Haldeman looked at 10 years' worth of Canadian malpractice data and found that the risk of an arterial dissection following chiropractic was *one per 5.85 million* cervical manipulations.[145] In other words, very, very small. In 2002, Haldeman's team further noted that strokes triggered by arterial dissection can come from other things, not just chiropractic manipulations, and thus should be viewed as random, unpredictable complications of any neck movement.[146] Any sudden or unusual head or neck movement can trigger an arterial dissection and stroke, Haldeman told me, including a car accident or just tipping one's head back to the sink at a hairdresser's. If, unbeknownst to either the patient or the practitioner, an arterial dissection is already quietly underway—a process that can take hours or even days—any sudden jerk of the head may be the final insult that leads to problems.[147, 148]

An interesting 2008 study by Toronto researchers tried again to tease apart the purported association between chiropractic care and vertebral artery dissection and stroke. They did find an association. But they *also* found strong associations between these tragic events and visits to primary care doctors just before the event, which makes sense. If you have neck pain from an arterial dissection in progress, you'll probably go to a doctor, either a mainstream physician or a chiropractor.[149]

Other studies have documented that serious side effects from spinal manipulation of the neck are rare.[150, 151] But the debate continues. In a pair of opinion pieces in June 2012 in the *British Medical Journal*, one camp argued that neck chiropractic is "unnecessary and inadvisable," and the other, that "manipulation benefits people with neck pain."[152, 153]

So the odds are that neck chiropractic is safe. But when it comes to *my* ridiculously fragile neck, I'm cautious. I wouldn't want to be that one in 5.85 million.

DIET, VITAMINS, AND HERBALS: DON'T GET YOUR HOPES UP

Eating a healthy diet is a cornerstone of good health, but there are a few specific dietary habits that may be extra important if you have chronic pain. The most obvious, especially if you have inflammatory pain such as arthritis, is to follow what health guru—and purveyor of dietary supplements—Andrew Weil calls the "Anti-inflammatory Diet."[154]

An anti-inflammatory diet means eating all the usual fruits and veggies but also getting the right ratio of polyunsaturated fatty acids (PUFAs). These are the omega-3s, which come from fatty, cold-water fish; walnuts; canola, soy, and flaxseed oil; and the omega-6s, which come chiefly from corn and safflower oils. Earlier in human history, we ate pretty close to a 50–50 ratio of omega-6 to omega-3 fatty acids. Now, we consume way too many omega-6s and too few omega-3s.[155] Most fast food, for instance, is loaded with the former and lacking in the latter. The goal is to fix this balance by increasingly omega-3s. Why? Because omega-6s increase inflammation and omega-3s decrease it. In the body, omega-6 fatty acids are converted to chemical substances that rev up the immune system and inflammatory process. This is great for fighting infections, but bad for problems like arthritis. Omega-6s also boost blood clotting, which is terrific if you're bleeding to death, but not so good in terms of creating blood clots that can lead to heart attacks or strokes.

Some data suggest that fish oils—from real fish or supplements—may help combat the inflammation of rheumatoid arthritis (RA). One observational survey looked at rheumatoid arthritis patients taking at least 1,200 milligrams a day of fish oil. The oil contained eicosapentaenoic acid and docosahexaenoic acid. Almost 60 percent of the patients reported decreases in pain and were able to discontinue use of NSAIDs.[156] But fish oil supplements vary significantly in quality, so buyer beware.[157]

Vitamin D

This is the famous "sunshine" vitamin, so named because our bodies synthesize it in response to sunlight. In truth, vitamin D is a misnomer. It's really a hormone, and it has long been proposed as a pain reliever, as well as a way to protect bones against osteoporosis and resulting fractures that can cause pain. Vitamin D also may protect against a condition called osteomalacia, a softening of the bones that can lead to widespread bone pain.[158]

In 2010, after reviewing more than 1,000 published studies, the Institute of Medicine (IOM) issued new recommendations for daily vitamin D intake, at levels some endocrinologists (the specialists who treat osteoporosis, osteomalacia, and vitamin D deficiency) found puzzling.[159] The new IOM recommendations called for 600 international units (IUs) a day for adults, with 800 a day for adults 71 and over. (The highest safe dose of vitamin D, according to the Institute of Medicine, is 4,000 IUs a day.) But whether 600 to 800 IUs a day is really enough, especially for people who live in less sunny, Northern latitudes, is a subject for debate. After the IOM released its new guidelines, the Endocrine Society questioned whether they were adequate because many Americans are deficient in vitamin D.

So in 2011, the Endocrine Society came out with its own new guidelines.[160] These called for babies to take 400 to 1,000 IUs a day; for children aged 1 to 18 to take 600 to 1,000 IUs; and for adults over 18 to take 1,500 to 2,000 a day. Even these recommendations, however, may be open to question, in part because there are so little data on vitamin D and pain.[161] One 2010 European study—based on questionnaires sent through the mail—did suggest that men whose vitamin D levels were low were more likely to report chronic pain, specifically musculoskeletal pain.[162] But mailed questionnaires are not as reliable as randomized studies.

And randomized, controlled clinical trials of vitamin D are hard to come by. There was a German review of four studies in 2010, but those studies weren't methodologically good enough to allow firm conclusions.[163] More encouraging was a 2011 study by researchers at Washington University in St. Louis. They found that extra vitamin D relieved joint and muscle pain in a specific situation—women with breast cancer who were taking drugs called aromatase-inhibitors.[164] Studies in 2011 in India and Turkey also suggested that high doses of vitamin D may relieve chronic pain in arthritis patients.[165, 166] A 2012 systematic review and meta-analysis involving a total of 215,757 people by South Korean researchers showed higher levels of vitamin D from food or sunshine were associated with lower risk of developing rheumatoid arthritis and lower severity of disease, but these were observational not treatment data.[167]

A randomized, controlled Italian trial in 2012 showed that high-dose vitamin D may relieve menstrual cramps.[168] And a small 2012 case study (with no control group) from Emory University showed that giving vitamin D to veterans with chronic pain improved pain scores, sleep, general health, and social functioning.[169] A 2012 California study of nearly 500 people with multiple sclerosis (MS) showed that higher vitamin D levels were associated with lower risk of new symptoms and disability, though this was not a treatment study.[170] And what of the alleged benefit that vitamin D can prevent painful fractures? A large 2012 analysis of 11 studies involving more than 31,000 people showed vitamin D supplementation was somewhat effective at preventing fractures.[171, 172]

Despite the paucity of research data, some pain specialists are convinced by their clinical experience that high doses of vitamin D can help selected pain patients. John Pereira, a pain specialist at the University of Calgary, told me he has given "many thousands" of IUs of vitamin D to some chronic pain patients, with encouraging results, though he noted that, as with all hormones, there are potential risks as well.[173] Michael Holick, a professor of medicine, physiology, and biophysics at Boston University Medical Center, also uses high-dose vitamin D in pain patients and consults with several vitamin D supplement manufacturers. Patients with osteomalacia, he told me, get "dramatic improvement" with 50,000 IUs of vitamin D once a week for eight weeks, followed by maintenance therapy of 50,000 IUs every other week.[174, 175] He told me he has even given 10,000 units a day to healthy adults for five months with no toxicity.

But there have been reports of adverse side effects with high doses. A 2010 study of older women showed that those getting a very high dose—500,000 IUs once a year—actually broke *more* bones than those getting placebo. It's unclear why, though it's possible that women in the high-dose group felt better and were thus more mobile, which led to their falling, and breaking bones, more often.[176, 177]

Scientists are also still debating whether a particular type of vitamin D—D2 or D3—is any better than the other. A few years ago, researchers thought D3 was better. But now, it seems to be a draw. In 2011, a Cochrane Collaboration review of 50 studies involving 94,148 patients did find that D3, but not D2, was linked to a lower risk of overall mortality. But these researchers didn't look at chronic pain specifically.[178] Other studies say it makes virtually no difference which form a person takes. Or even whether the vitamin is consumed as a supplement or in vitamin D-fortified orange juice.[179, 180] Finally, there's some debate about the accuracy of blood tests for vitamin D (25 hydroxy vitamin D). Newer assays, although they are approved by the US Food and Drug Administration, are fairly inaccurate and may lead to an overestimate of vitamin D deficiency.[181]

My take-home message? It makes sense to take vitamin D supplements at the doses recommended by the Endocrine Society. The benefits seem to outweigh any harms.

Other Supplements

Beyond vitamin D, other supplements, too, have been tried for chronic pain relief. The best known is the combination known as glucosamine-chondroitin. Too bad it doesn't work.

In 2006, a team led by researchers from the University of Utah reported in the *New England Journal of Medicine* on a carefully designed project called the GAIT study. The researchers randomly assigned 1,583 people with symptomatic knee osteoarthritis to receive daily one of the following five regimens: 1,500 milligrams of glucosamine, 1,200 milligrams of chondroitin sulfate, both glucosamine and chondroitin sulfate together, 200 milligrams of celecoxib (Celebrex), or placebo for 24 weeks. All participants were allowed to take up to 4,000 milligrams daily of acetaminophen in addition if they needed it.[182] Overall, glucosamine and chondroitin failed to meet the predetermined threshold of reducing pain by at least 20 percent, though a subgroup of patients with moderate-to-severe knee pain did benefit somewhat. In 2008, the researchers reported further that the same doses of glucosamine and chondroitin also didn't stop the loss of cartilage in people with knee osteoarthritis.[183] In 2010, a two-year follow-up confirmed these earlier results.[184]

Quite disappointing. Whether used alone or together for osteoarthritis, glucosamine and chondroitin simply don't work, except possibly for a subgroup of people with moderate to severe disease, concluded a 2009 report from the Agency for Healthcare Research and Quality.[185]

Other Dietary Interventions for Pain

Ginger comes from a plant called *Zingiber officinale* and is widely used in Asian, Indian, and Arabic traditional medicine for pain and other problems. A British review of eight studies came to the tentative conclusion that ginger can act as an anti-inflammatory agent and can help relieve various types of pain.[186] Iranian researchers have found that ginger can potentiate the pain-relieving potency of morphine.[187] Researchers from Georgia found that consuming either raw or heat-treated ginger can modestly reduce muscle pain.[188] But frankly, the overall evidence is skimpy.

Soy. There's also not much evidence that soy protein can reduce chronic pain. Three studies in rodents suggest it might help with inflammatory pain, and a study in people with osteoarthritis pain was also encouraging, especially for men. But more research is needed.[189, 190, 191, 192]

Turmeric. This spice, a staple in Ayurvedic (traditional Indian) medicine and a prime ingredient in curry, is a potential inflammatory pain reducer. In studies at the University of Arizona, endocrinologist Janet Funk has shown that turmeric can slow joint inflammation in animals, suggesting it may be useful for arthritis.[193, 194] But, again, more research is needed.

Peppermint. Long known as a folk remedy for gastrointestinal problems, peppermint may help by activating a specific anti-pain channel called TRPM8 in the bowel. Australian researchers showed in 2011 that peppermint seems to inhibit pain sensations such as those triggered by capsaicin, the active ingredient in hot peppers.[195]

Others. A few other herbal pain remedies are popular, though hard evidence, again, is lacking. Among those are feverfew (from evening primrose), gamma linolenic acid (GLA) from evening primrose, ASUs (avocado-soybean unsaponifiables), and boswellia (frankincense). A Canadian review found that other herbals—*Harpagophytum procumbens* (devil's claw), *Salix alba,* and *Capsicum frutescens*—may reduce low back pain more than placebo.[196] There *is* some preliminary evidence that injections of vitamin B12 may help reduce pain, but the jury is still out.[197, 198] All of which leaves us in an unsatisfying place. There are, alas, few miracles to be had from the health food store.

Plain Water. The data are preliminary. But a 2012 Dutch study suggests that drinking more water daily—about six extra 8-ounce glasses—may reduce the pain of recurrent headaches, though adding this amount of water had no effect on the number of days a person experienced at least moderate headache.[199] (And it can be dangerous to consume *too* much water—the result can be hyponatremia, or low sodium levels in the blood, which can be life-threatening.)

MAGNETS AND PULSED ELECTROMAGNETIC FIELDS: CAVEAT EMPTOR

There are two things that nonmedical professionals generally think of as magnet therapy—static magnets, like the kind you put on your refrigerator, for which there is little evidence of efficacy for chronic pain; and pulsed electromagnetic field therapy (PEMF), for which there is lots of hype and a tiny bit of scientific research.[200]

Static magnets (also known as permanent magnets) have been used for centuries for pain control and other health purposes. In the United States, static magnets are now a booming multimillion-dollar industry, with magnets strapped on as belts, wraps, bracelets, and necklaces, or even put in mattress pads.[201] There is no convincing evidence from rigorous studies that this kind of therapy relieves pain of any type, according to the National Center for Complementary and Alternative Medicine, although it's conceivable that the magnets studied so far have been too weak to show an effect.[202] Still, the evidence is so weak that in 1999, Operation Cure All, a law enforcement and consumer education campaign sponsored by the Federal Trade Commission, blasted sellers of magnet therapies for making totally unsubstantiated claims.[203]

For chronic pelvic pain, for instance, a 2002 study comparing real and fake magnets suggested that magnets might reduce pain if worn continuously for four weeks. But the people in this study could easily have figured out whether they were getting the real or the fake magnets, raising the possibility of a placebo effect.[204] (This was not rocket science—if a metal pin placed nearby moved toward the magnet, it was real.) A double-blind, placebo-controlled 2003 study of magnetic insoles for people with painful diabetic neuropathy in the feet showed some improvement in pain, tingling, and burning sensations. But that study was not very convincing, either. It took three to four months for even this slight effect to be noticed.[205]

A separate 2003 randomized, controlled study of magnetic insoles for plantar heel pain found no difference between the folks who got magnetic insoles and those who got fakes: Everybody got better after eight weeks.[206] It was much the same story with pain from carpal tunnel syndrome. A 2002 double-blind, placebo-controlled, randomized trial showed that static magnets placed on the wrist for 45 minutes significantly reduced pain. But so did the fake magnets.[207] A 2004 randomized, controlled, six-month trial compared two types of real magnetic mattress pads with fake pads and usual care in people with fibromyalgia. The groups using the real pads had some improvements in pain scores, but the differences were not significant.[208]

Another 2004 study, this one by British researchers, found some benefit to magnetic bracelets for people with hip and knee osteoarthritis, but the researchers wondered whether this was a placebo effect.[209] In 2007, a randomized, double-blind study of 165 patients by Tufts University researchers compared postoperative pain in people who had real or fake magnets placed over their surgical incisions. The people getting the real magnets actually had more pain than the people getting the fakes.[210]

There was better news from a different randomized, double-blind study in 2007, but it was not much better. In this study, researchers at the National Institutes of Health found a possible small beneficial effect of the magnets in people with low back pain, provided the magnets were sufficiently strong and were used for five weeks at a time.[211] In 2007, British researchers tried to settle the matter with a meta-analysis of pooled data from nine placebo-controlled trials. They found no evidence of effectiveness of magnet therapy for pain reduction, although the results for people with osteoarthritis pain were just tantalizing enough, they said, that more study is warranted.[212]

This discouraging story should not be surprising because scientists have no idea how static magnets might affect the body. There have been hypotheses—that the magnets might affect nerve function, change the balance between normal cell death and cell growth, change blood flow to tissues, or increase body temperature in the area where the magnet is placed. But so far, there's just too little evidence.[213]

Far more controversial than static magnets is pulsed electromagnetic field therapy (PEMF), which is being marketed aggressively on the Internet and on television. In PEMF, a magnetic field is generated on or near the body. Because this magnetic field is pulsating (i.e., not stable or constant), there is the possibility that electrical fields are induced in the body. It's also possible that the magnetic field itself may have some biological effects.[214]

In one area of medicine—healing broken bones—there is fairly clear evidence that PEMF may help. Scientists think that the cells that promote bone healing may grow and organize themselves better when exposed to a magnetic field. Since the late 1950s, in fact, researchers have steadily documented that electrical currents can stimulate bone growth.[215, 216, 217, 218, 219, 220, 221, 222]

But some research has been contradictory. In 2001, for instance, an observational study of 48 high-risk patients who had spinal fusion surgery showed that adding pulsed electromagnetic field stimulation after surgery yielded a better success rate.[223] But a 2008 study came to the opposite conclusion, though it did find that PEMF was safe.[224]

For chronic pain specifically, the picture is also mixed. In 1993, Connecticut researchers found that PEMF reduced pain and increased functionality in people with osteoarthritis of the knee and in 1994 showed that it works for osteoarthritis in the neck, too.[225, 226] Other studies on knee osteoarthritis have also been encouraging.[227, 228, 229] But there have been discouraging studies, too.

For fibromyalgia and chronic, localized musculoskeletal pain, PEMF delivered transcranially through a headset reduced pain a bit in fibromyalgia patients, but the results were not statistically significant.[230] More important, a systematic review of five randomized controlled trials in

2006 concluded that PEMF does *not* significantly reduce the pain of knee osteoarthritis.[231] Obviously, the bottom line on complementary medicine as a whole is mixed. But so is the bottom line on *Western* treatments for chronic pain.

For me, the trick has been taking an integrative, open-minded approach to both—choosing carefully a treatment to try, assessing honestly whether it seems to help, and combining complementary and Western treatments in an ad hoc, individually tailored way. If everything helps a little, combining treatments might help a lot.

CHAPTER 13

Exercise

The Real Magic Bullet

OVERVIEW

It was July 1, 2008. I was standing at the entrance to the Outpatient Center at Chestnut Hill/New England Baptist Hospital in Boston—better known as "boot camp"—and I was petrified. I had been in excruciating neck pain multiple times a day for more than six months. The burning, searing pain—it felt like my nerve was on fire—ran straight from the lower part of my neck across to my left shoulder, along the way triggering muscle spasms so severe that my head was chronically tipped to the left, a problem called *cervical dystonia*, or, alternatively, *torticollis*.

I had had MRIs, which showed bone spurs, arthritically degenerating vertebrae, and spondylolisthesis, a condition in which one vertebra slides out of position over another. In addition, the tiny, almost-invisible nerves in the facet joints of my neck vertebrae were so chronically inflamed that the slightest wrong move was unbearable. I had trudged from doctor to doctor looking for relief. I had taken several weeks off from work. I had tried opioids, NSAIDs, acupuncture, meditation, massage, and physical therapy. I couldn't walk the dog, lest she jerk suddenly on her leash and send my neck into agony. I couldn't even put on toenail polish—it hurt too much to bend over and crane my neck to see my toes. I was losing hope.

Peeking in the door at boot camp, I could see four or five physical therapists hovering over back and neck patients who were really going at it, doing impressively strenuous exercises on dozens of machines. Back extensions. Rotary torso twists. Lat pull-downs. Leg presses. Seated rows. Arm bikes. Even, to my astonishment, a crazy-looking exercise in which patients filled colorful plastic milk cartons with weights and lifted them to shelves at various heights—precisely the kind of move that would send my neck and shoulders into spasm. No way was I going to do this. First of all, it would hurt like crazy. Second, given what a mess my neck was, I was sure that one false move would cause a bone spur to slice through my spinal cord, turning me into a quadriplegic. Catastrophizing? Not me! It was just plain common sense: Pain equals damage. Therefore, any movement that triggered more pain was going to make me worse.

Enter Dr. James Rainville, a friendly spine and rehabilitation specialist who, along with Lisa Childs, a soft-spoken physical therapist, set up the New England Baptist boot camp more than 20 years ago. It has been a mecca for pain patients like me ever since. And a testimonial to the real unsung heroes of rehab—physical therapists. The Rainville credo, now backed by numerous studies is that, counterintuitive as it sounds, pain does *not* equal tissue damage. In fact, by and large, exercise not only does not cause harm, it can decrease pain and improve function and mobility, even if you're older.[1, 2, 3, 4, 5, 6, 7]

"To date, there is no scientific evidence that activity and exercises are harmful, or that pain-inducing activity must be avoided," Rainville says.[8] Indeed, empirical evidence to the contrary suggests that activity and exercise that challenge physical impairments actually result in an improvement in chronic back pain. Even "aggressive" exercise—that's Rainville's word—does not raise the risk of more back problems in the future. To the contrary, current medical literature suggests that exercise has either a neutral effect or may slightly reduce risk of future back injuries.[9] In other words, people with chronic low back pain, he stressed, should get out and "exercise, run, ski [and] play sports as they desire."[10]

To be sure, this is not absolute. In acute situations, if you're having chest pain from a heart attack or angina, for instance, *that* pain *does* signal that there's probably damage to heart tissue from insufficient blood supply. So it's unwise to exercise if you think you're having a heart attack. (Call 911.) That said, with very few exceptions, exercise may be the single best thing you can do for the most common chronic non-cancer pain problems—arthritis, fibromyalgia, and chronic low back pain. Some studies show that exercise can reduce back pain between 10 and 60 percent, though other data suggest that's a bit optimistic.[11, 12, 13] No one knows exactly why exercise should help, but the leading theory is that it desensitizes a hyperactive nervous system.

In 2008, *Consumer Reports* magazine surveyed more than 14,000 subscribers who had had back pain the previous year and asked them what had helped the most. Exercise was the top-rated measure to help relieve back pain, the magazine announced in September 2011, with 58 percent of respondents adding that they wished they had done even more exercises.[14]

For many years, Rainville's group, including Childs and New England Baptist rehabilitation medicine physician Carol Hartigan, was one of the few teams willing to put to the test the idea that exercise might do more good than harm. The prevailing sentiment in the old days was that rest—weeks and weeks in bed, if necessary—was the safest and most effective treatment for pain. Today, the opposite view—"Rest is rust"—holds sway. Now, nurses get heart surgery patients up and walking as soon as possible. Hip replacement patients are dragged out of bed to walk, with help, in a day or two. Even cancer patients with numbing fatigue are now told to get up and move around. The new view, as Australian researchers put it in a 1999 paper, is that bed rest is not only unnecessary for low back pain but may actually increase disability.[15] A 2005 Cochrane Collaboration review nailed it down further: Randomized, controlled studies of people with low back pain show that those told to rest in bed have *more* pain than those told to stay active.[16]

To be sure, chronic pain usually hurts worse when you move, acknowledges Jennifer Schneider, author of *Living with Chronic Pain*. "So people don't move. They quit exercising," she told me.[17] A 2011 study by Australian and Dutch researchers who pooled data from 18 other studies documented this common, downward slide.[18] But the problem is, the less you exercise, the more deconditioned you get. So when you do have to move, it hurts even more. The only long-term solution is to keep your muscles strong, Schneider acknowledged to me, and she should know—she's not only a pain and addiction medicine specialist in Tucson, Arizona, but a longtime chronic pain patient herself.

The epidemiological evidence for exercise as a preventive measure is overwhelming: The more a person exercises, the less likely he or she is to wind up with back pain. In 1997, Danish researchers tracked 640 school children over 25 years and found that those who were physically active for at least three hours a week had a lower lifetime risk of back pain.[19] In 1998, Finnish researchers studied 498 adults and found that the fittest people had the lowest risk of back problems.[20] In 1999, British researchers studied 2,715 adults without back pain and found that it was not physical activity that increased the risk of low back pain later on—but poor health and being overweight.[21] And in a 2011 study of 46,533 adults, Norwegian researchers found that among young and middle-aged people, the prevalence of chronic pain was 10 to 12 percent lower for exercisers. The difference was even bigger—a whopping 21 to 38 percent—among women aged 65 or older and, with slightly less dramatic numbers, among older men, too.[22]

Yes, it's hard to work exercise into a busy schedule, especially if you don't feel well. But you shouldn't use busyness as an excuse. "When people say to me, 'I'm just too busy,' I will say to them respectfully, 'I'm really busy, too, but I fit it into my life because it's an absolute priority,'" says Carolyn Bernstein, a migraine patient herself and author of *The Migraine Brain*.[23] "If I don't get my exercise, I'm going to lose out on that piece of wellness." The point is to get yourself into as good shape as you possibly can. That won't get rid of migraines, she acknowledges. But it will make your body better able to handle them.[24]

I am living proof. Thanks largely to boot camp and a wonderful physical therapist, Susan Lattanzi in Watertown, MA, my neck pain today is virtually gone—knock on wood—even though my latest MRI showed the same damage as when my pain began. I'm back to competing in swim meets, going to the gym, kayaking—and putting on that toenail polish.

LOW BACK PAIN

While exercise is beneficial for many, if not most, kinds of chronic non-cancer pain, the most research has been done on three conditions—low back pain, arthritis, and fibromyalgia—and we'll take a closer look at all of them. The biggest of these is chronic low back pain, as the Institute of Medicine (IOM) noted in its 2011 report *Relieving*

Pain in America. It found that more than 28 percent of all people in chronic pain have pain in their lower backs; another 15 percent have pain in their necks.[25] While many episodes of back pain disappear in a month or so, for many other people, the problem becomes chronic. Not surprisingly, back pain is also one of the country's most expensive medical conditions. Spending on it grew from $7.9 billion in 1987 to $17.5 billion in 2000; low back pain contributed almost 3 percent to the total increase in national healthcare spending in that period. Estimates are even higher today—$30 billion. And the incidence is rising.

For the record, back pain can be devilishly tricky to diagnose because it can be caused by many different things—strained or spasming muscles, arthritis, degenerating discs in the spine, compressed spinal nerves, or herniated discs, to name but a few. (Herniated discs occur when there is a tear in the ring surrounding the discs that separate vertebrae; the tear allows the soft inner part of the disc to bulge out and secrete toxic, inflammatory chemicals and, in the worst case, even press on the spinal cord itself.) Even more confusing, people with severe back pain may not show serious structural problems on imaging scans. And many people with terrible scans report no pain at all. Doctors can't explain it. Understandably, people with chronic low back pain often avoid exercise out of fear, the specific fear that exercise, indeed any movement at all, will make their pain worse. This fear is known as kinesiophobia, and Rainville and others have tackled it head on.[26, 27, 28, 29]

Their findings have been fascinating. When the researchers analyzed the behavior of people with back pain, they found that the more fear people had about moving, the more pain they reported *during* activity.[30] But if people can be nudged to get over this fear—with some gentle coaching—surprising things happen. In a 1993 study, for instance, Rainville compared 42 disabled low back pain patients who stuck to an intensive reconditioning program and 30 with similar pain who dropped out. The people who hung in and completed the exercise program were those *who were able to change their beliefs.* In other words, they did a reality test of their fears and found that they could move around after all. Their functioning improved, even if the pain itself did not immediately improve.

In 2002, a Dutch trial of 1,572 people with low back pain similarly found that the people most likely to still be in pain six months later were the ones clinging most tightly to their fear of movement. Other studies agree.[31, 32, 33, 34] It's not easy, of course, to change such beliefs. But it can be done. In the late 1990s, Australian researchers spent $10 million on a three-year effort—on prime-time TV—to convince people with back pain not to fear physical activity. It worked. People with back pain, and doctors as well, changed their long-held beliefs, as gauged by pre- and postcampaign questionnaires.[35]

As for the evidence that exercise reduces chronic back pain? The data are so extensive that we can present only the highlights here. In 1992, Swedish researchers randomized 103 low back pain sufferers to a carefully graded exercise program or usual care. All were blue-collar workers on sick leave for disability. The people who got exercise training returned to work much faster than those who did not.[36] A 2000 study by Finnish scientists came to similar conclusions.[37] So did a 2004 Dutch review of data from 14 randomized controlled trials, a 2005 Swiss study, as well as a 2010 review of nine studies involving 1,520 people and a 2010 Dutch review of 61 studies involving 6,390 people.[38, 39, 40, 41] More recently, a 2011 Italian study of 261 people with chronic low back pain showed that those who stuck with a 12-month physical activity program wound up with significantly improved overall health, as well as significant pain improvement, compared to 310 similar patients who did not.[42]

So, the idea that exercise overall improves pain is settled science. The question then becomes: What kind of exercise helps most? This is a bit trickier. One answer, some research shows, is strength training, also called resistance training or weightlifting. A 2003 review by Irish researchers of 16 randomized controlled trials involving 1,730 people with chronic low back pain found that strength training is a particularly effective way to reduce pain.[43] On the other hand, a 2008 review found that, while lumbar strengthening exercise is more effective than no treatment, it may not be better than other exercise programs.[44] Other data show that a somewhat similar approach—exercises to boost lumbar stabilization—is moderately effective at improving pain and function, but isn't necessarily better than a general exercise program.[45]

Another question is how hard to exercise with chronic back pain. It turns out that intensity—exercising really hard, or, as researchers put it, doing "high-dose" exercise—is good. Researchers from Dalhousie University in Canada found that intensive exercise with stretching and strengthening is good for improving both pain and function. Ideally, they said, exercise sessions should last more than 20 minutes and be tailored to each individual.[46, 47]

So where does aerobic exercise like running or biking fit into pain rehab? It's not totally clear. In a 2011 study of Kosovo power plant workers, male and female, researchers found that people randomly assigned to high-intensity aerobic exercise (treadmill walking, stationary cycling, or stair climbing) wound up with significantly less pain, disability, and anxiety three months later than those assigned to some type of passive treatment such as ultrasound, heat, or electrical stimulation.[48] Aerobic exercise also has the added benefit of increased overall fitness.[49] On the other hand, Hong Kong researchers, in a different randomized trial, found that adding aerobic exercise to physiotherapy did not increase improvement of pain or disability in people with low back pain.[50]

People with chronic back pain often wonder whether they would get more relief from joining supervised exercise classes than from exercising alone at home. Some data, including a 1997 study of 74 women, all aged 57 with chronic low back pain, suggest that group exercise classes help people stick with the program better. They also take less sick leave and make less use of health services.[51] But a 2011 randomized study of 301 people came to more wishy-washy conclusions, as did a 2010 review of 42 studies involving 8,243 people with low back pain.[52, 53]

For what it's worth, I found the group setting at boot camp motivating in and of itself, and very reassuring because of the presence of physical therapists. Finally, if exercising in a gym seems too tough or not enough fun, there's always water therapy—exercising in a pool. There's considerable evidence that aquatic exercise can reduce low back pain.[54]

Increasingly, people with back pain are turning not just to traditional exercise but to yoga, the 4,000-year-old Indian practice that combines meditation and mindful breathing with specific poses (asanas) and movements. (Pilates, too, which also focuses on controlled movements, breathing and core strengthening, can reduce low back pain, according to a 2011 analysis of seven other studies.[55])

By some estimates, the number of Americans doing yoga has exploded from 4 million in 2001 to as many as 20 million in 2011.[56] Yoga is now one of the 10 most popular complementary and alternative approaches to health, a 2007 government survey showed.[57] But yoga cuts both ways.

While there's growing evidence that yoga can help significantly with low back pain, there's also increasing evidence of yoga-induced injuries.

First, the positive news. In a 2005 West Virginia University study, 42 people with chronic low back pain were randomized to yoga or an education program for 16 weeks. The yoga group had more reductions in pain intensity, functional disability, and use of pain medications.[58] Another West Virginia University study in 2009 came to similar conclusions.[59] A 2007 review of a wide variety of treatments for low back pain also found at least "fair" evidence that yoga can help.[60] Yoga research had a veritable banner year in 2011. In one 2011 randomized trial, British researchers compared yoga to usual care in 313 adults with chronic low back pain. The group doing 12 classes of yoga over three months had better back *function* at three, six, and 12 months later, although the two groups wound up with similar scores on back *pain*.[61]

In a 2011 American study, researchers from the Group Health Research Institute in Seattle randomized 228 adults with chronic low back pain to 12 once-a-week yoga classes, conventional stretching exercise, or a self-care book.[62] At the end of the study, the yoga group did better in terms of function and the "bothersomeness" of pain. But 15 percent of the yoga group, like 17 percent of the stretching group, suffered mild to moderate adverse effects, including, in one yoga case, a herniated disk. Only 2 percent of the self-care book group reported problems. In 2011, there were also reviews in which data from numerous studies were analyzed systematically. In one such review of seven randomized clinical trials, five showed clear reductions in pain for yoga compared to usual care in people with chronic low back pain.[63] Another 2011 review, this one involving 10 studies, showed similar results.[64] And in yet another 2011 review of 13 studies, Duke University researchers also found that yoga yielded improvements in pain, fatigue, and functional disability.[65] A meta-analysis in 2012 similarly found that yoga can be useful for many pain conditions, including low back pain.[66, 67]

But there are dangers to yoga as well, as *New York Times* science writer William J. Broad has documented.[68] In a January 2012 magazine piece, Broad quoted a prominent yoga teacher who has seen so many yoga injuries that he now thinks the vast majority of people should give up yoga because it's too likely to cause harm.[69] Citing studies from major medical journals, Broad noted that certain poses in particular—including those that overstretch the neck—can be dangerous.

The value of exercise for people in the throes of acute, as opposed to chronic, back pain is less clear. Dutch scientists writing in 1993 found that exercise did not help people in acute back pain.[70] A more recent Cochrane Collaboration review of 23 randomized controlled studies involving 3,676 workers also found that if a person has acute low back pain, exercise may not speed the return to work.[71] On the other hand, Norwegian researchers reported in 1999 that even with acute low back pain, people who exercise have fewer recurrences than those who don't.[72] And in 2001, Australian researchers found that with a first episode of acute low back pain, people who exercise are less likely than those who don't to have a recurrence a year later.[73]

For acute low back pain, then, the jury is still out. But for chronic pain, the verdict is in: Exercise helps. In fact, there is now so much evidence for the efficacy of exercise for low back pain that we as taxpayers should stop paying for more studies and focus instead on getting people moving. If we simply apply what we already know, wrote Eric L. Hurwitz, an epidemiologist at the University of Hawaii, in a 2011 commentary for *The Spine Journal*, we could prevent a substantial amount of chronic low back pain and reduce the public health burden, personal suffering, and the costs associated with all this misery.[74]

ARTHRITIS

Arthritis, which is a grab bag of more than 100 diseases, afflicts more than 50 million Americans today and by 2030, is expected to impact 67 million.[75] It comes in two major forms. Osteoarthritis, or wear-and-tear arthritis, is the most common, and is characterized by the breakdown of cartilage in the joints, which causes bones to rub against each other painfully. Rheumatoid arthritis is a systemic, inflammatory problem that can affect multiple organs but attacks the joints as well.[76] Not surprisingly, because both forms of arthritis are so painful, exercise is often the last thing that people want to do—especially if they have gained weight, as many do, because of inactivity. And for years, doctors didn't push it, either, assuming that exercise, especially high-intensity workouts like running or jogging, could be harmful.[77, 78] But that thinking has changed dramatically, thanks to a groundswell of studies showing that exercise—including exercise done in water—can be good medicine for arthritis.

Let's take the rheumatoid form first. One of the leaders in this field is Zuzana de Jong, a rheumatologist at Leiden University Medical Center in the Netherlands. Except in severe cases, her research shows, long-term, high intensity, weight-bearing exercise is both safe and effective for many people with rheumatoid arthritis.[79] A 2003 study by de Jong and colleagues involving 309 patients showed that those randomly assigned to an intensive exercise program called Rheumatoid Arthritis Patients in Training (RAPIT) wound up with significant improvements. The exercisers sweated their way through 75-minute strength and endurance training twice a week, and kept at it for an impressive two years. By and large, they did not suffer increased damage to joints, as gauged by X-rays, except for those who had a lot of damage in the large joints to begin with (a finding they confirmed in 2005).[80, 81] The exercisers also improved in cardiovascular fitness, an important finding because people with arthritis who remain inactive lose fitness.[82]

Equally important, a second 2003 study by the de Jong team showed that, contrary to what naysayers might think, people with rheumatoid arthritis not only can stick with an exercise program, they come to love it. In this study, the team looked at 146 people in the RAPIT program. By the end of the program, 81 percent were still attending classes and 78 percent said they would strongly recommend it to other rheumatoid arthritis patients.[83] Even more impressive, a follow-up 18 months later showed that the majority of patients in the original exercise group were *still* hard at it, exercising intensely, albeit a bit less frequently.[84] Their continued exercise preserved their gains in muscle strength without making their arthritis worse.

In a series of papers in 2004, the Dutch team again analyzed data from the RAPIT participants. In one study, they found that patients randomized to the intensive exercise program were able to slow down their rate of bone loss, a significant finding because people with rheumatoid arthritis are at greater than normal risk of osteoporosis and bone fractures.[85] In another study, they found that two years of intensive, weight-bearing exercise did not cause progression of joint damage in the *small* joints of the hands and feet and might even protect the joints in the feet.[86] A 2009 study by a different team from Leiden University reviewed eight studies and concluded that both aerobic exercise and strength training can improve pain and physical function without causing damage.[87] Similarly, in 2010, a French team analyzed 14 randomized controlled trials involving 1,040 people and found that aerobic training is safe, reduces pain, and improves overall quality of life in people with rheumatoid arthritis, a finding confirmed by other researchers in 2011.[88, 89]

Exercise helps people with osteoarthritis, too. As with low back pain, osteoarthritis pain responds well to exercising in water.[90, 91, 92] But you don't have to splash around to get better—dry land exercise also reduces osteoarthritis pain. A North Carolina study of aerobic exercise and strength training in people aged 60 or more with knee osteoarthritis (the FAST trial) showed that either type of exercise yields improvements in both pain and disability—strong enough results to recommend that exercise be prescribed as a regular part of treatment.[93]

A different team of North Carolina researchers found in the so-called ADAPT trial that for overweight or obese people over 60 with knee osteoarthritis, a combination of modest weight loss plus moderate exercise yielded more improvement in pain and function than either intervention alone.[94] But you do have to stick with it to maintain improvements from exercise. A 2010 Dutch study of people with knee or hip osteoarthritis found that, after five years of follow-up, the people who kept exercising had less pain and better functioning than people who did not.[95]

FIBROMYALGIA

Fibromyalgia, once dismissed as psychogenic, is increasingly recognized as a complex medical disorder with biological and psychological components. It is characterized by chronic, widespread musculoskeletal pain, allodynia (increased pain with simple touch or pressure), and "tender points" on at least 11 out of 18 defined spots on the body, according to the International Association for the Study of Pain.[96, 97] It is believed to be caused in part by changes in pain sensitivity in the central nervous system. Like low back pain and arthritis, fibromyalgia is common, with more than 5 million sufferers in the United States alone and 200 million worldwide.[98, 99] For unclear reasons, it affects vastly more women than men.[100] People with fibromyalgia often have insomnia, fatigue, anxiety, depression, gastrointestinal symptoms, and headaches.

Curiously, these symptoms occur without any obvious inflammation or damage to tissues, although researchers at McGill University have documented anatomical changes in the brain in fibromyalgia patients—a kind of accelerated aging process, though whether these changes are the cause or the effect of fibromyalgia is unclear.[101, 102] There are some remedies that doctors can offer, including antidepressants, drugs such as Neurontin (gabapentin) and Lyrica (pregabalin), stress management, and cognitive-behavior therapy. But of all the things that can help, exercise is particularly crucial, according to Don Goldenberg, chief of rheumatology at Newton-Wellesley Hospital in Massachusetts and a leading fibromyalgia researcher. "Exercise is one of the best things, perhaps even the best thing" a person with fibromyalgia can do to decrease pain, improve mood, and function and restore quality of life, Goldenberg emphasized to me.[103]

It's not clear exactly *why* exercise helps so much, but researchers think that it may work by reducing inflammation, a major contributor to fibromyalgia pain.[104] To be sure, people with fibromyalgia often feel too lousy to hit the gym,[105] and it can be tough to convince a person with fibromyalgia to begin regular exercise.[106] But it pays off.[107] In a randomized, 16-week study from Brazil, for instance, both patients who were assigned to a walking program and those who were assigned to muscle-strengthening exercises fared much better than the folks in the control group, who did nothing. By the end of the study, 80 percent of the control group was still taking pain medication, compared to 47 percent in the walking group and 41 percent in the strengthening group.[108] Even for people who are couch potatoes to begin with, doing some form of physical activity at least 30 minutes a day for five to seven days a week yields significant results: fewer deficits in function and less pain, according to researchers from Johns Hopkins University.[109] And you can accumulate these exercise minutes in short bursts—they don't have to be done all at once.

Of the various types of exercise that help people with fibromyalgia, aerobic exercise is one of the most effective. In a 2006 review of

46 studies involving 3,035 fibromyalgia patients, researchers at Oregon Health and Sciences University found that the strongest evidence was in support of aerobic exercise.[110] It doesn't have to be at killer levels of intensity, the Oregon team added. The pain and fatigue of fibromyalgia get better with even low- to moderate-intensity exercise.

Researchers from the University of Saskatchewan reviewed 34 studies on exercise and fibromyalgia in 2006 for the Cochrane Library and again in 2008 for the *Journal of Rheumatology*.[111, 112] They, too, found solid evidence for aerobic exercise—this time, at the more intense levels recommended by the American College of Sports Medicine. Aerobic exercise not only improves cardiorespiratory fitness but reduces pain at numerous tender "pressure points," they found.[113] Ideally, this aerobic exercise should be done two or three times a week.[114] The evidence for aerobic exercise in people with fibromyalgia is so convincing that guidelines of both the American Pain Society and the Association of the Scientific Medical Societies in Germany now give it their strongest recommendation.[115] And you don't have to hit the treadmill. In 2006, Spanish researchers found that exercise in warm, waist-high water relieved pain and improved health-related quality of life in women with fibromyalgia.[116] In 2009, Swedish researchers came to similar conclusions.[117] So did German researchers, who pooled data from 10 randomized, controlled trials involving 1,446 people.[118]

And then there's tai chi, one of the gentlest exercise programs in the world. Tai chi is an ancient Chinese mind–body practice that began as a martial art. It combines slow, gentle, graceful movements with deep breathing and relaxation.[119, 120] Like yoga, tai chi has been growing in popularity.[121] Although it has not been studied as much as yoga for chronic pain relief, tai chi does appear to be a promising approach for people with osteoarthritis, rheumatoid arthritis, low back pain, and fibromyalgia, says Peter Wayne, research director of the Osher Center for Integrative Medicine at Harvard Medical School.[122]

A small, pilot study in 2003 from Savannah, Georgia, showed that people with fibromyalgia who participated in twice-weekly tai chi classes for six weeks improved their scores significantly on a widely used test, the Fibromyalgia Impact Questionnaire.[123]

But the clincher was a well-designed, randomized, 12-week Boston study published in 2010 in the *New England Journal of Medicine*.[124]

Led by researchers from Tufts University, Boston University, and Newton-Wellesley Hospital, the study randomly assigned 66 people with fibromyalgia to either twice-weekly group tai chi lessons or a control group, which got twice-weekly wellness education and stretching. The tai chi group, whose classes were taught by a tai chi master with 20 years of experience, showed clinically significant improvements, not just in pain, but also in mood, quality of life, and sleep. The effects were still present six months later. These results are striking, applauded three specialists who wrote an editorial in the *Journal* accompanying the tai chi study.[125]

INSPIRATION FOR COUCH POTATOES: HOW SWIMMING SAVED SUSAN HELMRICH

I met Susan Helmrich, 55, a swimmer, PhD epidemiologist, wife and mother, licensed wellness coach, and three-time cancer survivor in April 2011 in Mesa, Arizona. We were choking down a pitiful pre-race breakfast of soggy bagels and little packets of jelly, packing in the calories for that day's events at the US Masters Swimming Nationals, where we were both competing. I did respectably. Susan was amazing. She came in second in her age group in the 1,650-yard freestyle (the meet's longest event), finished third in the 500-yard freestyle, and placed honorably in a handful of other events.[126]

Susan was just 20 months out of the hospital following one of modern medicine's most gruesome operations—a Whipple procedure, which is basically a partial evisceration in which surgeons removed the head of her pancreas, a portion of the bile duct, the gallbladder, and the duodenum. The goal of that operation was to get rid of the neuroendocrine pancreatic cancer with which Susan had been diagnosed. She had already lost the superior lobe of her right lung to cancer and, 34 years earlier, as a newly minted college grad, had lost her vagina and her entire reproductive system to a rare cancer caused by diethylstilbestrol (DES), the treacherous drug many women, including Susan's mother, were given during pregnancy to prevent miscarriage. Susan's hero, to this day, is Dr. Albert Herbst, the lead author of a groundbreaking article in the April 22, 1971, issue of the *New England Journal of Medicine* that, for the first time, linked rare vaginal cancers in young women to the

DES their mothers took during pregnancy.[127] Susan eventually sued the drug maker, Eli Lilly, and won a modest settlement.

After her DES experience, she was determined, as she put it, "to prevent drug disasters like this from ever happening again."[128] So she went to graduate school, earning a master's in epidemiology from the Harvard School of Public Health and a PhD in epidemiology from the University of California, Berkeley. But it wasn't even Susan's battles with cancer that impressed me most during our days in Arizona. It was that Susan was swimming her heart out despite severe, chronic pain from sciatica—pain in the lower back and leg caused by compression of or damage to spinal nerves.

Over breakfast, she had told me matter-of-factly, her pain right at that moment was a 6 on a scale of 10, which she said was normal for her. "It's unbelievable," she says, trying to describe it. "It's shooting pain, burning, it goes down to my foot. It's unbearable." She had never had sciatica before her Whipple. Nobody knows for sure what happened, but she thinks the surgeons either nicked a spinal nerve or somehow placed her in an awkward position that damaged the nerve during the surgery. She can't take opioid drugs for the pain because they cause constipation, and constipation would be a serious problem for her because she's already missing part of her colon. (Surgeons used her colon tissue to construct a new vagina to replace the one they removed because of the vaginal cancer.) She can't take nonsteroidal anti-inflammatory drugs (NSAIDs), either, because they are too irritating to what's left of her digestive system.

"Swimming is the only thing that makes me feel better," she told me. "It's the only time I'm not in pain. It's being horizontal and being weightless. There's no pressure on my nerve. I really think exercise has saved my life three times."

The first time was during her first surgery for vaginal cancer. She had swum on the boys' team in high school—this was in the old days, before Title IX fully kicked in—and, as a 21-year-old Syracuse University graduate, was super fit, coming off the best athletic year of her life. In fact, it was probably because she was in such great shape that she was able to withstand the 10½-hour surgery. Swimming probably saved her life again after the surgery at age 42, for her lung cancer. Knowing that she lived for swimming and needed all the lung power she could get, surgeons initially removed just the tumor. But they didn't get clean margins, so she had to go back and have the whole superior left lobe removed. Once again, she bounced back fast, getting back in the pool as soon as possible. "No one can believe it," she grinned as she told me, "but I can do laps without a breath." (I can't, and I have two lungs.)

Today, 34 years after her first cancer, without a lung, without all the innards that most people have, she swims. And swims and swims—almost three miles almost every day. No longer a full-time epidemiologist, she passes on her expertise about living with pain and illness as a wellness coach. Her message is simple: "I would be dead without exercise."

CHAPTER 14

The Way Forward

PAIN CARE: A FUNDAMENTAL HUMAN RIGHT

As a journalist for nearly 40 years now, I have watched with awe and admiration as people with AIDS, people with breast cancer, people with disabilities slowly awakened from their silence and their isolation. I have stood, notebook in hand, as sick men and women—once faceless statistics—took to the streets, to arcane scientific conferences, and to the bustling halls of Congress to make people pause and hear their stories. To insist that their humanity be taken seriously.

I have seen haggard men help hang AIDS quilts in cities around the world to remind the still-lucky, the still-healthy, that behind all the statistics were people with lives worth valuing. I have seen tired women walk miles to raise money for breast cancer, some still wearing the headscarves from chemotherapy that became their personal badges of courage, some carrying pictures of friends and sisters and mothers and daughters who had lost their lives to the disease.

It is time now for people in chronic pain to shed *their* stigma and *their* hopelessness. They—we—too, can stand up to legislators and demand serious money for pain research. They—we—too, can insist that medical schools teach pain. They—we—too, can insist on seeing doctors who believe them.

Fixing the chronic pain crisis in America is, as the Institute of Medicine so aptly acknowledged, nothing short of a "moral imperative."[1] For one academic year a while ago, I was a fellow in medical ethics at Harvard Medical School. I learned that in medical ethics, there are four basic principles: beneficence, nonmaleficence, autonomy, and justice.

The failure to treat chronic pain violates all four.[2] Treating pain well is an example of *beneficence*, or doing good, which means the failure to do so violates this principle. Failure to relieve pain also causes harm, a violation of the second principle, *nonmaleficence* ("doing no harm"). Untreated pain can also destroy a person's right to and capacity for self-determination, thus, to some extent, violating the third principle, *autonomy*. Failure to treat pain also violates the fourth principle, *justice*. It is unfair to ignore the humanitarian and financial costs of undertreated pain.

Better pain management is already beginning to be viewed as a fundamental human right. In 2010, delegates to the International Association for the Study of Pain conference in Montreal issued a declaration stating just that.[3] Once pain management is truly viewed as a fundamental right, failure to provide it can become grounds for lawsuits under negligence law, criminal law, and elder abuse, as well as grounds for professional misconduct, as three leading pain physicians—Frank Brennan, Daniel Carr, and Michael Cousins—argued in an influential 2007 paper.[4]

There have already been some lawsuits. In 2001, a California physician was successfully sued under the state's elder-abuse statute for not providing adequate pain treatment to an 85-year-old dying patient (*Bergman v. Chin*). The patient's family was awarded $1.5 million.[5] Two years later, another physician was successfully sued for inadequate pain management (*Tomlinson v. Bayberry Care Center*).[6]

The right to adequate pain management is also implicitly built into an explicit right—the right to the highest obtainable level of physical and mental health. This right is formally codified in the International Covenant of Economic, Social and Cultural Rights, which was enacted in the 1960s and went into effect on January 3, 1976.[7]

A number of countries have approved this covenant, though the United States has not, in part because of a longstanding American aversion to signing international agreements. (President Jimmy Carter did sign the covenant in October 1977, but Congress never ratified it.) Under the covenant, countries must ensure that all their people have access to essential medications, as defined by the World Health

Organization (WHO). Since 1977, the WHO list of such medicines has included morphine. Even today, however, access to morphine is extremely limited or completely nonexistent in many parts of the world.

IS FAILURE TO TREAT PAIN "TORTURE BY OMISSION"?

There's an even more powerful argument for better pain care: that failure to adequately address pain borders on "torture by omission."[8] Two international treaties—the International Covenant on Civil and Political Rights and the "Torture Convention" (Convention Against Torture and Other Cruel, Inhuman or Degrading Treatment or Punishment)— both of which the United States *has* ratified (in 1992 and 1994, respectively), address this issue, at least implicitly. Both conventions condemn torture per se, which is defined as intentionally causing severe suffering with a specific objective such as to get a confession or information. The conventions also condemn cruel, inhuman, and degrading treatment, without regard to intention or motive.

This implies that countries have an *obligation* to protect people from torture and cruel treatment, said Diederik Lohman, a senior researcher in the health and human rights division of Human Rights Watch, an international, independent organization. "When people are experiencing severe suffering from treatable pain because doctors don't have access to inexpensive medications—morphine costs only pennies per dose—or have never been taught how to use the medications, at that point, you may be able to say that the country is failing to protect patients with pain from preventable suffering," he said.[9]

In February 2013, a United Nations report specifically declared that certain forms of abuse in healthcare settings "may cross a threshold of mistreatment that is tantamount to torture or cruel, inhuman or degrading treatment or punishment."[10] Specifically, the UN report said that countries' drug control laws should recognize the "indispensible [*sic*] nature of narcotic and psychotropic drugs for the relief of pain and suffering" and that countries should review national laws and administrative procedures "to guarantee adequate availability of those medicines for legitimate medical uses."

Kathleen Foley, a leading pain control activist and neurologist at Memorial Sloan-Kettering Cancer Center in New York, puts it more bluntly: Inadequate pain care constitutes "cruel, degrading and inhuman treatment. It is thus torture by omission."[11, 12, 13]

WHY IS THERE NO INSTITUTE ON PAIN AT THE NATIONAL INSTITUTES OF HEALTH?

When the Institute of Medicine, at the request of Congress, convened its blue-ribbon committee to assess chronic pain in America, I learned that there was one thing the committee was told it could *not* do—the one thing that might have made the most sense: recommend that Congress authorize the creation of an Institute on Pain at the National Institutes of Health.

As a practical and political matter, if there is no NIH institute dedicated to a particular disease, that disease is essentially disenfranchised. It is an orphan, nobody's responsibility. Officially, lack of money was cited as the reason for not allowing the IOM to recommend a pain institute. And that's valid, to a point. Setting up an institute on pain at NIH would mean taking money away from someplace else. Which means asking, explained John Loeser, a neurosurgeon at the University of Washington, "What are we going to un-fund to do something about the abysmal world of pain sufferers?"[14] Not a political hot potato that anyone wants to touch.

But the money excuse is getting weaker as the economy grows stronger. Since the IOM committee was convened, at least one new center (a *center* is one bureaucratic notch below an institute) *has* been set up at NIH, financial crisis or no financial crisis. This suggests that the biggest barrier to a more robust federal commitment to better pain management is not lack of money, but lack of political will. And the political will *could* be there, if people with chronic pain forced the issue: One hundred million Americans in chronic pain is a *lot* of people, a *lot* of votes, and a *lot* of potential pressure on Congress.

Absent a real pain institute, or even a "center," what we are left with are two small government entities, and both are weak. One is the new Inter-agency Pain Research Coordinating Committee (IPRCC), which was mandated as part of the Affordable Care Act (often called

"Obamacare") in 2010.[15] It has had a slow start. In July 2010, Kathleen Sebelius, the secretary of the Department of Health and Human Services, signed the charter establishing the committee. In the fall of 2010, the NIH posted a notice in the *Federal Register* calling for nominations to the committee. But it was not until February 2012 that the members of the committee, to be chaired by Story Landis, director of the National Institute of Neurological Disorders and Stroke, were announced.[16]

The members—pain experts—come from disparate agencies within the government including, the Veterans Administration, the Department of Defense, the US Food and Drug Administration, the National Institute of Dental and Craniofacial Research (part of NIH), the Centers for Disease Control and Prevention, the Agency for Healthcare Research and Quality, and the military.[17, 18, 19, 20] Six outside pain researchers and six people from advocacy groups were also appointed to the committee.

But the committee doesn't have much of a budget, and no line item— just enough money to pay travel expenses for committee members.[21] Worse, the law requires only that the committee meet at least once a year. And the secretary of HHS, by law, has to review "the necessity of the Committee" only once every two years.[22] Theoretically, the minute this committee's existence is deemed unnecessary, this effort, minimal as it is, disappears.

The other federal entity is the Pain Consortium, a group of the directors who head five NIH institutes. It, too, is chaired by Story Landis. But again, there is no significant budget or staff.

In other words, despite the Institute of Medicine report, the government is still doing almost nothing to address the chronic pain crisis. Which means it will be up to advocacy groups such as the Pain Action Alliance to Implement a National Strategy (PAAINS) to push the government to do what it should.[23]

REQUIRING MEDICAL SCHOOLS TO TEACH PAIN

Beyond the moral and political issues, medical schools should teach pain simply because patients need doctors to understand it. Nine hours of pain education, on average, over four years of medical school is obviously not enough for a problem that afflicts 100 million Americans, some severely. But medical education, as we've seen, is still largely a feudal system. To introduce significant pain education would mean that some entrenched professors would have to start teaching pain themselves or cede class time so other professors could.

One way to force medical schools to teach pain would be to test graduating medical graduates on their knowledge of pain. Those who flunk simply wouldn't get a license to practice medicine. "If you test for it, that will force medical schools to teach it," says Scott Fishman, an anesthesiologist who heads the division of pain medicine at the University of California, Davis.[24]

Meaningful testing would involve putting detailed questions about chronic pain and pain management on the licensing and certification exams that graduating medical students take.[25] This is a momentous task, but easier than it once would have been. Since 1992, there has been one national medical exam for MDs, the United States Medical Licensing Examination, and the Common Osteopathic Medical Licensing Examination (COMPLEX) for osteopaths. (This replaced different exams in different states.)[26] Beefing up these two exams is a lot easier than it would have been under the state-by-state system.

Some efforts are underway to do this, according to Lisa Robin, who heads governmental relations for the Federation of State Medical Boards, the group that administers the exam in partnership with the National Board of Medical Examiners. (A separate organization writes the exam for osteopathic doctors.)

But in revamping medical education, it will be important not just to teach more neurobiology, but the whole biopsychosocial process of pain. "Pain is a different type of topic than other medical topics," says Daniel Carr, an anesthesiologist who heads the Program in Pain Research, Education & Policy at Tufts University.[27] "If you jam four hours of pain into an already-jammed curriculum and just focus on biology, all you do is indoctrinate medical students into the same, old intellectualized world of ions and receptors," said Carr. And that would take students further away from the emotional, messy environment of pain. "That's like trying to get your head around the meaning of a cathedral by studying bricks," he said. Young doctors have to be taught to be "more comfortable dealing with the emotional distress and chaos of pain."

I'd go even further. I am convinced that it's impossible to understand intense pain until you've felt it yourself. Precisely because pain is so subjective and triggers such strong emotions, I think medical schools should follow the Johns Hopkins model of subjecting students to brief, experimental pain in the lab and getting them to process their emotional and physical responses.

Another way to get medical schools to do a better job of teaching pain is to work through the Liaison Committee on Medical Education,[28] the group that sets academic standards and accredits medical schools. This committee doesn't tell medical schools exactly what or how to teach, but it can insist on standards for what medical students should learn. The committee, ultimately, wields a big stick: withdrawing accreditation.

The same applies to the Accreditation Council for Graduate Medical Education, the group that accredits the postgraduate (three-year residency) programs that young physicians must participate in.[29] It also applies to the Accreditation Council for Continuing Medical Education, which accredits the refresher courses that practicing physicians must take in order to keep their licenses current and maintain specialty certification.[30]

In other words, we could use the power of tests, licensing, and accreditation to compel the medical education system to do better. We can also use publicity to highlight programs that *are* doing a good job, including the 12 schools named in 2012 by NIH as "centers of excellence" and "hubs" for the development, evaluation, and distribution of pain management curricula.[31]

Hospitals, too, can do more, though they're doing better than they used to. In 2001, the Joint Commission on Accreditation of Healthcare Organizations, now known as the Joint Commission, established standards for pain management in the roughly 4,400 hospitals it oversees.[32] (In addition to hospitals, the Joint Commission accredits ambulatory care centers, long-term care facilities and other healthcare organizations.) Without accreditation, a hospital can lose federal Medicare and Medicaid funds, which would be financially ruinous. The Joint Commission standards say that hospitals have an obligation to assess and manage a patient's pain. If a hospital does not comply on pain as well as a number of other standards, the Joint Commission can take away accreditation.

Unfortunately, there are no good data on whether the Joint Commission's pain standards have made a difference.[33] To compel the government and medical schools to do a better job with pain will require, as the IOM report noted, a true "cultural transformation in the way pain is viewed and treated."[34] That will be hard, but not impossible.

MOVING ON

Not long ago, I spoke with a young Massachusetts man, Andrew Chatzky, whose chronic headaches ultimately prompted him to join a pain support group, the first time in his life he had ever done such a thing. Upon joining the group, the leader asked what he hoped to get out of it. "Just one and a half hours a month where I don't have to hide that I am in pain," he told me.[35]

That doesn't seem like much. But to him and other people in severe, chronic pain, even just a few hours being with other people who understand chronic pain can help.

Ultimately, for people who live with chronic pain, the goal is to live life as fully as possible despite the pain. This means many things.

It means exercise. It means using opioids and other powerful drugs if you need them, and using them responsibly. It means getting whatever mental health support you need, not because emotions are causing your pain but because emotional distress is *part* of pain.

It probably means putting together your own program of healing—integrating the best of Western *and* complementary medicine. Some hospitals and pain clinics integrate all this for patients, but many do not, which means you may have to do it yourself. But think of it this way: If you find five things that each help a little, with luck you may make a significant dent in your pain.

Most profoundly, living fully despite chronic pain may mean acceptance: That chronic pain may be something you have to deal with every day. That you may never find the underlying reason for the pain, or the perfect cure. That you may have to make big adjustments in your life—doing what you still can and letting go of the rest.

That is not easy, obviously. But isn't that, basically, what life is all about?

ACKNOWLEDGMENTS

This book began to feel real after my very first phone call to my agent, Jim Levine of Levine Greenberg, gathered steam thanks to my dear friend, anthropologist/author Sally Merry, who guided me to Oxford University Press, and came to miraculous fruition thanks to my terrific Oxford editor, Abby Gross, and her energetic team.

Neuroscientist Cathy Bushnell, formerly at McGill University, now at the National Institutes of Health, and Kathy Kreiter get the credit for involving the International Association for the Study of Pain (IASP) as a co-publisher. The first Cathy was also "kind" enough to let her graduate student, at my request, subject me to pain tests in her lab to see how long I could keep my hand in ice water without screaming. IASP editor-in-chief Maria Adele Giamberardino coordinated the expert—and remarkably speedy—scientific vetting of all my chapters.

My semi-voluntary team of readers heroically read and commented chapter by chapter on early versions of the book. They include Alice Dungan Bouvrie, my swimming buddy who also distracted me regularly with good food and wine; Nils Bruzelius, my wonderful former science editor at the *Boston Globe*; Elaine Kaplan Dolph, my sister-in-law, who actually read the exercise chapter twice; University of Wisconsin pain policy analyst Aaron Gilson; Carey Goldberg, Globe friend, now WBUR/ Commonhealth blog cohost and science writer par excellence; Diane Kaplan, my perceptive step-daughter; Christina Spellman, head of the Mayday Fund; and Cindy Steinberg, a most inspiring patient advocate. In a class by herself is Pat McCaffrey, an MIT-trained biologist who co-runs Harvard's Pain Research Forum and who may have both a broader and a deeper understanding of pain than anyone in the world. She fact-checked every word, in record time.

Two other people in particular kept me sane and on track. One is my ever-patient research assistant, Amanda Paolitto, who must have said, "Just hit 'edit undo'" a hundred times. It is to her credit that my thousands of endnotes are formatted right and correlate to the proper places in the text. The other is Victor Salvucci, my unflappable computer guru who responded to my distress calls days, nights, and weekends. My webmeister Steve Bennett was also invaluable and creative, as was my nephew-in-law, Andy Dolph, who helped me make the audio/video talk that goes with this book.

A special thanks, too, to Stew Leavitt, the tireless PhD science writer who puts out the beautifully written, meticulously fair, weekly newsletter *Pain Treatment Topics*.

During the five years that I worked on this book, I interviewed more than 200 scientists, physicians, lawyers, and policy analysts either in person or by phone—many of them, poor souls, over and over again. I also badgered them frequently with endless "Did-I-get-this-right?" emails.

I thank them all, of course, but a few in particular became heroes to me. One is June Dahl, another is Kathy Foley, and another, Myra Christopher. June Dahl, a neuroscientist-pharmacologist at the University of Wisconsin, is a charming, white-haired lady—and "lady" is the perfect word—who works 24/7 and answered my endless emails with even more endless essays. She has slogged away for three decades trying to fix the state and federal laws and regulations that govern opioids and probably knows more than anyone about how these drugs both help and hurt. If I were president of the United States, I'd put her in charge of this whole mess—and, even at 82, she'd probably take the job.

Kathy Foley, an attending neurologist at Memorial-Sloan Cancer Center in New York, has long been *the* leading voice in palliative care in this country and abroad. She has enormous political courage. In a calm, soft-spoken voice, dressed in her pearls and dignified suits, her blond hair perfectly coiffed, she stands up time and again in front of skeptical audiences and says what most pain doctors won't admit: that failure to treat pain better, when the wherewithal to do so exists, is nothing less than torture.

Myra Christopher, a friendly, Midwestern people magnet who could network in her sleep, is a bioethicist at the Center for Practical Bioethics in Kansas City and was a member of the Institute of Medicine committee that wrote the blockbuster report on chronic pain in 2011. Since then, she has assigned herself the unenviable task of professional nudge, forming a small army of activists called PAAINS trying, despite formidable odds, to turn the IOM recommendations into reality.

As a longtime health columnist for the *Boston Globe*, I have turned to Dan Carr, a Tufts University anesthesiologist and another hero, as my go-to source for decades for clear, quick ("Help! I'm on deadline!") information on pain. Dan is a deeply caring man who's always too busy to explain things but does so anyway. Perry Fine, a University of Utah anesthesiologist, is also one of the most caring physicians I have ever met and has saved the lives of countless, suicidal pain patients with judicious use of opioids. His Utah colleagues Dick Chapman, David Bradshaw, and Lynn Webster were also very helpful.

Jeff Mogil, a McGill pain geneticist, is not only brilliant but incredibly organized, feeding me links to important papers mere minutes after I asked and tirelessly fact-checking my successive attempts to portray pain genetics accurately. He is a science writer's dream.

Joe Martin, the former dean of Harvard Medical School, was encouraging from the outset. John Loeser, a University of Washington neurosurgeon, guided me patiently by phone as I tried to visualize the intricacies of neurosurgery. Scott Fishman, a University of California, Davis neuroscientist sent me such a nice email after reviewing one of my chapters that I taped it to my bookcase. Cliff Woolf, a pain geneticist at Children's Hospital in Boston, was also repeatedly helpful and encouraging.

Vania Apkarian, Dan Barth, Mark Blumenthal, David Boorsook, Tim Brennan, Gary Brenner, Roger Chou, James Cleary, Mark Cooper, Ron Dubner, Kenneth Craig, John Kusiak, Lisa Loram, Michael Moskowitz, Anne Z. Murphy, Mary O'Connor, Phillip Pizzo, Donald Price, Kenneth Prkachin and Petra Schweinhardt, and Irene Tracey also spent more time with me than they really had. So did Inna Belfer, Fernando Cervero, Luda Diatchenko, Deb Gordon, Jerome Groopman, Ru-Rong Ji, William Maixner, Anne Louise Oaklander, Yoram Shir, Kathleen Sluka, Roland Staud, Larry Tabak, Steve Waxman, Julie Wieseler, and Hubert Yin.

If I remained befuddled by the devilishly complicated overlap of gender, hormones, and pain, it was not because Karen Berkley,

Roger Fillingim, Michael S. Gold, Joel Greenspan, Frank Keefe, Linda LeResche, Jon Levine, and Richard Traub didn't do their best to teach me.

Charles Berde, Celeste Johnston, Neil Schechter, and Lonnie Zeltzer pored over piles of heartbreaking research on undertreatment of children's pain with me. I can never give enough thanks to Jill Lawson, the mother of little Jeffrey Lawson, the baby who died after heart surgery without anesthesia, for the hours she spent with me reliving those awful days.

I loved the interviews I had with researchers for the chapter on the mind–body in pain. Sean Mackey was just plain cool, sharing his excitement about neurofeedback. Sara Lazar inspired me with her work on meditation for pain. Ajay Wasan was a goldmine of information on pain and depression, as was Kurt Kroenke. Ted Kaptchuk was, as always, the undisputed master of placebo effects in pain. Penney Cowan, Rob Edwards, Tim Gard, Randy Gollub, Bob Jamison, Mark Jensen, Marco Loggia, Stephen Morley, David Patterson, and Russ Portenoy were also extremely generous with their time.

Navigating my way through the opioid mess was the toughest part of this book. I am grateful to Andrew Kolody for taking the time to talk to me repeatedly, even though we disagreed. I'm also grateful for my conversations with Mark Collen, Carol Garner, Howard Heit, Diane Hoffman, Janice Kauffman, David Ropeik, Robert Twillman, and Michael Von Korff.

Neuroscientist Linda Watkins was the first researcher to let me spend days in her lab with her postdocs and their little white rats—an invaluable introduction into how immune (glial) immune cells ramp up pain. Doug Fields was also hugely helpful on this, as were Joyce De Leo and Michael Costigan.

The mysteries of marijuana chemistry and policy came into focus for me thanks to Don Abrams, J. Hampton Atkinson, Mark Blumenthal, Lyle Craker, Michael Cutler, Rick Doblin, Steven Gust, Raphael Mechoulam, Edgar Alfonso Romero-Sandoval, Ethan Russo, Mark Ware, and numerous patients, including Marcy Duda and Beth McCauley.

Spine surgeon Stephen Parazin was a wonderful explainer and fact-checker, despite a daunting travel schedule. Alvaro Pascual-Leone, to whom I've turned for years to explain transcranial magnetic stimulation, came through once again. Gary Bennett awed me with his knowledge of chemotherapy-induced pain. Conversations with Allan Basbaum, Steven P. Cohen, Charles Serhan, Min Zhou, and Mark Zylka were also exciting and helpful.

I'm also grateful to Joanne Gaffney, Scott Haldeman, Mike Holick, Vitaly Napadow, John Pereira, Pamela Pettinati, Bruce Pomeranz, and Peter Wayne for their insights into alternative pain treatments. And to Diederik Lohman and Lisa Robin for explaining aspects of international law and regulatory policies.

Jim Rainville not only let me, as a patient with a very bad neck, into his famous "boot camp," but cheerfully pointed me to a treasure trove of scientific papers on exercise for pain control. Carolyn Bernstein and Don Goldenberg, also strong believers in exercise, not only pointed me to research, but have taken good care of the people I referred to them.

Even more important, of course, are the pain patients, whose stories still haunt and inspire me. Hyrum Neizer, the truck driver with excruciating headaches who nearly committed suicide. Pam Costa, the awesome psychologist in constant pain because of a genetic mutation. The Blocker family, whose daughter, Ashlyn, is endangered because her genetic mutation means she never feels pain. Paul Konowitz, the ear, nose, and throat surgeon, who struggled with opioid dependence during his battle with chronic pain. And I'll never forget Tom Fersch, the director of sales for the New York Mets who was dying of cancer in considerable pain, nor the inspirational Susan Helmrich, who has swum her way to a wonderful life despite three types of cancer and chronic pain.

My own healers, physical therapists Susan Lattanzi and Lisa Childs, neurologist Deepak Tandon and his team at New England Baptist Hospital, and acupuncturist Jen Evans, were phenomenal.

Most of all, I can never properly thank my son, Mike Fowler, my daughter-in-law, Robin Just, and my grandsons, Owen and Hugo, for all their support and love.

But the absolute best is my husband, my biggest supporter and my best friend, Ken Kaplan. A psychiatrist who had been teaching mindfulness mediation for pain relief long before I even met him, Ken is the most compassionate person I have ever known. I am incredibly lucky to have him in my life.

Resources for Chronic Pain Patients

American Academy of Medical Acupuncture
American Academy of Pain Medicine
American Cancer Society
American Chiropractic Association
American Chronic Pain Association
American Osteopathic Association
American Physical Therapy Association (please go to http://www.moveforwardpt.com/Default.aspx)
Arthritis Foundation
CancerCare
National Center for Complementary and Alternative Medicine
National Fibromyalgia and Chronic Pain Association
National Hospice Foundation
National Vulvodynia Association
Pain Research Forum
Pain Treatment Topics newsletter (http://pain-topics.org)
US Pain Foundation

NOTES

CHAPTER 1

1. Institute of Medicine, Committee on Advancing Pain Research, Care, and Education. (2011). *Relieving pain in America: A blueprint for transforming prevention, care, education and research* (pp. 2–6). Prepublication copy. Washington, DC: National Academies Press.
2. Census Bureau Call Center (personal communication, September 23, 2011).
3. Tsang, A., Von Korff, M., Lee, S., Alonso, J., Karam, E., Angermeyer, M. C., et al. (2008). Common chronic pain conditions in developed and developing countries: Gender and age differences and comorbidity with depression-anxiety disorders. *The Journal of Pain, 9*(10), 883–891.
4. Brown, A. (2012, April 7). Chronic pain rates shoot up until Americans reach late 50s. Retrieved from http://www.gallup.com/poll/154169/Chronic-Pain-Rates-Shoot-Until-Americans-Reach-Late-50s.aspx
5. Portenoy, R. K., Ugarte, C., Fuller, I., & Haas, G. (2004). Population-based survey of pain in the United States: Differences among white, African American, and Hispanic subjects. *The Journal of Pain, 5*(6), 317–328.
6. Institute of Medicine, Committee on Advancing Pain Research, Care, and Education. (2011). *Relieving pain in America: A blueprint for transforming prevention, care, education and research* (pp. 2–6). Prepublication copy. Washington, DC: National Academies Press.
7. Krueger, A. B., & Stone, A. A. (2008). Assessment of pain: A community-based diary survey in the USA. *The Lancet, 371*(9623), 1519–1525.
8. Breivik, H., Collett, B., Ventafridda, V., Cohen, R., & Gallacher, D. (2006). Survey of chronic pain in Europe: Prevalence, impact on daily life, treatment. *European Journal of Pain, 10*(4), 287–333.
9. R. Portenoy (personal communication, September 3, 2008).
10. Breivik, H., Collett, B., Ventafridda, V., Cohen, R., & Gallacher, D. (2006). Survey of chronic pain in Europe: Prevalence, impact on daily life, treatment. *European Journal of Pain, 10*(4), 287–333.
11. L. Webster (personal communication, March 22, 2012).

12. Institute of Medicine, Committee on Advancing Pain Research, Care, and Education. (2011). *Relieving pain in America: A blueprint for transforming prevention, care, education and research* (pp. 2–27). Prepublication copy. Washington, DC: National Academies Press.
13. Institute of Medicine, Committee on Advancing Pain Research, Care, and Education. (2011). *Relieving pain in America: A blueprint for transforming prevention, care, education and research* (pp. 2–29). Prepublication copy. Washington, DC: National Academies Press.
14. Breslau, N., Schultz, L., Lipton, R., Peterson, E., & Welch, K. M. A. (2012). Migraine headaches and suicide attempt. *Headache: The Journal of Head and Face Pain, 52*(5), 723–731.
15. International Association for the Study of Pain. (2012, August 28). Unrelieved pain is a major global healthcare problem. Retrieved from http://www.iasp-pain.org/AM/Template.cfm?Section=Press_Release&Template=/CM/ContentDisplay.cfm&ContentID=2908
16. H. Heit (personal communication, September 20, 2011).
17. P. Konowitz (personal communication, November 15, 2009).
18. D. Biro (personal communication, September 19, 2011).
19. M. Cooper (personal communication, Sept. 29, 2011).
20. K. Binkley (personal communication, September 18, 2011).
21. Lamas, D., & Rosenbaum, L. (2012). Painful inequities—Palliative care in developing countries. *New England Journal of Medicine, 366*(3), 199–201.
22. Institute of Medicine, Committee on Advancing Pain Research, Care, and Education. (2011). *Relieving pain in America: A blueprint for transforming prevention, care, education and research* (pp. 4–17). Prepublication copy. Washington, DC: National Academies Press.
23. J. Martin (personal communication, October 4, 2011).
24. M. Zylka (personal communication, November 2, 2011).
25. Watt-Watson, J., McGillion, M., Hunter, J., Choiniere, M., Clark, A. J., Dewar, A., et al. (2009). A survey of prelicensure pain curricula in health science faculties in Canadian universities. *Pain Research & Management, 14*(6), 439–444.
26. Briggs, E. V., Carr, E. C. J., & Whittaker, M. S. (2011). Survey of undergraduate pain curricula for healthcare professionals in the United Kingdom. *European Journal of Pain, 15*(8), 789–795.
27. J. Prescott (personal communication, October 19, 2011).
28. Mezei, L., Murinson, B. B., & Johns Hopkins Pain Curriculum Development Team. (2011). Pain education in North American medical schools. *The Journal of Pain, 12*(12), 1199–1208.
29. Institute of Medicine, Committee on Advancing Pain Research, Care, and Education. (2011). *Relieving pain in America: A blueprint for transforming prevention, care, education and research* (pp. 4–14). Prepublication copy. Washington, DC: National Academies Press.
30. Blumenthal, D., Gokhale, M., Campbell, E. G., & Weissman, J. S. (2001). Preparedness for clinical practice: Reports of graduating residents at academic health centers. *Journal of the American Medical Association, 286*(9), 1027–1034.

31. Upshur, C. C., Luckmann, R. S., & Savageau, J. A. (2006). Primary care provider concerns about management of chronic pain in community clinic populations. *Journal of General Internal Medicine, 21*(6), 652–655.
32. Association of American Medical Colleges. (2006). Medical school graduation questionnaire: All schools report. Retrieved from https://www.aamc.org/download/90062/data/gq-2006.pdf
33. Association of American Medical Colleges. (2010). GQ Medical school graduation questionnaire: All schools summary report. Retrieved from https://www.aamc.org/download/140716/data/2010_gq_all_schools.pdf
34. Association of American Medical Colleges. (2011). GQ Medical school graduation questionnaire: All schools summary report. Retrieved from https://www.aamc.org/download/263712/data/gq-2011.pdf
35. O'Rorke, J. E., Chen, I., Genao, I., Panda, M., & Cykert, S. (2007). Physicians' comfort in caring for patients with chronic nonmalignant pain. *American Journal of Medical Sciences, 333*(2), 93–100.
36. J. Loeser (personal communication, September 16, 2011).
37. Murinson, B. B., Nenortas, E., Mayer, R. S., Mezei, L., Kozachik, S., Nesbit, S., et al. (2011). A new program in pain medicine for medical students: Integrating core curriculum knowledge with emotional and reflective development. *Pain Medicine, 12*, 186–195.
38. American Association of Nurse Anesthetists, American Academy of Pain Medicine, American Headache Society, American Pain Foundation, American Pain Society, American Society of Anesthesiologists, et al. (2011, June 29). *Consumers, health professionals and advocates join to hail release of landmark Institute of Medicine report on advancing pain research, care and education.* Statement released at the Institute of Medicine press conference, Washington, DC.
39. Burgoyne, D. S. (2007). Prevalence and economic implications of chronic pain. *Managed Care, 16*(2 Supplement 3), 2–4.
40. Pletcher, M. J., Kertesz, S. G., Kohn, M. A., & Gonzales, R. (2008). Trends in opioid prescribing by race/ethnicity for patients seeking care in US emergency departments. *Journal of the American Medical Association, 299*(1), 70–78.
41. Institute of Medicine, Committee on Advancing Pain Research, Care, and Education. (2011). *Relieving pain in America: A blueprint for transforming prevention, care, education and research* (pp. C.1–C.45). Prepublication copy. Washington, DC: National Academies Press.
42. Institute of Medicine, Committee on Advancing Pain Research, Care, and Education. (2011). *Relieving pain in America: A blueprint for transforming prevention, care, education and research* (pp. 2–33). Prepublication copy. Washington, DC: National Academies Press.
43. Institute of Medicine, Committee on Advancing Pain Research, Care, and Education. (2011). *Relieving pain in America: A blueprint for transforming prevention, care, education and research* (p. C-4). Prepublication copy. Washington, DC: National Academies Press.
44. Y. Shir (personal communication, November 12, 2009).

45. National Institutes of Health. (n.d.). The NIH Almanac—Appropriations (section 2). Retrieved from http://www.nih.gov/about/almanac/appropriations/part2.htm

46. National Institutes of Health Research Portfolio Online Reporting Tools (RePORT). (2012, February 13). Estimates of funding for various research, condition, and disease categories (RCDC). Retrieved from http://report.nih.gov/rcdc/categories/

47. R. Myles (personal communication, February 23, 2012).

48. R. Myles (personal communication, October 19, 2012).

49. Porter, L. (2012, October 22). *Federally-funded pain research portfolio.* Slides presented at the Second Meeting of the Interagency Pain Research Coordinating Committee, Bethesda, MD. Retrieved from http://videocast.nih.gov/pastevents.asp

50. D. Bradshaw (personal communication, September 20, 2011).

51. D. Bradshaw (personal communication, February 23, 2012).

52. National Institutes of Health Research Portfolio Online Reporting Tools (RePORT). (2012, February 13). Estimates of funding for various research, condition, and disease categories (RCDC). Retrieved from http://report.nih.gov/rcdc/categories/

53. National Institutes of Health. (n.d.). The NIH Almanac: Appropriations (section 2). Retrieved March 15, 2012, from http://www.nih.gov/about/almanac/appropriations/part2.htm

54. L. Porter (personal communication, February 22, 2012).

55. J. Kusiak (personal communication, September 26, 2011).

56. National Institutes of Health Research Portfolio Online Reporting Tools (RePORT). (2012, February 13). Estimates of funding for various research, condition, and disease categories (RCDC). Retrieved from http://report.nih.gov/rcdc/categories/

57. National Institutes of Health. (n.d.). The NIH Almanac: Appropriations (section 2). Retrieved March 15, 2012, from http://www.nih.gov/about/almanac/appropriations/part2.htm

58. R. Saner (personal communication, September 22, 2011).

59. S. Report No. 112-84 at 114 (2012).

60. S. Fishman (personal communication, October 10, 2011).

61. P. Pizzo (personal communication, September 22, 2011).

62. K. Foley (personal communication, September 21, 2011.)

63. C. Steinberg (personal communication, September 22, 2011).

64. Institute of Medicine, Committee on Advancing Pain Research, Care, and Education. (2011). *Relieving pain in America: A blueprint for transforming prevention, care, education and research* (pp. 2–7). Prepublication copy. Washington, DC: National Academies Press.

65. Rawal, N. (2007). Postoperative pain treatment for ambulatory surgery. *Best Practice & Research Clinical Anaesthesiology, 21*(1), 129–148.

66. Schug, S. A., & Chong, C. (2009). Pain management after ambulatory surgery. *Current Opinion in Anaesthesiology, 22*(6), 738–743.

67. Institute of Medicine, Committee on Advancing Pain Research, Care, and Education. (2011). *Relieving pain in America: A blueprint for transforming*

prevention, care, education and research (pp. 1–25). Prepublication copy. Washington, DC: National Academies Press.

68. Kehlet, H., Jensen, T. S., & Woolf, C. J. (2006). Persistent postsurgical pain: Risk factors and prevention. *The Lancet, 367*(9522), 1618–1625.

69. Wu, C. L., & Raja, S. N. (2011). Treatment of acute postoperative pain. *The Lancet, 377*(9784), 2215–2225.

70. Institute of Medicine, Committee on Advancing Pain Research, Care, and Education. (2011). *Relieving pain in America: A blueprint for transforming prevention, care, education and research* (pp. 2–7). Prepublication copy. Washington, DC: National Academies Press.

71. Green, C. R., Hart-Johnson, T., & Loeffler, D. R. (2011). Cancer-related chronic pain: Examining quality of life in diverse cancer survivors. *Cancer, 117*(9), 1994–2003.

72. Deandrea, S., Montanaari, M., Moja, L., & Apolone, G. (2008). Prevalence of undertreatment in cancer pain. A review of published literature. *Annals of Oncology, 19*(12), 1985–1991.

73. Institute of Medicine, Committee on Advancing Pain Research, Care, and Education. (2011). *Relieving pain in America: A blueprint for transforming prevention, care, education and research* (pp. 2–5). Prepublication copy. Washington, DC: National Academies Press.

74. C. Woolf (personal communication, September 26, 2011).

75. Tracey, I., & Bushnell, M. C. (2009). How neuroimaging studies have challenged us to rethink: Is chronic pain a disease? *The Journal of Pain, 10*(11), 1113–1120.

CHAPTER 2

1. International Association for the Study of Pain. (n.d.). IASP taxonomy: Pain. Retrieved from http://www.iasp-pain.org/Content/NavigationMenu/GeneralResourceLinks/PainDefinitions/default.htm

2. Institute of Medicine, Committee on Advancing Pain Research, Care, and Education. (2011). *Relieving pain in America: A blueprint for transforming prevention, care, education and research* (pp. 1–17). Prepublication copy. Washington, DC: National Academies Press.

3. Melzack, R. (2005). Evolution of the neuromatrix theory of pain. The Prithvi Raj lecture: Presented at the third World Congress of World Institute of Pain, Barcelona, 2004. *Pain Practice, 5*(2), 85–94.

4. Institute of Medicine, Committee on Advancing Pain Research, Care, and Education. (2011). *Relieving pain in America: A blueprint for transforming prevention, care, education and research* (pp. 1–18). Prepublication copy. Washington, DC: National Academies Press.

5. deCharms, R. C., Maeda, F., Glover, G. H., Ludlow, D., Pauly, J. M., Soneji, D., et al. (2005). Control over brain activation and pain learned by using real-time functional MRI. *Proceedings of the National Academy of Sciences, 102*(51), 18626–18631.

6. Thernstrom, M. (2010). *The pain chronicles: Cures, myths, mysteries, prayers, diaries, brain scans, healing, and the science of suffering* (p. 5). New York: Farrar, Straus and Giroux.

7. Scarry, E. (1985). *The body in pain: The making and unmaking of the world* (p. 7). New York: Oxford University Press.

8. Von Hehn, C. A., Baron, R., & Woolf, C. (2012). Deconstructing the neuropathic pain phenotype to reveal neural mechanisms. *Neuron, 73*(4), 638–652.

9. Andrews, N. (2012, July 9). Moving pain treatments forward: NIH Pain Consortium Symposium. Retrieved from http://www.painresearchforum.org/news/17877-moving-pain-treatments-forward-nih-pain-consortium-symposium

10. C. Woolf (personal communication, July 16, 2012).

11. Costigan, M., Scholz, J., & Woolf, C. J. (2009). Neuropathic pain: A maladaptive response of the nervous system to damage. *Annual Review of Neuroscience, 32*, 1–32.

12. Scholz, J., & Woolf, C. J. (2002). Can we conquer pain? [Review]. *Nature Neuroscience, 5* (Supplement), 1062–1067.

13. Brenner, G. J., & Woolf, C. J. (2007). Mechanisms of chronic pain. In D. E. Longnecker, D. L. Brown, M. F. Newman, & W. M Zapol (Eds.), *Anesthesiology* (pp. 2000–2019). New York: McGraw Hill Companies.

14. Brenner, G. J., & Woolf, C. J. (2007). Mechanisms of chronic pain. In D. E. Longnecker, D. L. Brown, M. F. Newman, & W. M Zapol (Eds.), *Anesthesiology* (pp. 2000–2019). New York: McGraw Hill Companies.

15. Costigan, M., Scholz, J., & Woolf, C. J. (2009). Neuropathic pain: A maladaptive response of the nervous system to damage. *Annual Review of Neuroscience, 32*, 1–32.

16. Haanpää, M., & Treede, R. D. (2010). Diagnosis and classification of neuropathic pain. *PAIN: Clinical Updates, 18*(7), 1–6.

17. Braz, J. M., Sharif-Naeini, R., Vogt, D., Kriegstein, A., Alvarez-Buylia, A., Rubenstein, J. L., et al. (2012). Forebrain GABAergic neuron precursors integrate into adult spinal cord and reduce injury-induced neuropathic pain. *Neuron, 74*(4), 663–675.

18. G. Brenner (personal communication, October 28, 2010).

19. Fishman, S., & Berger, L. (2001). *The war on pain* (p. 118). New York: HarperCollins.

20. Woolf, C. J., & Ma, Q. (2007). Nociceptors—noxious stimulus detectors. *Neuron, 55*, 353–364.

21. Brenner, G. J., & Woolf, C. J. (2007). Mechanisms of chronic pain. In D. E. Longnecker, D. L. Brown, M. F. Newman, & W. M. Zapol (Eds.), *Anesthesiology* (pp. 2000–2019). New York: McGraw Hill Companies.

22. Patapoutian, A., Tate, S., & Woolf, C. J. (2009). Transient receptor potential channels: Targeting pain at the source. *Nature Reviews Drug Discovery, 8*, 55–68.

23. Bohlen, C. J., Chesler, A. T., Sharif-Naeini, R., Medzihradszky, K. F., Zhou, S., King, D., et al. (2011). A heteromeric Texas coral snake toxin targets acid-sensing ion channels to produce pain. *Nature, 479*(7373), 410–414.

24. Talkington, M. (2011, November 18). Lone star snakes reveal unexpected role for acid-sensing channels in pain. Retrieved from http://www.painresearchforum.org/search/site/Lone%20Star%20Snakes

25. Wortman, M. (2012). Where does it hurt? Researchers are getting to the molecular details of pain's circuitry to answer the question with real specificity. *Howard Hughes Medical Institute Bulletin, 25*(1), 32–33, 48.

26. Miller, A. N., & Long, S. B. (2012). Crystal structure of the human two-pore domain potassium channel K2P1 [Abstract]. *Science, 335*(6067), 432–436.

27. Brohawn, S. G., del Marmol, J., & MacKinnon, R. (2012). Crystal structure of the human K2P TRAAK, a lipid-and mechano-sensitive K+ ion channel [Abstract]. *Science, 335*(6067), 436–441.

28. Kim, S. E., Coste, B., Chadha, A., Cook, B., & Patapoutian, A. (2012). The role of Drosophila Piezo in mechanical nociception [Abstract]. *Nature, 483*(7388), 209–212.

29. Coste, B., Xiao, B., Santos, J. S., Syeda, R., Grandl, J., Kim, S. E., et al. (2012). Piezo proteins are pore-forming subunits of mechanically activated channels. *Nature, 483*(7388), 176–181.

30. Talkington, M. (2012, February 23). Novel ion channel senses painful touch. Retrieved from http://www.painresearchforum.org/news/13812-novel-ion-channel-senses-painful-touch?search_term=novel%20ion%20channel

31. Porreca, F. (2011, October 17). Cancer biology seminar series: Descending modulatory circuits and cancer pain [Video file]. Retrieved from http://streaming.biocom.arizone.edu/people/?id=11499

32. Beecher, H. K. (1956). Relationship of significance of wound to pain experienced. *Journal of the American Medical Association, 161*(17), 1609–1613.

33. von Mourik, O. (2006, April 2). Penfield's homunculus and the mystery of phantom limbs. Retrieved from http://journalism.nyu.edu/publishing/archives/annotate/node/270

34. G. Brenner (personal communication, March 13, 2012).

35. NOVA online. (n.d.). Secrets of the mind: Brain-mapping pioneers. Retrieved from http://www.pbs.org/wgbh/nova/mind/prob_pio.html

36. Blakeslee, S., & Blakeslee, M. (2007). *The body has a mind of its own: How body maps in your brain help you do (almost) everything better* (pp. 17–22). New York: Random House.

37. Ramachandran, V. S., Rogers-Ramachandran, D., & Stewart, M. I. (1992). Perceptual correlates of massive cortical reorganization. *Science, 258*(5085), 1159–1160.

38. Apkarian, A. V., Sosa, Y., Sonty, S., Levy, R. M., Harden, R. N., Parrish, T. B., et al. (2004). Chronic back pain is associated with decreased prefrontal and thalamic gray matter density. *Journal of Neuroscience, 24*(46), 10410–10415.

39. Latremoliere., & Woolf, C. (2009). Central sensitization: A generator of pain hypersensitivity by central neural plasticity [Critical review]. *The Journal of Pain, 10*(9), 895–926.

40. Brenner, G. J., & Woolf, C. J. (2007). Mechanisms of chronic pain. In D. E. Longnecker, D. L. Brown, M. F. Newman, & W. M. Zapol (Eds.), *Anesthesiology* (pp. 2000–2019). New York: McGraw Hill Companies.

41. Woolf, C. J. (2007). Central sensitization: Uncovering the relation between pain and plasticity. *Anesthesiology, 106*(4), 864–867.
42. Woolf, C. J. (2010, September). *Central sensitization: How plasticity produces pain*. Lecture presented at the 13th World Congress on Pain, Montreal, Canada.
43. Apkarian, A. V., Baliki, M. N., & Geha, P. Y. (2009). Towards a theory of chronic pain. *Progress in Neurobiology, 87,* 81–97.
44. Apkarian, A. V., Bushnell, M. C., Treede, R. D., & Zubieta, J. K. (2005). Human brain mechanisms of pain perception and regulation in health and disease. *European Journal of Pain, 9*(4), 463–484.
45. Gottschalk, A., Smith, D. S., Jobes, D. R., Kennedy, S. K., Lally, S. E., Noble, V. E., et al. (1998). Preemptive epidural analgesia and recovery from radical prostatectomy: A randomized controlled trial. *Journal of the American Medical Association, 279*(14), 1076–1082.
46. L. Watkins (personal communication, October 28, 2009).
47. Tracey, I., & Bushnell, M. C. (2009). How neuroimaging studies have challenged us to rethink: Is chronic pain a disease? *The Journal of Pain, 10*(11), 1113–1120.
48. Brown, J. E., Chatterjee, N., Younger, J., & Mackey, S. (2011). Towards a physiology-based measure of pain: Patterns of human brain activity distinguish painful from non-painful thermal stimulation. *PLoS ONE, 6*(9), e24124.
49. White, T. (2011, September 13). Does that hurt? Objective way to measure pain being developed at Stanford [Press release]. Retrieved from http://med.stanford.edu/ism/2011/september/pain.html
50. S. Mackey (personal communication, April 14, 2012).
51. Miller, G. (2009, January). Brain scans of pain raise questions for the law. *Science, 323,* 195.
52. White, T. (2011, September 13). Does that hurt? Objective way to measure pain being developed at Stanford [Press release]. Retrieved from http://med.stanford.edu/ism/2011/september/pain.html
53. Apkarian, A. V., Sosa, Y., Sonty, S., Levy, R. M., Harden, R. N., Parrish, T. B., et al. (2004). Chronic back pain is associated with decreased prefrontal and thalamic gray matter density. *Journal of Neuroscience, 24*(46), 10410–10415.
54. Kuchinad, A., Schweinhardt, P., Seminowicz, D. A., Wood, P. B., Chizh, B. A., & Bushnell, M. C. (2007). Accelerated brain gray matter loss in fibromyalgia patients: Premature aging of the brain? *Journal of Neuroscience, 27*(15), 4004–4007.
55. Seminowicz, D. A., Labus, J. S., Bueller, J. A., Tillisch, K., Naliboff, B. D., & Bushnell, M. C. (2010). Regional gray matter density changes in brains of patients with irritable bowel syndrome. *Gastroenterology, 139*(1), 48–57.
56. Schmidt-Wilcke, T., Leinisch, E., Straube, A., Kampfe, N., Draganski, B., Diener, H. C., et al. (2005). Gray matter decrease in patients with chronic tension type headache. *Neurology, 65,* 1483–1486.

57. Da Silva, A. F., Becerra, L., Pendse, G., Chizh, B., Tully, S., & Borsook, D. (2008). Colocalized structural and functional changes in the cortex of patients with trigeminal neuropathic pain. *PLoS ONE, 3*(10), e3396.
58. Draganski, B., Moser, T., Lummel, N., Ganssbauer, S., Bogdahn, U., Haas, F., et al. (2006). Decrease of thalamic gray matter following limb amputation. *Neuroimage, 31*(3), 951–957.
59. Wrigley, P. J., Gustin, S. M., Macey, P. M., Nash, P. G., Gandevia, S. C., Macefield, V. G., et al. (2009). Anatomical changes in human motor cortex and motor pathways following complete thoracic spinal cord injury. *Cerebral Cortex, 19*(1), 224–232.
60. Younger, J. W., Chu, L. F., D'Arcy, N. T., Trott, K. E., Jastrzab, L. E., & Mackey, S. C. (2011). Prescription opioid analgesics rapidly change the human brain. *PAIN, 152*(8), 1803–1810.
61. Tracey, I., & Bushnell, M. C. (2009). How neuroimaging studies have challenged us to rethink: Is chronic pain a disease? *The Journal of Pain, 10*(11), 1113–1120.
62. G. Scherr (personal communication, October 13, 2010).
63. G. Scherr (personal communication, February 5, 2012).
64. Schweinhardt, P., Kuchinad, A., Pukall, C. F., & Bushnell, M. C. (2008). Increased gray matter density in young women with chronic vulvar pain. *PAIN, 140*(3), 411–419.
65. Nikolajsen, L., Brandsborg, B., Lucht, U., Jensen, T. S., & Kehlet, H. (2006). Chronic pain following total hip arthroplasty: A nationwide questionnaire study. *Acta Anaesthesiologica Scandinavica, 50*, 495–500.
66. Rodriguez-Raecke, R., Niemeier, A., Ihle, K., Ruether, W., & May, A. (2009). Brain gray matter decrease in chronic pain is the consequence and not the cause of pain. *Journal of Neuroscience, 29*(44), 13746–13750.
67. Gwilym, S. E., Filippini, N., Douaud, G., Carr, A. J., & Tracey, I. (2010). Thalamic atrophy associated with painful osteoarthritis of the hip is reversible after arthroplasty: A longitudinal voxel-based-morphometric study. *Arthritis & Rheumatism, 62*(10), 2930–2940.
68. Seminowicz, D. A., Wideman, T. H., Naso, L., Hatami-khoroushahi, Z., Fallatah, S., Ware, M. A., et al. (2011). Effective treatment of chronic low back pain in humans reverses abnormal brain anatomy and function. *Journal of Neuroscience, 31*(20), 7540–7550.
69. Graceley, R. H., Geisser, M. E., Giesecke, T., Grant, M. A. B., Petske, F., Williams, D. A., et al. (2004). Pain catastrophizing and neural responses to pain among persons with fibromyalgia. *Brain, 127*, 835–843.
70. Baliki, M. N., Chialvo, D. R., Geha, P. Y., Levy, R. M., Harden, R. N., Parrish, T. B., et al. (2006). Chronic pain and the emotional brain: Specific brain activity associated with spontaneous fluctuations of intensity of chronic back pain. *Journal of Neuroscience, 26*(47), 12165–12173.
71. Apkarian, A. V., Bushnell, M. C., Treede, R. D., & Zubieta, J. K. (2005). Human brain mechanisms of pain perception and regulation in health and disease. *European Journal of Pain, 9*(4), 463–484.

72. Schweinhardt, P., Glynn, C., Brooks, J., McQuay, H., Jack, T., Chessell, I., et al. (2006). An fMRI study of cerebral processing of brush-evoked allodynia in neuropathic pain patients. *Neuroimage*, *32*(1), 256–265.
73. Apkarian, A. V., Baliki, M. N., & Geha, P. Y. (2009). Towards a theory of chronic pain. *Progress in Neurobiology*, *87*, 81–97.
74. D. Borsook (personal communication, July 1, 2010).
75. DaSilva, A. F., Becerra, L., Pendse, G., Chizh, B., Tully, S., & Borsook, D. (2008). Colocalized structural and functional changes in the cortex of patients with trigeminal neuropathic pain. *PLoS ONE*, *3*(10), e3396.
76. Borras, M. C., Becerra, L., Ploghaus, A., Gostic, J. M., DaSilva, A., Gonzalez, R. G., et al. (2004). fMRI measurement of CNS responses to naloxone infusion and subsequent mild noxious thermal stimuli in healthy volunteers. *Journal of Neurophysiology*, *91*(6), 2723–2733.
77. Borsook, D. (2012, August). *Imaging opioid effects on the brain—from preclinical to postclinical.* Paper presented at the International Association for the Study of Pain's 14th World Congress on Pain, Milan, Italy. Abstract retrieved from http://www.abstracts2view.com/iasp/sessionindex.php
78. Langford, D. J., Bailey, A. L., Chanda, M. L., Clarke, S. E., Drummond, T. E., Echols, S., et al. (2010). Coding of facial expressions of pain in the laboratory mouse. *Nature Methods*, *7*, 447–449.
79. Keating, S. C. J., Thomas, A. A., Flecknell, P. A., & Leach, M. C. (2012). Evaluation of EMLA cream for preventing pain during tattooing of rabbits: Changes in physiological, behavioural and facial expression responses. *PLoS ONE*, *7*(9), e44437.
80. Ashraf, A. B., Lucey, S., Cohn, J. F., Chen, T., Ambadar, Z., Prkachin, K., et al. (2009). The painful face—pain expression recognition using active appearance models. *Image and Vision Computing*, *27*(12), 1788–1796.
81. K. Prkachin (personal communication, October 21, 2010).
82. Kappesser, J., Williams, A. C., & Prkachin, K. (2006). Testing two accounts of pain underestimation. *PAIN*, *124*(1–2), 109–116.
83. Melzack, R. (n.d.). The McGill Pain Questionnaire. Retrieved from http://www.cebp.nl/?NODE=154
84. D. Price (personal communication, October 21, 2010).
85. R. Staud (personal communication, September 21, 2010).
86. R. Jamison (personal communication, February 14, 2011).
87. Marceau, L. D., Link, C., Jamison R. N., & Carolan, S. (2007). Electronic diaries as a tool to improve pain management: Is there any evidence? *Pain Medicine*, *8*(Supplement s3), S101–S109.
88. Jamison, R. N., Raymond, S. A., Levine, J. G., Slawsby, E. A., Nedeljkovic, S. S., & Katz, N. P. (2001). Electronic diaries for monitoring chronic pain: 1-year validation study. *PAIN*, *91*(3), 277–285.
89. Scholz, J., Mannion, R. J., Hord, D. E., Griffin, R. S., Rawal, B., Zheng, H., et al. (2009). A novel tool for the assessment of pain: Validation in low back pain. *PLoS Medicine*, *6*(4), e1000047.
90. Prkachin, K. M., & Craig, K. D. (1995). Expressing pain: The communication and interpretation of facial pain signals. *Journal of Nonverbal Behavior*, *19*(4), 191–205.

91. Prkachin, K. M., Solomon, P., Hwang, T., & Mercer, S. R. (2001). Does experience influence judgments of pain behaviour? Evidence from relatives of pain patients and therapists. *Pain Research & Management, 6*(2), 105–112.
92. K. Prkachin (personal communication, October 21, 2010).
93. Kappesser, J., Williams, A. C., & Prkachin, K. (2006). Testing two accounts of pain underestimation. *PAIN, 124*(1–2), 109–116.
94. Martel, M. O., Thibault, P., & Sullivan, M. J. (2011). Judgments about pain intensity and pain genuineness: The role of pain behavior and judgmental heuristics. *The Journal of Pain, 12*(4), 468–475.
95. K. Craig (personal communication, October 26, 2010).

CHAPTER 3

1. Nielsen, C. S., Staud, R., & Price, D. D. (2009). Individual differences in pain sensitivity: Measurement, causation and consequences. *The Journal of Pain, 10*(3), 231–237.
2. M. Rowbotham (personal communication, November 11, 2010).
3. Thyregod, H. G., Rowbotham, M. C., Peters, M., Possehn, J., Berro, M., & Petersen, K. L. (2007). Natural history of pain following herpes zoster. *PAIN, 128*, 148–156.
4. National Diabetes Information Clearinghouse. (2009, February). What are diabetic neuropathies? Retrieved from http://diabetes.niddk.nih.gov/dm/pubs/neuropathies/index.aspx
5. O'Hare, J. A., Abuaisha, F., & Geoghegan, M. (1994). Prevalence and forms of neuropathic morbidity in 800 diabetics [Abstract]. *Irish Journal of Medical Science, 163*(3), 132–135.
6. J. Mogil (personal communication, September 24, 2012).
7. C. Woolf (personal communication, February 15, 2012).
8. Alvan, G., Bechtel, P., Iselius, L., & Gundert-Remy, U. (1990). Hydroxylation polymorphisms of debrisoquine and mephenytoin in European populations. *European Journal of Clinical Pharmacology, 39*(6), 533–537.
9. P. Costa (personal communication, November 11, 2010).
10. J. & T. Blocker (personal communication, November 6, 2010).
11. Weiss, J., Pyrski, M., Jacobi, E., Bufe, B., Willnecker, V., Schick, B., et al. (2011). Loss-of-function mutations in sodium channel Nav1.7 cause anosmia. *Nature, 472*, 186–190.
12. J. & T. Blocker (personal communication, November 6, 2010).
13. Cox, J. J., Reimann, F., Nicholas, A. K., Thornton, G., Roberts, E., Springell, K., et al. (2006). An *SCN9A* channelopathy causes congenital inability to experience pain. *Nature, 444*, 894–898.
14. R. Staud (personal communication, October 21, 2010).
15. S. Waxman (personal communication, September 25, 2012).
16. Faber, C. G., Hoeijmakers, J. G. J., Ahn, H. S., Cheng, X., Han, C., Choi, J. S., et al. (2012). Gain of function Nav1.7 mutations in idiopathic small fiber neuropathy. *Annals of Neurology, 71*(1), 26–39.

17. Reimann, F., Cox, J. J., Belfer, A., Diatchenko, L., Zaykin, D. V., McHale, D. P., et al. (2010). Pain perception is altered by a nucleotide polymorphism in SCN9A. *Proceedings of the National Academy of Sciences, 107*(11), 5148–5153.
18. P. Costa (personal communication, November 11, 2010).
19. S. Waxman (personal communication, November 4, 2010).
20. Drenth, J. P. H., te Morsche, R. H. M., Guillet, G., Taieb, A., Kirby, R. L., & Jansen, J. B. M. J. (2005). SCN9A mutations define primary erythermalgia as a neuropathic disorder of voltage gated sodium channels. *The Journal of Investigative Dermatology, 124*, 1333–1338.
21. Legroux-Crespel, E., Sassolas, B., Guillet, G., Kupfer, I., Dupre, D., & Misery, L. (2003). Treatment of familial erythermalgia with the association of lidocaine and mexiletine. *Annales de Dermatologie et de Vénéréologie, 130*(4), 429–433.
22. Fischer, T. A., Gilmore, E. S., Estacion, M., Eastman, E., Taylor, S., Melanson, M., et al. (2009). A novel Nav 1.7 mutation producing carbamazepine-responsive erythromelalgia. *Annals of Neurology, 65*(6), 733–741.
23. Cummins, T. R., Dib-Hajj, S. D., & Waxman, S. G. (2004). Electrophysiological properties of mutant Nav 1.7 sodium channels in a painful inherited neuropathy. *Journal of Neuroscience, 24*(38), 8232–8236.
24. Dib-Hajj, S. D., Cummins, T. R., Black, J. A., & Waxman, S. G. (2010). Sodium channels in normal and pathological pain. *Annual Review of Neuroscience, 33*, 325–347.
25. Dib-Hajj, S. D., Cummins, T. R., Black, J. A., & Waxman, S. G. (2007). From genes to pain: Nav 1.7 and human pain disorders. *Trends in Neuroscience, 30*(11), 555–563.
26. Black, J. A., Nikolajsen, L., Kroner, K., Jensen, T. S., & Waxman, S. G. (2008). Multiple sodium channel isoforms and mitogen-activated protein kinases are present in painful human neuromas. *Annals of Neurology, 64*(6), 644–653.
27. S. Waxman (personal communication, September 25, 2012).
28. Mogil, J. S., Wilson, S. G., Bon, K., Lee, S. E., Chung, K., Raber, P., et al. (1999). Heritability of nociception I: Responses of 11 inbred mouse strains on 12 measures of nociception. *PAIN, 80*(1), 67–82.
29. Mogil, J. S. (1999). The genetic mediation of individual differences in sensitivity to pain and its inhibition. *Proceedings of the National Academy of Sciences, 96*, 7744–7751.
30. MacGregor, A. J., Andrew, T., Sambrook, P. N., & Spector, T. D. (2004). Structural, psychological and genetic influences on low back and neck pain: A study of adult female twins. *Arthritis Care & Research, 51*(2), 160–167.
31. Norbury, T. A., MacGregor, A. J., Urwin, J., Spector, T. D., & McMahon, S. B. (2007). Heritability of responses to painful stimuli in women: A classical twin study. *Brain, 130*, 3041–3049.
32. Nielsen, C. S., Stubhaug, A., Price, D. D., Vassend, O., Czajkowski, N., & Harris, J. R. (2008). Individual differences in pain sensitivity: Genetic and environmental contributions. *PAIN, 136*(1), 21–29.
33. Hartvigsen, J., Nielsen, J., Kyvik, K. O., Fejer, R., Vach, W., Iachine, I., et al. (2009). Heritability of spinal pain and consequences of

spinal pain: A comprehensive genetic epidemiologic analysis using a population-based sample of 15,328 twins ages 20–71 years. *Arthritis Care and Research, 61*(10), 1343–1351.

34. Markkula, R., Jarvinen, P., Leino-Arjas, P., Koskenvuo, M., Kalso, E., & Kaprio, J. (2009). Clustering of symptoms associated with fibromyalgia in a Finnish twin cohort. *European Journal of Pain, 13*(7), 744–750.

35. Mogil, J. S. (1999). The genetic mediation of individual differences in sensitivity to pain and its inhibition. *Proceedings of the National Academy of Sciences, 96,* 7744–7751.

36. Spector, T. D., & MacGregor, A. J. (2004). Risk factors for osteoarthritis: Genetics. *Osteoarthritis and Cartilage, 12*(Supplement 1), 39–44.

37. J. Mogil (personal communication, September 24, 2012).

38. Talkington, M. (2011, October 17). Epigenetic downregulation of GABA signaling perpetuates pain. Retrieved from http://www.pain-researchforum.org/news/10272-epigenetic-downregulation-gaba-signaling-perpetuates-pain

39. Zhang, Z., Cai, Y. Q., Zou, F., Bie, B., & Pan, Z. Z. (2011). Epigenetic suppression of GAD65 expression mediates persistent pain. *Nature Medicine, 17*(11), 1448–1455.

40. Langford, D. J., Bailey, A. L., Chanda, M. L., Clarke, S. E., Drummond, T. E., Echols, S., et al. (2010). Coding of facial expressions of pain in the laboratory mouse. *Nature Methods, 7,* 447–449.

41. Mogil, J. (2012, February). *The nature and nurture of pain.* Paper presented at the 10th International Association for the Study of Pain Research Symposium, Miami Beach, FL.

42. Costigan, M., Belfer, I., Griffin, R. S., Dai, F., Barrett, L. B., Coppola, G., et al. (2010). Multiple chronic pain states are associated with a common amino acid-changing allele in KCNS1. *Brain, 133*(9), 2519–2527.

43. Neely, G. G., Hess, A., Costigan, M., Keene, A. C., Goulas, S., Langeslag, M., et al. (2010). A genome-wide *Drosophila* screen for heat nociception identifies α2δ3 as an evolutionarily conserved pain gene. *Cell, 143*(4), 628–638.

44. M. Moskowitz (personal communication, November 29, 2010).

45. Gardner, K. L. (2006). Genetics of migraine: An update. *Headache: The Journal of Head and Face Pain, 46*(Supplement 1), S19–S24.

46. Anttila, V., Stefansson, H., Kallela, M., Todt, U., Terwindt, G. M., Calafato, M. S., et al. (2010). Genome-wide association study of migraine implicates a common susceptibility variant on 8q22.1 [Letter]. *Nature Genetics, 42,* 869–873.

47. Tegeder, I., Costigan, M., Griffin, R. S., Abele, A., Belfer, I., Schmidt, H., et al. (2006). GTP cyclohydrolase and tetrahydrobiopterin regulate pain sensitivity and persistence. *Nature Medicine, 12*(11), 1269–1277.

48. Tegeder, I., Adolph, J., Schmidt, H., Woolf, C. J., Geisslinger, G., & Lotsch, J. (2008). Reduced hyperalgesia in homozygous carriers of a GTP cyclohydrolase 1 haplotype. *European Journal of Pain, 12*(8), 1069–1077.

49. Cromie, W. J. (2006, November 16). Sensitivity to pain explained. *Harvard University Gazette*. Retrieved from http://news.harvard.edu/gazette/story/2006/11/sensitivity-to-pain-explained

50. Lotsch, J., Belfer, I., Kirchhof, A., Mishra, B. K., Max, M. B., Doehring, A., et al. (2007). Reliable screening for a pain-protective haplotype in the GTP cyclohydrolase 1 gene (GCH1) through the use of 3 or fewer single nucleotide polymorphisms. *Clinical Chemistry*, 53(6), 1010–1015.

51. L. Diatchenko (personal communication, November 5, 2010).

52. W. Maixner (personal communication, November 1, 2010).

53. Maixner, W. (2012, February). *Unraveling persistent pain conditions with genetic and phenotypic biomarkers*. Paper presented at the 10th International Association for the Study of Pain Research Symposium, Miami Beach, FL.

54. Tchivileva, I. E., Lim, P. F., Smith, S. B., Slade, G. D., Diatchenko, L., McLean, S. A., et al. (2010). Effect of catechol-O-methyltransferase polymorphism on response to propranolol therapy in chronic musculoskeletal pain: A randomized, double-blind, placebo-controlled, crossover pilot study. *Pharmacogenetics and Genomics*, 20(4), 239–248.

55. Light, K. C., Bragdon, E. E., Grewen, K. M., Brownley, K. A., Girdler, S. S., & Maixner, W. (2009). Adrenergic dysregulation and pain with and without acute beta-blockage in women with fibromyalgia and temporomandibular disorder. *The Journal of Pain*, 10(5), 542–552.

56. Emery, E. C., Young, G. T., Berrocoso, E. M., Chen, L., & McNaughton, P. A. (2011). HCN2 ion channels play a central role in inflammatory and neuropathic pain. *Science*, 333(6048), 1462–1466.

57. University of Cambridge. (2011, September 9). Gene that controls chronic pain identified. Research lays groundwork for the development of new, targeted pain medications [Press release]. Retrieved from http://www.bbsrc.ac.uk/news/health/2011/110909-pr-gene-that-controls-pain.aspx

58. Bond, C., LaForge, K.S., Tian, M., Melia, D., Zhang, S., Borg, L., et al. (1998). Single-nucleotide polymorphism in the human mu opioid receptor gene alters B-endorphin binding and activity: Possible implications for opiate addiction. *Proceedings of the National Academy of Sciences*, 95(16), 9608–9613.

59. Pan, Y-X. (2005). Diversity and complexity of the mu opioid receptor gene: Alternative pre-mRNA splicing and promoters. *DNA and Cell Biology*, 24(11), 736–750.

60. Walter, C., & Lotsch, J. (2009). Meta-analysis of the relevance of the OPRM1 118A> G genetic variant for pain treatment. *PAIN*, 146, 270–275.

61. University of North Carolina at Chapel Hill. (2011, November 10). Large-scale jaw pain study sheds light on pain disorders [Press release]. Retrieved from http://uncnews.unc.edu/content/view/4910/71/

62. Slade, G. D., Bair, E., By, K., Mulkey, F., Baraian, C., Rothwell, R., et al. (2011). Study methods, recruitment, sociodemographic findings, and demographic representativeness in the OPPERA study. *The Journal of Pain*, 12(11 Supplement), T12–T26.

CHAPTER 4

1. Ayroles, J. F., Carbone, M. A., Stone, E. A., Jordan, K. W., Lyman, R. F., Magwire, M. M., et al. (2009). Systems of genetics of complex traits in *Drosophila melanogaster*. *Nature Genetics*, *41*(3), 305.

2. I. Belfer (personal communication, March 7, 2012).

3. Unruh, A. M. (1996). Gender variations in clinical pain experience [Abstract]. *PAIN*, *65*(2–3), 123–167.

4. Fillingim, R. B., King, C. D., Ribeiro-Dasilva, M. C., Rahim-Williams, B., & Riley, J. L., III. (2009). Sex, gender, and pain: A review of recent clinical and experimental findings. *The Journal of Pain*, *10*(5), 447–485.

5. Aubrun, F., Salvi, N., Coriat, P., & Riou, B. (2005). Sex-and age-related differences in morphine requirements for postoperative pain relief [Abstract]. *Anesthesiology*, *103*(1), 156–160.

6. LeResche, L. (2011). Defining gender disparities in pain management. *Clinical Orthopaedics and Related Research*, *469*(7), 1871–1877.

7. Tsang, A., Von Korff, M., Lee, S., Alonso, J., Karam, E., Angermeyer, M. C., et al. (2008). Common chronic pain conditions in developed and developing countries: Gender and age differences and comorbidity with depression-anxiety disorders. *The Journal of Pain*, *9*(10), 883–891.

8. Fillingim, R. B., King, C. D., Ribeiro-Dasilva, M. C., Rahim-Williams, B., & Riley, J. L., III. (2009). Sex, gender, and pain: A review of recent clinical and experimental findings. *The Journal of Pain*, *10*(5), 447–485.

9. Bennett, M. I., Lee, A. J., Smith, B. H., & Torrance, N. (2006). The epidemiology of chronic pain of predominantly neuropathic origin: Results from a general population survey [Abstract]. *The Journal of Pain*, *7*(4), 281–289.

10. National Institute of Neurological Disorders and Stroke. NINDS complex regional pain syndrome information page. Retrieved June 6, 2013, from http://www.ninds.nih.gov/disorders/reflex_sympathetic_dystrophy/reflex_sympathetic_dystrophy.htm

11. de Mos, M., De Bruijn, A. G. J., Huygen, F., Dieleman, J. P., Stricker, B. H., & Sturkenboom, M. (2007). The incidence of complex regional pain syndrome: A population-based study [Abstract]. *PAIN*, *129*(1–2), 12–20.

12. Hall, G. C., Carroll, D., Parry, D., & McQuay, H. J. (2006). Epidemiology and treatment of neuropathic pain: The UK primary care perspective. *PAIN*, *122*(1–2), 156–162.

13. Fillingim, R. B., King, C. D., Ribeiro-Dasilva, M. C., Rahim-Williams, B., & Riley, J. L., III. (2009). Sex, gender, and pain: A review of recent clinical and experimental findings. *The Journal of Pain*, *10*(5), 447–485.

14. Srikanth, V. K., Fryer, J. L., Zhai, G., Winzenberg, T. M., Hosmer, D., & Jones, G. (2005). A meta-analysis of sex differences prevalence, incidence and severity of osteoarthritis [Abstract]. *Osteoarthritis and Cartilage*, *13*(9), 769–781.

15. Christmas, C., Crespo, C. J., Franckowiak, S. C., Bathon, J. M., Bartlett, S. J., & Andersen, R. E. (2002). How common is hip pain among older adults?

Results from the third national health and nutrition examination survey. *The Journal of Family Practice, 51*(4), 345–348.

16. Fillingim, R. B., King, C. D., Ribeiro-Dasilva, M. C., Rahim-Williams, B., & Riley, J. L., III. (2009). Sex, gender, and pain: A review of recent clinical and experimental findings. *The Journal of Pain, 10*(5), 447–485.

17. Fillingim, R. B., King, C. D., Ribeiro-Dasilva, M. C., Rahim-Williams, B., & Riley, JL., III. (2009). Sex, gender, and pain: A review of recent clinical and experimental findings. *The Journal of Pain, 10*(5), 447–485.

18. Fillingim, R. B., King, C. D., Ribeiro-Dasilva, M. C., Rahim-Williams, B., & Riley, J. L., III. (2009). Sex, gender, and pain: A review of recent clinical and experimental findings. *The Journal of Pain, 10*(5), 447–485.

19. Sandler, R. S. (1990). Epidemiology of irritable bowel syndrome in the United States [Abstract]. *Gastroenterology, 99*(2), 409–415.

20. M. Gold (personal communication, April 25, 2012).

21. Fillingim, R. B., King, C. D., Ribeiro-Dasilva, M. C., Rahim-Williams, B., & Riley, J. L., III. (2009). Sex, gender, and pain: A review of recent clinical and experimental findings. *The Journal of Pain, 10*(5), 447–485.

22. Darnall, B. D. (n.d.). Sex/gender disparity in pain and pain treatment: Closing the gap and meeting women's treatment needs. Retrieved from http://www.forgrace.org/images/uploads/Gender_Disparities_in_Pain_feature.pdf

23. Ruau, D., Liu, L. Y., Clark, J. D., Angst, M. S., & Butte, A. J. (2012). Sex differences in reported pain across 11,000 patients captured in electronic medical records. *The Journal of Pain, 13*(3), 228–234.

24. W. Maixner (personal communication, November 1, 2010).

25. H. Bursztajn (personal communication, October 20, 2010).

26. Mogil, J. S., & Chanda, M. L. (2005). The case for the inclusion of female subjects in basic science studies of pain. *PAIN, 117*(1–2), 1–5.

27. Wizemann, T. M., & Pardue, M-L. (Eds.). (2001). *Exploring the biological contributions to human health: Does sex matter?* Washington, DC: National Academies Press.

28. Fillingim, R. B., King, C. D., Ribeiro-Dasilva, M. C., Rahim-Williams, B., & Riley, J. L., III. (2009). Sex, gender, and pain: A review of recent clinical and experimental findings. *The Journal of Pain, 10*(5), 447–485.

29. Greenspan, J. D., Craft, R. M., LeResche, L., Arendt-Nielsen, L., Berkley, K. J., Fillingim, R. B., et al. (2007). Studying sex and gender differences in pain and analgesia: A consensus report. *PAIN, 132*, S26–S45.

30. K. Berkley (personal communication, October 5, 2010).

31. Levine, F. M., & De Simone, L. L. (1991). The effects of experimenter gender on pain report in male and female subjects [Abstract]. *PAIN, 44*(1), 69–72.

32. Gijsbers, K., & Nicholson, F. (2005). Experimental pain thresholds influenced by sex of experimenter. *Perceptual and Motor Skills, 101*(3), 803–807.

33. Fillingim, R. B., Browning, A. D., Powell, T., & Wright, R. A. (2002). Sex differences in perceptual and cardiovascular responses to pain: The influence

of a perceived ability manipulation [Abstract]. *The Journal of Pain*, 3(6), 439–445.

34. Racine, M., Tousignant-Laflamme, Y., Kloda, L. A., Dion, D., Dupuis, G., & Choiniere, M. (2012). A systematic literature review of 10 years of research on sex/gender and experimental pain perception—part I: Are there really differences between men and women? *PAIN*, 153(3), 602–618.

35. Fillingim, R. B., King, C. D., Ribeiro-Dasilva, M. C., Rahim-Williams, B., & Riley, J. L., III. (2009). Sex, gender, and pain: A review of recent clinical and experimental findings. *The Journal of Pain*, 10(5), 447–485.

36. Fillingim, R. B., King, C. D., Ribeiro-Dasilva, M. C., Rahim-Williams, B., & Riley, J.L., III. (2009). Sex, gender, and pain: A review of recent clinical and experimental findings. *The Journal of Pain*, 10(5), 447–485.

37. Fillingim, R. B., King, C. D., Ribeiro-Dasilva, M. C., Rahim-Williams, B., & Riley, J. L., III. (2009). Sex, gender, and pain: A review of recent clinical and experimental findings. *The Journal of Pain*, 10(5), 447–485.

38. Sarlani, E., Grace, E. G., Reynolds, M. A., & Greenspan, J. D. (2004). Sex differences in temporal summation of pain and aftersensations following repetitive noxious mechanical stimulation. *PAIN*, 109(1), 115–123.

39. Sarlani, E., & Greenspan, J. D. (2002). Gender differences in temporal summation of mechanically evoked pain [Abstract]. *PAIN*, 97(1), 163–169.

40. Racine, M., Tousignant-Laflamme, Y., Kloda, L. A., Dion, D., Dupuis, G., & Choiniere, M. (2012). A systematic literature review of 10 years of research on sex/gender and experimental pain perception—part 2: Do biopsychosocial factors alter pain sensitivity differently in women and men? *PAIN*, 153(3), 619–635.

41. J. Greenspan (personal communication, October 20, 2010).

42. Paulson, P. E., Minoshima, S., Morrow, T. J., & Casey, K. L. (1998). Gender differences in pain perception and patterns of cerebral activation during noxious heat stimulation in humans [Abstract]. *PAIN*, 76(1–2), 223–229.

43. Naliboff, B. D., Berman, S., Chang, L., Derbyshire, S. W. G., Suyenobu, B., Vogt, B. A., et al. (2003). Sex-related differences in IBS patients: Central processing of visceral stimuli. *Gastroenterology*, 124(7), 1738–1747.

44. Maleki, N., Linnman, C., Brawn, J., Burstein, R., Becerra, L., & Borsook, D. (2012). Her versus his migraine: Multiple sex differences in brain function and structure. *Brain*, 135(8), 2546–2559.

45. Berman, S. M., Naliboff, B. D., Suyenobu, B., Labus, J. S., Stains, J., Bueller, J. A., et al. (2006). Sex differences in regional brain response to aversive pelvic visceral stimuli [Abstract]. *American Journal of Physiology-Regulatory, Integrative and Comparative Physiology*, 291(2), R268–R276.

46. Weisse, C. S., Sorum, P. C., & Dominguez, R. E. (2003). The influence of gender and race on physicians' pain management decisions. *The Journal of Pain*, 4(9), 505–510.

47. Raftery, K. A., Smith-Coggins, R., & Chen, A. H. M. (1995). Gender-associated differences in emergency department pain management [Abstract]. *Annals of Emergency Medicine*, 26(4), 414–421.

48. Hoffmann, D. E., & Tarzian, A. J. (2001). The girl who cried pain: A bias against women in the treatment of pain. *The Journal of Law, Medicine & Ethics*, 28, 13–27.

49. Fishbain, D. A., Goldberg, M., Meagher, B. R., Steele, R., & Rosomoff, H. (1986). Male and female chronic pain patients categorized by DSM-III psychiatric diagnostic criteria [Abstract]. *PAIN*, 26(2), 181–197.

50. A. Oaklander (personal communication, October 6, 2010).

51. Di Cecco, R., Patel, U., & Upshur, R. E. (2002). Is there a clinically significant gender bias in post-myocardial infarction pharmacological management in the older (>60) population of a primary care practice? *BMC Family Practice*, 3, 8.

52. Fowler, R. A., Sabur, N., Li, P., Juurlink, D. N., Pinto, R., Hladunewich, M. A., et al. (2007). Sex-and age-based differences in the delivery and outcomes of critical care. *Canadian Medical Association Journal*, 177(12), 1513–1519.

53. Calderone, K. L. (1990). The influence of gender on the frequency of pain and sedative medication administered to postoperative patients. *Sex Roles*, 23(11), 713–725.

54. Schulman, K. A., Berlin, J. A., Harless, W., Kerner, J. F., Sistrunk, S., Gersh, B. J., et al. (1999). The effect of race and sex on physicians' recommendations for cardiac catheterization [Abstract]. *The New England Journal of Medicine*, 340(8), 618–626.

55. Daly, C., Clemens, F., Lopez Sendon, J. L., Tavazzi, L., Boersma, E., Danchin, N., et al. (2006). Gender differences in the management and clinical outcome of stable angina [Abstract]. *Circulation*, 113(4), 490–498.

56. Roger, V. L., Farkouh, M. E., Weston, S. A., Reeder, G. S., Jacobsen, S. J., Zinsmeister, A. R., et al. (2000). Sex differences in evaluation and outcome of unstable angina [Abstract]. *The Journal of the American Medical Association*, 283(5), 646–652.

57. M. O'Connor (personal communication, April 6, 2012).

58. O'Connor, M. I. (2011). Implant survival, knee function and pain relief after TKA. *Clinical Orthopaedics and Related Research*, 469(7), 1846–1851.

59. Borkhoff, C. M., Hawker, G. A., Kreder, H. J., Glazier, R. H., Mahomed, N. N., & Wright, J. G. (2008). The effect of patients' sex on physicians' recommendations for total knee arthroplasty. *Canadian Medical Association Journal*, 178(6), 681–687.

60. Chen, E. H., Shofer, F. S., Dean, A. J., Hollander, J. E., Baxt, W. G., Robey, J. L., et al. (2008). Gender disparity in analgesic treatment of emergency department patients with acute abdominal pain. *Academic Emergency Medicine*, 15(5), 414–418.

61. Cleeland, C. S., Gonin, R., Hatfield, A. K., & Edmonson, J. H. (1994). Pain and its treatment in outpatients with metastatic cancer [Abstract]. *The New England Journal of Medicine*, 330(9), 592–596.

62. Breitbart, W., Rosenfeld, B. D., Passik, S. D., McDonald, M. V., Thaler, H., & Portenoy, R. K. (1996). The undertreatment of pain in ambulatory AIDS patients [Abstract]. *PAIN*, 65(2–3), 243–249.

63. Hamberg, K., Risberg, G., Johansson, E. E., & Westman, G. (2002). Gender bias in physicians' management of neck pain: A study of the answers in a Swedish national examination [Abstract]. *Journal of Women's Health & Gender-Based Medicine, 11*(7), 653–666.

64. J. Levine (personal communication, September 21, 2010).

65. Klein, M. M., Downs, H. M., & Oaklander, A. L. (2010, September). *Normal innervation in distal-leg skin biopsies: Evidence of superabundance in youth, subsequent axonal pruning, plus new diagnostic recommendations.* A Works in Progress paper presented at the 135th Annual Meeting of the American Neurological Association, San Francisco, CA.

66. Racine, M., Tousignant-Laflamme, Y., Kloda, L.A., Dion, D., Dupuis, G., & Choiniere, M. (2012). A systematic literature review of 10 years of research on sex/gender and experimental pain perception—part 2: Do biopsychosocial factors alter pain sensitivity differently in women and men? *PAIN, 153*(3), 619–635.

67. Lipton, R. B., Stewart, W. F., Diamond, S., Diamond, M. L., & Reed, M. (2001). Prevalence and burden of migraine in the United States: Data from the American migraine study II [Abstract]. *Headache: The Journal of Head and Face Pain, 41*(7), 646–657.

68. Stewart, W. F., Lipton, R. B., Celentano, D. D., & Reed, M. L. (1992). Prevalence of migraine headache in the United States—relation to age, income, race, and other sociodemographic factors [Abstract]. *The Journal of the American Medical Association, 267*(1), 64–69.

69. LeResche, L. (1997). Epidemiology of temporomandibular disorders: Implications for the investigation of etiologic factors [Abstract]. *Critical Reviews in Oral Biology & Medicine, 8*(3), 291–305.

70. LeResche, L., Mancl, L. A., Drangsholt, M. T., Saunders, K., & Korff, M. V. (2005). Relationship of pain and symptoms to pubertal development in adolescents [Abstract]. *PAIN, 118*(1–2), 201–209.

71. LeResche, L., Mancl, L. A., Drangsholt, M. T., Saunders, K., & Korff, M. V. (2005). Relationship of pain and symptoms to pubertal development in adolescents [Abstract]. *PAIN, 118*(1–2), 201–209.

72. Cicero, T. J., Nock, B., O'Connor, L., & Meyer, E. R. (2002). Role of steroids in sex differences in morphine-induced analgesia: Activational and organizational effects. *Journal of Pharmacology and Experimental Therapeutics, 300*(2), 695–670.

73. L. Zeltzer (personal communication, August 31, 2010).

74. W. Maixner (personal communication, February 8, 2012).

75. Ji, Y., Murphy, A. Z., & Traub, R. J. (2003). Estrogen modulates the visceromotor reflex and responses of spinal dorsal horn neurons to colorectal stimulation in the rat [Abstract]. *The Journal of Neuroscience, 23*(9), 3908–3915.

76. LeResche, L., Saunders, K., Von Korff, M. R., Barlow, W., & Dworkin, S. F. (1997). Use of exogenous hormones and risk of temporomandibular disorder pain [Abstract]. *PAIN, 69*(1–2), 153–160.

77. LeResche, L., Saunders, K., Von Korff, M. R., Barlow, W., & Dworkin, S. F. (1997). Use of exogenous hormones and risk of temporomandibular disorder pain [Abstract]. *PAIN, 69*(1–2), 153–160.
78. Musgrave, D. S., Vogt, M. T., Nevitt, M. C., & Cauley, J. A. (2001). Back problems among postmenopausal women taking estrogen replacement therapy: The study of osteoporotic fractures [Abstract]. *Spine, 26*(14), 1606–1612.
79. Brynhildsen, J. O., Björs, E., Skarsgård, C., & Hammar, M. L. (1998). Is hormone replacement therapy a risk factor for low back pain among postmenopausal women? [Abstract]. *Spine, 23*(7), 809–813.
80. Fillingim, R. B., & Edwards, R. R. (2001). The association of hormone replacement therapy with experimental pain responses in postmenopausal women. *PAIN, 92*(1–2), 229–234.
81. Ockene, J. K., Barad, D. H., Cochrane, B. B., Larson, J. C., Gass, M., Wassertheil-Smoller, S., et al. (2005). Symptom experience after discontinuing use of estrogen plus progestin. *The Journal of the American Medical Association, 294*(2), 183–193.
82. Lichten, E. M., Lichten, J. B., Whitty, A., & Pieper, D. (1996). The confirmation of a biochemical marker for women's hormonal migraine: The depo-estradiol challenge test [Abstract]. *Headache: The Journal of Head and Face Pain, 36*(6), 367–371.
83. M. Gold (personal communication, April 25, 2012).
84. Aloisi, A. M., Bachiocco, V., Costantino, A., Stefani, R., Ceccarelli, I., Bertaccini, A., et al. (2007). Cross-sex hormone administration changes pain in transsexual women and men [Abstract]. *PAIN, 132*(Supplement 1), S60–S67.
85. LeResche, L., Mancl, L., Sherman, J. J., Gandara, B., & Dworkin, S. F. (2003). Changes in temporomandibular pain and other symptoms across the menstrual cycle [Abstract]. *PAIN, 106*(3), 253–261.
86. F. Cervero (personal communication, September 8, 2010).
87. Fillingim, R. B., & Gear, R. W. (2004). Sex differences in opioid analgesia: Clinical and experimental findings. *European Journal of Pain, 8*(5), 413–42.
88. Sarton, E., Olofsen, E., Romberg, R., den Hartigh, J., Kest, B., Nieuwenhuijs, D., et al. (2000). Sex differences in morphine analgesia: An experimental study in healthy volunteers [Abstract]. *Anesthesiology, 93*(5), 1245–1254.
89. Stoffel, E. C., Ulibarri, C. M., Folk, J. E., Rice, K. C., & Craft, R. M. (2005). Gonadal hormone modulation of mu, kappa, and delta opioid antinociception in male and female rats [Abstract]. *The Journal of Pain, 6*(4), 261–274.
90. Fillingim, R. B., & Gear, R. W. (2004). Sex differences in opioid analgesia: Clinical and experimental findings. *European Journal of Pain, 8*(5), 413–42.
91. M. Gold (personal communication, April 25, 2012).
92. Fillingim, R. B., & Gear, R. W. (2004). Sex differences in opioid analgesia: Clinical and experimental findings. *European Journal of Pain, 8*(5), 413–42.

93. Loyd, D. R., Wang, X., & Murphy, A. Z. (2008). Sex differences in μ-opioid receptor expression in the rat midbrain periaqueductal gray are essential for eliciting sex differences in morphine analgesia. *The Journal of Neuroscience, 28*(52), 14007–14017.

94. Wang, X., Traub, R. J., & Murphy, A. Z. (2006). Persistent pain model reveals sex difference in morphine potency. *American Journal of Physiology: Regulatory, Integrative and Comparative Physiology, 291*, R300–R306.

95. Society for Neuroscience. (2007, May). Brain briefings: Gender and pain. Retrieved from http://www.sfn.org/siteobjects/published/0000BDF20 016F63800FD712C30FA42DD/0000BDF2000006250112C47B4702 8AD6/file/BrainBriefings_May2007.pdf

96. Cepeda, M. S., & Carr, D. B. (2003). Women experience more pain and require more morphine than men to achieve a similar degree of analgesia. *Anesthesia & Analgesia, 97*(5), 1464–1468.

97. R. W. Gear (personal communication, September 22, 2010).

98. Niesters, M., Dahan, A., Kest, B., Zacny, J., Stijnen, T., Aarts, L., et al. (2010). Do sex differences exist in opioid analgesia? A systematic review and meta-analysis of human experimental and clinical studies. *PAIN, 151*(1), 61–68.

99. Niesters, M., Dahan, A., Kest, B., Zacny, J., Stijnen, T., Aarts, L., et al. (2010). Do sex differences exist in opioid analgesia? A systematic review and meta-analysis of human experimental and clinical studies. *PAIN, 151*(1), 61–68.

100. Niesters, M., Dahan, A., Kest, B., Zacny, J., Stijnen, T., Aarts, L., et al. (2010). Do sex differences exist in opioid analgesia? A systematic review and meta-analysis of human experimental and clinical studies. *PAIN, 151*(1), 61–68.

101. Niesters, M., Dahan, A., Kest, B., Zacny, J., Stijnen, T., Aarts, L., et al. (2010). Do sex differences exist in opioid analgesia? A systematic review and meta-analysis of human experimental and clinical studies. *PAIN, 151*(1), 61–68.

102. Miaskowski, C., & Levine, J. D. (1999). Does opioid analgesia show a gender preference for females? *Pain Forum, 8*(1), 34–44.

103. Gear, R. W., Miaskowski, C., Gordon, N. C., Paul, S. M., Heller, P. H., & Levine, J. D. (1996). Kappa–opioids produce significantly greater analgesia in women than in men [Abstract]. *Nature Medicine, 2*(11), 1248–1250.

104. Gear, R. W., Gordon, N. C., Heller, P. H., Paul, S., Miaskowski, C., & Levine, J. D. (1996). Gender difference in analgesic response to the kappa-opioid pentazocine [Abstract]. *Neuroscience Letters, 205*(3), 207–209.

105. Gear, R. W., Miaskowski, C., Gordon, N. C., Paul, S. M., Heller, P. H. & Levine, J. D. (1999). The kappa opioid nalbuphine produces gender- and dose-dependent analgesia and antianalgesia in patients with postoperative pain. *PAIN, 83*(2), 339–345.

106. J. Mogil (personal communication, April 5, 2012).

107. Mogil, J. S., Wilson, S. G., Chesler, E. J., Rankin, L., Nemmani, K. V. S., Lariviere, W. R., et al. (2003). The melanocortin-1 receptor gene mediates female-specific mechanisms of analgesia in mice and humans. *Proceedings of the National Academy of Sciences, 100*(8), 4867–4872.

108. Smith, Y. R., Stohler, C. S., Nichols, T. E., Bueller, J. A., Koeppe, R. A., & Zubieta, J-K. (2006). Pronociceptive and antinociceptive effects of estradiol through endogenous opioid neurotransmission in women [Abstract]. *The Journal of Neuroscience, 26*(21), 5777–5785.

109. Niesters, M., Dahan, A., Kest, B., Zacny, J., Stijnen, T., Aarts, L., et al. (2010). Do sex differences exist in opioid analgesia? A systematic review and meta-analysis of human experimental and clinical studies. *PAIN, 151*(1), 61–68.

CHAPTER 5

1. Schechter, N. L., & Allen, D. (1986). Physicians' attitudes toward pain in children [Abstract]. *Journal of Developmental and Behavioral Pediatrics, 7*(6), 350–354.

2. Chamberlain, D. B. (1991, May). *Babies don't feel pain: A century of denial in medicine.* Paper presented at the Second International Symposium on Circumcision, San Francisco, CA.

3. Swafford, L. I., & Allan, D. (1968). Pain relief in the pediatric patient. *Medical Clinics of North America, 52*(1), 133.

4. N. Schechter (personal communication, December 3, 2010).

5. C. Berde (personal communication, December 3, 2010).

6. J. Lawson (personal communication, December 2, 2010).

7. Lawson, J. R. (1988). Standards of practice and the pain of premature infants. *Zero to Three/The Bulletin of the National Center for Clinical Infant Programs, 9*(2), 1–5.

8. Eland, J. M., & Anderson, M. J. (1977). The experience of pain in children. In A. Jacox (Ed.), *Pain: A sourcebook for nurses and other health professionals* (pp. 453–476). Boston: Little, Brown, & Company.

9. Asprey, J. R. (1994). Postoperative analgesic prescription and administration in a pediatric population [Abstract]. *Journal of Pediatric Nursing, 9*(3), 150–157.

10. Perry, S., & Heidrich, G. (1982). Management of pain during debridement: A survey of US burn units [Abstract]. *PAIN, 13*(3), 267–280.

11. Beyer, J. E., DeGood, D. E., Ashley, L. C., & Russell, G. A. (1983). Patterns of postoperative analgesic use with adults and children following cardiac surgery [Abstract]. *PAIN, 17*(1), 71–81.

12. Mather, L., & Mackie, J. (1983). The incidence of postoperative pain in children [Abstract]. *PAIN, 15*(3), 271–282.

13. Schechter, N. L., Allen, D. A., & Hanson, K. (1986). Status of pediatric pain control: A comparison of hospital analgesic usage in children and adults [Abstract]. *Pediatrics, 77*(1), 11–15.

14. Fitzgerald, M., & Beggs, S. (2001). The neurobiology of pain: Developmental aspects [Abstract]. *The Neuroscientist, 7*(3), 246–257.
15. Fitzgerald, M., Millard, C., & McIntosh, N. (1989). Cutaneous hypersensitivity following peripheral tissue damage in newborn infants and its reversal with topical anaesthesia [Abstract]. *PAIN, 39*(1), 31–36.
16. Slater, R., Fabrizi, L., Worley, A., Meek, J., Boyd, S., & Fitzgerald, M. (2010). Premature infants display increased noxious-evoked neuronal activity in the brain compared to healthy age-matched term-born infants [Abstract]. *NeuroImage, 52*(2), 583–589.
17. Slater, R., Worley, A., Fabrizi, L., Roberts, S., Meek, J., Boyd, S., et al. (2010). Evoked potentials generated by noxious stimulation in the human infant brain [Abstract]. *European Journal of Pain, 14*(3), 321–326.
18. Andrews, K., & Fitzgerald, M. (1994). The cutaneous withdrawal reflex in human neonates: Sensitization, receptive fields, and the effects of contralateral stimulation [Abstract]. *PAIN, 56*(1), 95–101.
19. Fitzgerald, M., & Jennings, E. (1999). The postnatal development of spinal sensory processing. *Proceedings of the National Academy of Sciences, 96*(14), 7719–7722.
20. Marsh, D., Dickenson, A., Hatch, D., & Fitzgerald, M. (1999). Epidural opioid analgesia in infant rats II: Responses to carrageenan and capsaicin. *PAIN, 82*(1), 33–38.
21. Fitzgerald, M. (1991). Development of pain mechanisms. *British Medical Bulletin, 47*(3), 667–675.
22. Fitzgerald, M., & Walker, S. M. (2009). Infant pain management: A developmental neurobiological approach. *Nature Clinical Practice: Neurology, 5*(1), 35–50.
23. Anand, K. J. S., & Hickey, P. R. (1987). Pain and its effects in the human neonate and fetus. *New England Journal of Medicine, 317*(21), 1323.
24. Anand, K. J. S. (2001). Consensus statement for the prevention and management of pain in the newborn [Abstract]. *Archives of Pediatrics and Adolescent Medicine, 155*(2), 173–180.
25. Anand, K. J. S. (1998). Clinical importance of pain and stress in preterm neonates [Abstract]. *Biology of the Neonate, 73*(1), 1–9.
26. Anand, K. J., & Carr, D. B. (1989). The neuroanatomy, neurophysiology, and neurochemistry of pain, stress, and analgesia in newborns and children [Abstract]. *Pediatric Clinics of North America, 36*(4), 795–822.
27. Anand, K., Hall, R., Desai, N., Shephard, B., Bergqvist, L. L., Young, T. E., et al. (2004). Effects of morphine analgesia in ventilated preterm neonates: Primary outcomes from the NEOPAIN randomised trial. *The Lancet, 363*(9422), 1673–1682.
28. Anand, K. J. S., Aranda, J. V., Berde, C. B., Buckman, S. A., Capparelli, E. V., Carlo, W., et al. (2006). Summary proceedings from the neonatal pain-control group [Abstract]. *Pediatrics, 117*(3), S9–S22.
29. Anand, K., Johnston, C. C., Oberlander, T. F., Taddio, A., Tutag Lehr, V., & Walco, G. A. (2005). Analgesia and local anesthesia during invasive

procedures in the neonate [Abstract]. *Clinical Therapeutics, 27*(6), 844–876.

30. Carbajal, R., & Anand, K. (2008). Prevention of pain in neonates [Reply]. *The Journal of the American Medical Association, 300*(19), 2248–2249.

31. Fabrizi, L., Slater, R., Worley, A., Meek, J., Boyd, S., Olhede, S., & Fitzgerald, M. (2011). A shift in sensory processing that enables the developing human brain to discriminate touch from pain. *Current Biology, 21*(18), 1552–1558.

32. Johnston, C. (2010). *From the mouths of babes: What have we learned from studies of pain in neonates?* Paper presented at the International Association of Pain's 13th World Congress on Pain, Montreal, Canada.

33. Fitzgerald, M., & Koltzenburg, M. (1986). The functional development of descending inhibitory pathways in the dorsolateral funiculus of the newborn rat spinal cord [Abstract]. *Developmental Brain Research, 24*(1–2), 261–270.

34. Anand, K. J. S., & Hickey, P. R. (1987). Pain and its effects in the human neonate and fetus. *New England Journal of Medicine, 317*(21), 1321–1329.

35. Csontos, K., Rust, M., Hollt, V., Mahr, W., Kromer, W., & Teschemacher, H. J. (1979). Elevated plasma beta-endorphin levels in pregnant women and their neonates. *Life Sciences, 25*(10), 835–844.

36. Gautray, J. P., Jolivet, A., Viehl, J. P., & Guillemin, R. (1977). Presence of immunoassayable beta-endorphin in human amniotic fluid: Elevation in cases of fetal distress. *American Journal of Obstetrics and Gynecology, 129*(2), 211–212.

37. Emde, R. N, Harmon, R. J., Metcalf, D., Koenig, K. L., & Wagonfeld, S. (1971). Stress and neonatal sleep [Abstract]. *Psychosomatic Medicine, 33*(6), 491–497.

38. Talbert, L. M., Kraybill, E. N., & Potter, H. D. (1976). Adrenal cortical response to circumcision in the neonate [Abstract]. *Obstetrics and Gynecology, 48*(2), 208–210.

39. Williamson, P. S., & Williamson, M. L. (1983). Physiologic stress reduction by a local anesthetic during newborn circumcision. *Pediatrics, 71*(1), 36–40.

40. Taddio, A., Katz, J., Ilersich, A. L., & Koren, G. (1997). Effect of neonatal circumcision on pain response during subsequent routine vaccination [Abstract]. *The Lancet, 349*(9052), 599–603.

41. Taddio, A., Stevens, B., Craig, K., Rastogi, P., Ben-David, S., Shennan, A., et al. (1997). Efficacy and safety of lidocaine–prilocaine cream for pain during circumcision [Abstract]. *New England Journal of Medicine, 336*(17), 1197–1201.

42. Weisman, S. J., Bernstein, B., & Schechter, N. L. (1998). Consequences of inadequate analgesia during painful procedures in children [Abstract]. *Archives of Pediatrics and Adolescent Medicine, 152*(2), 147–149.

43. Zeltzer, L. K., & Krane, E. J. (2011). Pediatric pain management. In R. M. Kliegman, R. E. Behrmen, B. F. Stanton, N. Schor, & J. St. Geme (Eds.), *Nelson's textbook of pediatrics* (19th ed., p. 7). New York: Elsevier.

44. Anand, K. J., Sippell, W. G., & Aynsley-Green, A. (1987). Randomised trial of fentanyl anaesthesia in preterm babies undergoing surgery: Effects on the stress response. [Abstract]. *The Lancet, 1*(8524), 62–66.
45. Anand, K. J. S., Carr, D. B., & Mickey, P. R. (1987). Randomised trial of high-dose sufentanil anesthesia in neonates undergoing cardiac surgery: Hormonal and hemodynamic stress responses [Abstract]. *Anesthesiology, 67*(3), A501.
46. Berde, C. B., & Sethna, N. F. (2002). Analgesics for the treatment of pain in children. *New England Journal of Medicine, 347*(14), 1094–1103.
47. Cohen, M. M., Cameron, C. B., & Duncan, P. G. (1990). Pediatric anesthesia morbidity and mortality in the perioperative period [Abstract]. *Anesthesia & Analgesia, 70*(2), 160–167.
48. Zeltzer, L. K., & Krane, E. J. (2011). Pediatric pain management. In R. M. Kliegman, R. E. Behrmen, B. F. Stanton, N. Schor, & J. St. Geme (Eds.), *Nelson's textbook of pediatrics* (19th ed., p. 5). New York: Elsevier.
49. Berde, C. B., & Sethna, N. F. (2002). Analgesics for the treatment of pain in children. *New England Journal of Medicine, 347*(14), 1094–1103.
50. Anand, K. J. S., & Arnold, J. H. (1994). Opioid tolerance and dependence in infants and children [Abstract]. *Critical Care Medicine, 22*(2), 334–342.
51. Suresh, S., & Anand, K. J. S. (1998). Opioid tolerance in neonates: Mechanisms, diagnosis, assessment, and management [Abstract]. *Seminars in Perinatology, 22*(5), 425–433.
52. Berde, C. B., Lehn, B. M., Yee, J. D., Sethna, N. F., & Russo, D. (1991). Patient-controlled analgesia in children and adolescents: A randomized, prospective comparison with intramuscular administration of morphine for postoperative analgesia [Abstract]. *The Journal of Pediatrics, 118*(3), 460–466.
53. Berde, C. B., Lehn, B. M., Yee, J. D., Sethna, N. F., & Russo, D. (1991). Patient-controlled analgesia in children and adolescents: A randomized, prospective comparison with intramuscular administration of morphine for postoperative analgesia [Abstract]. *The Journal of Pediatrics, 118*(3), 460–466.
54. Zeltzer, L. K., & Krane, E. J. (2011). Pediatric pain management. In R. M. Kliegman, R. E. Behrmen, B. F. Stanton, N. Schor, & J. St. Geme (Eds.), *Nelson's textbook of pediatrics* (19th ed., p. 8). New York: Elsevier.
55. Zeltzer, L. K., & Krane, E. J. (2011). Pediatric pain management. In R. M. Kliegman, R. E. Behrmen, B. F. Stanton, N. Schor, & J. St. Geme (Eds.), *Nelson's textbook of pediatrics* (19th ed., p. 8). New York: Elsevier.
56. Johnston, C. (2010). *From the mouths of babes: What have we learned from studies of pain in neonates?* Paper presented at the International Association of Pain's 13th World Congress on Pain, Montreal, Canada.
57. Barr, R. G., Pantel, M. S., Young, S. N., Wright, J. H., Hendricks, L. A., & Gravel, R. (1999). The response of crying newborns to sucrose: Is it a "sweetness" effect? *Physiology & Behavior, 66*(3), 409–417.
58. Stevens, B., Yamada, J., & Ohlsson, A. (2010). Sucrose for analgesia in newborn infants undergoing painful procedures [Review]. *Cochrane Database of Systematic Reviews, 2010*(1), CD001069.

59. Akman, I. (2002). Sweet solutions and pacifiers for pain relief in newborn infants [Abstract]. *The Journal of Pain, 3*(3), 199–202.

60. Barr, R. G., Young, S. N., Wright, J. H., Gravel, R., & Alkawaf, R. (1999). Differential calming responses to sucrose taste in crying infants with and without colic [Abstract]. *Pediatrics, 103*(5), e68.

61. Johnston, C. (2010). *From the mouths of babes: What have we learned from studies of pain in neonates?* Paper presented at the International Association of Pain's 13th World Congress on Pain, Montreal, Canada.

62. Slater, R., Cornelissen, L., Fabrizi, L., Patten, D., Yoxen, J., Worley, A., et al. (2010). Oral sucrose as an analgesic drug for procedural pain in newborn infants: A randomised controlled trial [Abstract]. *The Lancet, 376*(9748), 1225–1232.

63. Johnston, C. (2010). *From the mouths of babes: What have we learned from studies of pain in neonates?* Paper presented at the International Association of Pain's 13th World Congress on Pain, Montreal, Canada.

64. Carbajal, R., Chauvet, X., Couderc, S., & Olivier-Martin, M. (1999). Randomised trial of analgesic effects of sucrose, glucose, and pacifiers in term neonates. *British Medical Journal, 319*(7222), 1393–1397.

65. Gray, L., Miller, L. W., Philipp, B. L., & Blass, E. M. (2002). Breastfeeding is analgesic in healthy newborns [Abstract]. *Pediatrics, 109*(4), 590–593.

66. Carbajal, R., Veerapen, S., Couderc, S., Jugie, M., & Ville, Y. (2003). Analgesic effect of breast feeding in term neonates: Randomised controlled trial. *British Medical Journal, 326*(7379), 1–5.

67. Johnston, C. C., Filion, F., Campbell-Yeo, M., Goulet, C., Bell, L., McNaughton, K., et al. (2009). Enhanced kangaroo mother care for heel lance in preterm neonates: A crossover trial [Abstract]. *Journal of Perinatology, 29*(1), 51–56.

68. Johnston, C. C., Filion, F., Campbell-Yeo, M., Goulet, C., Bell, L., McNaughton, K., et al. (2008). Kangaroo mother care diminishes pain from heel lance in very preterm neonates: A crossover trial. *BMC Pediatrics, 8*(1), 13.

69. Gray, L., Watt, L., & Blass, E. M. (2000). Skin-to-skin contact is analgesic in healthy newborns [Abstract]. *Pediatrics, 105*(1), e14.

70. Johnston, C. C., Abbott, F. V., Gray-Donald, K., & Jeans, M. E. (1992). A survey of pain in hospitalized patients aged 4–14 years [Abstract]. *The Clinical Journal of Pain, 8*(2), 154–163.

71. Jacob, E., & Puntillo, K. A. (2000). Variability of analgesic practices for hospitalized children on different pediatric specialty units [Abstract]. *Journal of Pain and Symptom Management, 20*(1), 59–67.

72. Ellis, J. A., O'Connor, B. V., Cappelli, M., Goodman, J. T., Blouin, R., & Reid, C. W. (2002). Pain in hospitalized pediatric patients: How are we doing? [Abstract]. *The Clinical Journal of Pain, 18*(4), 262–269.

73. Karling, M., RenströNewm, M., & Ljungman, G. (2002). Acute and postoperative pain in children: A Swedish nationwide survey [Abstract]. *Acta Paediatrica, 91*(6), 660–666.

74. Alexander, J., & Manno, M. (2003). Underuse of analgesia in very young pediatric patients with isolated painful injuries [Abstract]. *Annals of Emergency Medicine, 41*(5), 617–622.

75. Simons, S. H. P., van Dijk, M., Anand, K. S., Roofthooft, D., van Lingen, R. A., & Tibboel, D. (2003). Do we still hurt newborn babies? A prospective study of procedural pain and analgesia in neonates [Abstract]. *Archives of Pediatrics and Adolescent Medicine, 157*(11), 1058–1064.

76. Carbajal, R., Rousset, A., Danan, C., Coquery, S., Nolent, P., Ducrocq, S., et al. (2008). Epidemiology and treatment of painful procedures in neonates in intensive care units. *The Journal of the American Medical Association, 300*(1), 60–70.

77. Carbajal, R., Nguyen-Bourgain, C., & Armengaud, J. B. (2008). How can we improve pain relief in neonates? *Expert Review of Neurotherapeutics, 8*(11), 1617–1620.

78. Taylor, E. M., Boyer, K., & Campbell, F. A. (2008). Pain in hospitalized children: A prospective cross-sectional survey of pain prevalence, intensity, assessment and management in a Canadian pediatric teaching hospital. *Pain Research & Management: The Journal of the Canadian Pain Society, 13*(1), 25–32.

79. Harrison, D., Loughnan, P., & Johnston, L. (2006). Pain assessment and procedural pain management practices in neonatal units in Australia [Abstract]. *Journal of Paediatrics and Child Health, 42*(1-2), 6–9.

80. N. Schechter (personal communication, December 3, 2010).

81. Schechter, N. L., Allen, D. A., & Hanson, K. (1986). Status of pediatric pain control: A comparison of hospital analgesic usage in children and adults [Abstract]. *Pediatrics, 77*(1), 11–15.

82. Schechter, N. L., Zempsky, W. T., Cohen, L. L., McGrath, P. J., McMurtry, C. M., & Bright, N. S. (2007). Pain reduction during pediatric immunizations: Evidence-based review and recommendations. *Pediatrics, 119*(5), e1184–e1198.

83. Schechter, N. L., Bernstein, B. A., Zempsky, W. T., Bright, N. S., & Willard, A. K. (2010). Educational outreach to reduce immunization pain in office settings. *Pediatrics, 126*(6), e1514–e1521.

84. Schechter, N. L. (1989). The undertreatment of pain in children: An overview. *Pediatric Clinics of North America, 36*(4), 781–794.

85. Schechter, N. L. (2008). From the ouchless place to comfort central: The evolution of a concept. *Pediatrics, 122*(Supplement 3), S154–S160.

86. Harrison, D., Loughnan, P., & Johnston, L. (2006). Pain assessment and procedural pain management practices in neonatal units in Australia [Abstract]. *Journal of Paediatrics and Child Health, 42*(1-2), 6–9.

87. Wolfe, J., Grier, H. E., Klar, N., Levin, S. B., Ellenbogen, J. M., Salem-Schatz, S., et al. (2000). Symptoms and suffering at the end of life in children with cancer [Abstract]. *New England Journal of Medicine, 342*(5), 326–333.

88. Wolfe, J., Hammel, J. F., Edwards, K. E., Duncan, J., Comeau, M., Breyer, J., et al. (2008). Easing of suffering in children with cancer at the end of life: Is care changing? *Journal of Clinical Oncology, 26*(10), 1717–1723.

89. Schechter, N. L., Finley, G. A., Bright, N. S., Laycock, M., & Forgeron, P. (2010). ChildKind: A global initiative to reduce pain in children. *Pediatric Pain Letter*, 12(3), 26–30.
90. J. Lawson (personal communication, December 2, 2010.)

CHAPTER 6

1. Taylor, J. B. (2008). *My stroke of insight: A brain scientist's personal journey* (p. 17). New York: Viking.
2. Beecher, H. K. (1956). Relationship of significance of wound to pain experienced [Abstract]. *Journal of the American Medical Association*, 161(17), 1609–1613.
3. Wiech, K., Lin, C-S., Brodersen, K. H., Bingel, U., Ploner, M., & Tracey, I. (2010). Anterior insula integrates information about salience into perceptual decisions about pain. *Journal of Neuroscience*, 30(48), 16324–16331.
4. Lester, N., & Keefe, F. (1997). Coping with chronic pain. In A. Baum, S. Newman, J. Weinman, R. West, & C. McManus (Eds.), *Cambridge handbook of psychology, health and medicine* (pp. 87–90). Cambridge, UK: Cambridge University Press.
5. Keefe, F. J., Rumble, M. E., Scipio, C. D., Giordano, L. A., & Perri, L. C. M. (2004). Psychological aspects of persistent pain: Current state of the science. *The Journal of Pain*, 5(4), 195–211.
6. Institute of Medicine, Committee on Advancing Pain Research, Care, and Education. (2011). *Relieving pain in America: A blueprint for transforming prevention, care, education and research* (pp. 3–17). Prepublication copy. Washington, DC: National Academies Press.
7. van Middendorp, H., Lumley, M. A., Jacobs, J. W. G., Bijlsma, J. W. J., & Geenen, R. (2010). The effects of anger and sadness on clinical pain reports and experimentally-induced pain thresholds in women with and without fibromyalgia [Abstract]. *Arthritis Care & Research*, 62(10), 1370–1376.
8. Younger, J., Aron, A., Parke, S., Chatterjee, N., & Mackey, S., (2010). Viewing pictures of a romantic partner reduces experimental pain: Involvement of neural reward systems. *PloS One*, 5(10), e13309.
9. Reese, J. B., Somers, T. J., Keefe, F. J., Mosley-Williams, A., & Lumley, M. A. (2010). Pain and functioning of rheumatoid arthritis patients based on marital status: Is a distressed marriage preferable to no marriage? [Abstract]. *The Journal of Pain*, 11(10), 958–964.
10. Wasan, A. D., Sullivan, M. D., & Clark, M. R. (2010). Psychiatric illness, depression, anxiety, and somatoform pain disorders. In J. C. Ballantyne, J. P. Rathmell, and S. M. Fishman (Eds.), *Bonica's management of pain* (4th ed., pp. 393–417). Philadelphia: Lippincott, Williams, and Wilkins.
11. F. Keefe (personal communication, January 3, 2011.)
12. Engel, G. L. (1977). The need for a new medical model: A challenge for biomedicine. *Science*, 196(4286), 129–136.
13. Lumley, M. A., Cohen, J. L., Borszcz, G. S., Cano, A., Radcliffe, A. M., Porter, L. S., et al. (2011). Pain and emotion: A biopsychosocial review of recent research. *Journal of Clinical Psychology*, 67(9), 942–968.

14. Cole, S. W., Hawkley, L. C., Arevalo, J. M. G., & Cacioppo, J. T. (2011). Transcript origin analysis identifies antigen-presenting cells as primary targets of socially regulated gene expression in leukocytes. *Proceedings of the National Academy of Sciences, 108*(7), 3080–3085.
15. Narayan, M. C. (2010). Culture's effects on pain assessment and management. *The American Journal of Nursing, 110*(4), 38–47.
16. P. Cowan (personal communication, Oct. 18, 2010).
17. Foreman, J. (2006, February 6). Trick or treatment? *The Boston Globe*, p. C1.
18. Foreman, J. (2006, February 6). Trick or treatment? *The Boston Globe*, p. C1.
19. Benedetti, F., Mayberg, H. S., Wager, T. D., Stohler, C. S., & Zubieta, J-K. (2005). Neurobiological mechanisms of the placebo effect. *Journal of Neuroscience, 25*(45), 10390–10402.
20. Finniss, D. G., Kaptchuk, T. J., Miller, F., & Benedetti, F. (2010). Biological, clinical, and ethical advances of placebo effects. *The Lancet, 375*(9715), 686–695.
21. Jamison, R. N. (2011). Nonspecific treatment effects in pain medicine. *PAIN: Clinical Updates, 19*(2), 1–7.
22. Grelotti, D. J., & Kaptchuk, T. J. (2011). Placebo by proxy. *British Medical Journal, 343*, d4345.
23. T. Kaptchuk (personal communication, April 4, 2012).
24. Kong, J., Kaptchuk, T. J., Polich, G., Kirsch, I., & Gollub, R. L. (2007). Placebo analgesia: Findings from brain imaging studies and emerging hypotheses. *Reviews in the Neurosciences, 18*(3–4), 173–190.
25. Hrobjartsson, A., & Gotzsche, P. C. (2010). Placebo interventions for all clinical conditions. *Cochrane Database of Systematic Reviews, 2010*(1), CD003974.
26. Kaptchuk, T. J., Friedlander, E., Kelley, J. M., Sanchez, M. N., Kokkotou, E., Singer, J. P., et al. (2010). Placebos without deception: A randomized controlled trial in irritable bowel syndrome. *PloS One, 5*(12), e15591.
27. T. Kaptchuk (personal communication, December 29, 2010).
28. Finniss, D. G., Kaptchuk, T. J., Miller, F., & Benedetti, F. (2010). Biological, clinical, and ethical advances of placebo effects. *The Lancet, 375*(9715), 686–695.
29. Jensen, K. B., Kaptchuk, T. J., Kirsch, I., Lindstrom, K. M., Berna, C., Gollub, R. L., et al, (2012) Nonconscious activation of placebo and nocebo pain responses. *Proceedings of the National Academy of Sciences, 109*(39), 15959–15964.
30. Kong, J., Kaptchuk, T. J., Polich, G., Kirsch, I., & Gollub, R. L. (2007). Placebo analgesia: Findings from brain imaging studies and emerging hypotheses. *Reviews in the Neurosciences, 18*(3–4), 173–190.
31. Bingel, U., Wanigasekera, V., Wiech, K., Ni Mhuircheartaigh, R., Lee, M. C., Ploner, M., et al. (2011). The effect of treatment expectation on drug efficacy: Imaging the analgesic benefit of the opioid remifentanil [Abstract]. *Science Translational Medicine, 3*(70), 70ra14.
32. Gollub, R. L., & Kong, J. (2011). For placebo effects in medicine, seeing is believing [Abstract]. *Science Translational Medicine, 3*(70), 70ps5.

33. Wager, T. D., Rilling, J. K., Smith, E. E., Sokolik, A., Casey, K. L., Davidson, R. J., et al. (2004). Placebo-induced changes in fMRI in the anticipation and experience of pain [Abstract]. *Science, 303*(5661), 1162–1167.

34. Price, D. D., Craggs, J., Verne, G. N., Perlstein, W. M., & Robinson, M. E. (2007). Placebo analgesia is accompanied by large reductions in pain-related activity in irritable bowel syndrome patients [Abstract]. *PAIN, 127*(1), 63–72.

35. Koyama, T., McHaffie, J. G., Laurienti, P. J., & Coghill, R. C. (2005). The subjective experience of pain: Where expectations become reality [Abstract]. *Proceedings of the National Academy of Sciences, 102*(36), 12950–12955.

36. Porro, C. A., Baraldi, P., Pagnoni, G., Serafini, M., Facchin, P., Maieron, M., et al. (2002). Does anticipation of pain affect cortical nociceptive systems? [Abstract]. *The Journal of Neuroscience, 22*(8), 3206–3214.

37. R. Gollub (personal communication, January 5, 2011).

38. Levine, J. D., Gordon, N. C., & Fields, H. L. (1978). The mechanism of placebo analgesia. *The Lancet, 312*(8091), 654–657.

39. Petrovic, P., Kalso, E., Petersson, K. M., & Ingvar, M. (2002). Placebo and opioid analgesia—imaging a shared neuronal network [Abstract]. *Science, 295*(5560), 1737–1740.

40. Zubieta, J-K., Bueller, J. A., Jackson, L. R., Scott, D. J., Xu, Y., Koeppe, R. A., et al. (2005). Placebo effects mediated by endogenous opioid activity on μ-opioid receptors [Abstract]. *Journal of Neuroscience, 25*(34), 7754–7762.

41. Wager, T. D., Scott, D. J., & Zubieta, J-K. (2007). Placebo effects on human μ-opioid activity during pain. *Proceedings of the National Academy of Sciences, 104*(26), 11056–11061.

42. Zubieta, J-K., Yau, W. Y., Scott, D. J., & Stohler, C. S. (2006). Belief or need? Accounting for individual variations in the neurochemistry of the placebo effect [Abstract]. *Brain, Behavior, and Immunity, 20*(1), 15–26.

43. Benedetti, F., Arduino, C., & Amanzio, M. (1999). Somatotopic activation of opioid systems by target-directed expectations of analgesia [Abstract]. *The Journal of Neuroscience, 19*(9), 3639–3648.

44. Benedetti, F., Arduino, C., & Amanzio, M. (1999). Somatotopic activation of opioid systems by target-directed expectations of analgesia [Abstract]. *The Journal of Neuroscience, 19*(9), 3639–3648.

45. Pollo, A., Vighetti, S., Rainero, I., & Benedetti, F. (2003). Placebo analgesia and the heart. *PAIN, 102*(1), 125–133.

46. Benedetti, F., Amanzio, M., Rosato, R., & Blanchard, C. (2011). Nonopioid placebo analgesia is mediated by CB1 cannabinoid receptors. *Nature Medicine, 17*(10), 1228–1230.

47. Talkington, M. (2011, October). Endocannabinoids pitch in for placebo effect. Retrieved from http://www.painresearchforum.org/news/10 072-endocannabinoids-pitch-placebo-effect?search_term=Endocannabinoids%2

48. Pollo, A., Vighetti, S., Rainero, I., & Benedetti, F. (2003). Placebo analgesia and the heart. *PAIN, 102*(1–2), 125–133.

49. T. Kaptchuk (personal communication, February 18, 2011).
50. Ohayon, M. M., & Schatzberg, A. F. (2003). Using chronic pain to predict depressive morbidity in the general population. *Archives of General Psychiatry, 60*(1), 39–47.
51. Elman, I., Zubieta, J-K., & Borsook, D. (2011). The missing P in psychiatric training: Why it is important to teach pain to psychiatrists. *Archives of General Psychiatry, 68*(1), 12–20.
52. A. Wasan (personal communication, January 3, 2011).
53. Kroenke, K., Spitzer, R. L., Williams, J. B. W., Linzer, M., Hahn, S. R., deGruy, F. V., III, et al. (1994). Physical symptoms in primary care: Predictors of psychiatric disorders and functional impairment. *Archives of Family Medicine, 3*(9), 774.
54. Wasan, A. D., Sullivan, M. D., & Clark, M. R. (2010). Psychiatric illness, depression, anxiety, and somatoform pain disorders. In J. C. Ballantyne, J. P. Rathmell, and S. M. Fishman, (Eds.), *Bonica's management of pain* (4th ed., pp. 393–417). Philadelphia: Lippincott, Williams, and Wilkins.
55. Berna, C., Leknes, S., Holmes, E. A., Edwards, R. R., Goodwin, G. M., & Tracey, I. (2010). Induction of depressed mood disrupts emotion regulation neurocircuitry and enhances pain unpleasantness. *Biological Psychiatry, 67*(11), 1083–1090.
56. R. Jamison (personal communication, December 20, 2010).
57. Dersh, J., Mayer, T., Theodore, B. R., Polatin, P., & Gatchel, R. J. (2007). Do psychiatric disorders first appear preinjury or postinjury in chronic disabling occupational spinal disorders? [Abstract]. *Spine, 32*(9), 1045–1051.
58. The American Academy of Neurology. (2012). Migraine linked to increased risk of depression in women [Press release]. Retrieved from http://www.aan.com/press/?fuseaction=release.view&release=1033
59. Wasan, A. D., Sullivan, M. D., & Clark, M. R. (2010). Psychiatric illness, depression, anxiety, and somatoform pain disorders. In J. C. Ballantyne, J. P. Rathmell, and S. M. Fishman (Eds.), *Bonica's management of pain* (4th ed., pp. 393–417). Philadelphia: Lippincott, Williams, and Wilkins.
60. R. Jamison (personal communication, December 30, 2010).
61. Wasan, A. D., Sullivan, M. D., & Clark, M. R. (2010). Psychiatric illness, depression, anxiety, and somatoform pain disorders. In J. C. Ballantyne, J. P. Rathmell, and S. M. Fishman (Eds.), *Bonica's management of pain* (4th ed., pp. 393–417). Philadelphia: Lippincott, Williams, and Wilkins.
62. Wasan, A. D., Davar, G., & Jamison, R. (2005). The association between negative affect and opioid analgesia in patients with discogenic low back pain [Abstract]. *PAIN, 117*(3), 450–461.
63. Kroenke, K. (2005). Somatic symptoms and depression: A double hurt. *Primary Care Companion to the Journal of Clinical Psychiatry, 7*(4), 148–149.
64. Kroenke, K. (2003). The interface between physical and psychological symptoms. *The Primary Care Companion to the Journal of Clinical Psychiatry, 5*(Supplement 7), 11–18.
65. K. Kroenke (personal communication, December 30, 2010).

66. Giesecke, T., Gracely, R. H., Williams, D. A., Geisser, M. E., Petzke, F. W., & Clauw, D. J. (2005). The relationship between depression, clinical pain, and experimental pain in a chronic pain cohort. *Arthritis & Rheumatism, 52*(5), 1577–1584.

67. Meier, B. (2003). *Pain killer: A "wonder" drug's trail of addiction and death.* Emmaus, PA: Rodale Books.

68. Wasan, A. D., Sullivan, M. D., & Clark, M. R. (2010). Psychiatric illness, depression, anxiety, and somatoform pain disorders. In J. C. Ballantyne, J. P. Rathmell, and S. M. Fishman (Eds.), *Bonica's management of pain* (4th ed., pp. 393–417). Philadelphia: Lippincott, Williams, and Wilkins.

69. Bair, M. J., Robinson, R. L., Katon, W., & Kroenke, K. (2003). Depression and pain comorbidity: A literature review. *Archives of Internal Medicine, 163*(20), 2433–2445.

70. Urquhart, D. M., Hoving, J. L., Assendelft, W. J. J., Roland, M., & van Tulder, M. W. (2008). Antidepressants for non-specific low back pain. *Cochrane Database of Systematic Reviews, 2008*(1), CD001703.

71. Seidel, S., Aigner, M., Ossege, M., Pernicka, E., Wildner, B., & Sycha, T. (2010). Antipsychotics for acute and chronic pain in adults [Abstract]. *Journal of Pain and Symptom Management, 39*(4), 768–778.

72. Urquhart, D. M., Hoving, J. L., Assendelft, W. J. J., Roland, M., & van Tulder, M. W. (2008). Antidepressants for non-specific low back pain. *Cochrane Database of Systematic Reviews, 2008*(1), CD001703.

73. Lunn, M. P., Hughes, R. A., & Wiffen, P. J. (2009). Duloxetine for treating painful neuropathy or chronic pain [Abstract]. *Cochrane Database of Systematic Reviews, 2009*(4), CD007115.

74. Saarto, T., & Wiffen, P. J. (2005). Antidepressants for neuropathic pain [Abstract]. *Cochrane Database of Systematic Reviews, 2005*(3), CD005454.

75. Jackson, J. L., O Malley, P. G., & Kroenke, K. (2006). Antidepressants and cognitive-behavioral therapy for symptom syndromes. *CNS Spectrums, 11*(3), 212–222.

76. Kroenke, K., Bair, M. J., Damush, T. M., Wu, J., Hoke, S., Sutherland, J., et al. (2009). Optimized antidepressant therapy and pain self-management in primary care patients with depression and musculoskeletal pain. *The Journal of the American Medical Association, 301*(20), 2099–2110.

77. L. Zeltzer (personal communication, August 31, 2010).

78. Keefe, F. J., Lefebvre, J. C., Egert, J. R., Affleck, G., Sullivan, M. J., & Caldwell, D. S. (2000). The relationship of gender to pain, pain behavior, and disability in osteoarthritis patients: The role of catastrophizing. *PAIN, 87*(3), 325–334.

79. Edwards, R. R., Haythornthwaite, J. A., Sullivan, M. J., & Fillingim, R. B. (2004). Catastrophizing as a mediator of sex differences in pain: Differential effects for daily pain versus laboratory-induced pain. *PAIN, 111*(3), 335–341.

80. R. Portenoy (personal communication, September 10, 2009).

81. Sullivan, M. J. L., Bishop, S. R., & Pivik, J. (1995). The pain catastrophizing scale: Development and validation. *Psychological Assessment, 7*(4), 524–532.

82. Edwards, R. R., Bingham, C.O., III, Bathon, J., & Haythornthwaite, J. A. (2006). Catastrophizing and pain in arthritis, fibromyalgia, and other rheumatic diseases. *Arthritis Care & Research, 55*(2), 325–332.
83. Edwards, R. R., Kronfli, T., Haythornthwaite, J. A., Smith, M. T., McGuire, L., & Page, G. G. (2008). Association of catastrophizing with interleukin-6 responses to acute pain. *PAIN, 140*(1), 135–144.
84. Gracely, R. H., Geisser, M. E., Giesecke, T., Grant, M. A. B., Petzke, F., Williams, D. A., et al. (2004). Pain catastrophizing and neural responses to pain among persons with fibromyalgia [Abstract]. *Brain, 127*(4), 835–843.
85. Seminowicz, D. A., & Davis, K. D. (2006). Cortical responses to pain in healthy individuals depends on pain catastrophizing. *PAIN, 120*(3), 297–306.
86. Superio-Cabuslay, E., Ward, M. M., & Lorig, K. R. (1996). Patient education interventions in osteoarthritis and rheumatoid arthritis: A meta-analytic comparison with nonsteroidal anti-inflammatory drug treatment [Abstract]. *Arthritis & Rheumatism, 9*(4), 292–301.
87. Keefe, F. J., Abernethy, A. P., & Campbell, L. C. (2005). Psychological approaches to understanding and treating disease-related pain. *Annual Review of Psychology, 56*, 601–630.
88. Keefe, F. J., Caldwell, D. S., Williams, D. A., Gil, K. M., Mitchell, D., Robertson, C., et al. (1991). Pain coping skills training in the management of osteoarthritic knee pain: A comparative study. *Behavior Therapy, 21*(1), 49–62.
89. Benson, H., & Klipper, M. Z. (2000). *The relaxation response*. New York: HarperCollins.
90. Keefe, F. J., Rumble, M. E., Scipio, C. D., Giordano, L. A., & Perri, L. C. M. (2004). Psychological aspects of persistent pain: Current state of the science. *The Journal of Pain, 5*(4), 195–211.
91. Chou, R., & Huffman, L. (2007). Nonpharmacologic therapies for acute and chronic low back pain: A review of the evidence for an American Pain Society/American College of Physicians clinical practice guideline. *Annals of Internal Medicine, 147*(7), 492–504.
92. Gatchel, R. J., & Rollings, K. H. (2008). Evidence-informed management of chronic low back pain with cognitive behavioral therapy. *The Spine Journal, 8*, 40–44.
93. Burns, D. D. (1999). *Feeling good: The new mood therapy*. New York: Harper Paperbacks.
94. Keefe, F. J., Abernethy, A. P., & Campbell, L. C. (2005). Psychological approaches to understanding and treating disease-related pain. *Annual Review of Psychology, 56*, 601–630.
95. Turner, J. A., Mancl, L., & Aaron, L. A. (2006). Short-and long-term efficacy of brief cognitive-behavioral therapy for patients with chronic temporomandibular disorder pain: A randomized, controlled trial [Abstract]. *PAIN, 121*(3), 181–194.
96. Jackson, J. L., O'Malley, P. G., & Kroenke, K. (2006). Antidepressants and cognitive-behavioral therapy for symptom syndromes. *CNS Spectrums, 11*(3), 212–222.

97. Butler, A. C., Chapman, J. E., Forman, E. M., & Beck, A. T. (2006). The empirical status of cognitive-behavioral therapy: A review of meta-analyses [Abstract]. *Clinical Psychology Review, 26*(1), 17–31.
98. Morley, S., Eccleston, C., & Williams, A. (1999). Systematic review and meta-analysis of randomized controlled trials of cognitive behaviour therapy and behaviour therapy for chronic pain in adults, excluding headache. *PAIN, 80*(1–2), 1–13.
99. Morley, S., Williams, A., & Hussain, S. (2008). Estimating the clinical effectiveness of cognitive behavioural therapy in the clinic: Evaluation of a CBT informed pain management programme. *PAIN, 137*(3), 670–680.
100. S. Morley (personal communication, February 3, 2011).
101. Morley, S. (2011). Efficacy and effectiveness of cognitive behaviour therapy for chronic pain: Progress and some challenges. *PAIN, 152*(3), S99–S106.
102. Eccleston, C., Palermo, T. M., Williams, A. C., Lewandowski, A., & Morley, S. (2009). Psychological therapies for the management of chronic and recurrent pain in children and adolescents [Abstract]. *Cochrane Database of Systematic Reviews, 2009*(2), CD003968.
103. Macea, D. D., Gajos, K., Daglia Calil, Y. A., & Fregni, F. (2010). The efficacy of web-based cognitive behavioral interventions for chronic pain: A systematic review and meta-analysis [Abstract]. *The Journal of Pain, 11*(10), 917–929.
104. Jackson, J. L., O'Malley, P. G., & Kroenke, K. (2006). Antidepressants and cognitive-behavioral therapy for symptom syndromes. *CNS Spectrums, 11*(3), 212–222.
105. Jensen, M. P., Turner, J. A., & Romano, J. M. (2001). Changes in beliefs, catastrophizing, and coping are associated with improvement in multidisciplinary pain treatment. *Journal of Consulting and Clinical Psychology, 69*(4), 655–662.
106. Edwards, R. R., Bingham, C. O., III, Bathon, J., & Haythornthwaite, J. A. (2006). Catastrophizing and pain in arthritis, fibromyalgia, and other rheumatic diseases. *Arthritis Care & Research, 55*(2), 325–332.
107. Cepeda, M. S., Carr, D. B., Lau, J., & Alvarez, H. (2006). Music for pain relief [Abstract]. *Cochrane Database of Systematic Reviews, 2006*(2), CD004843.
108. Ford, G. K., Moriarty, O., McGuire, B. E., & Finn, D. P. (2008). Investigating the effects of distracting stimuli on nociceptive behaviour and associated alterations in brain monoamines in rats. *European Journal of Pain, 12*(8), 970–979.
109. M. Jensen & D. Patterson (personal communication, February 2, 2010).
110. Hoffman, H. G. (2004). Virtual-reality therapy. *Scientific American, 291*, 58–64.
111. Hoffman, H. G., Patterson, D. R., Magula, J., Carrougher, G. J., Zeltzer, K., Dagadakis, S., et al. (2004). Water-friendly virtual reality pain control during wound care [Abstract]. *Journal of Clinical Psychology, 60*(2), 189–195.

112. Hoffman, H. G., Patterson, D. R., & Carrougher, G. J. (2000). Use of virtual reality for adjunctive treatment of adult burn pain during physical therapy: A controlled study [Abstract]. *The Clinical Journal of Pain, 16*(3), 244–250.

113. Patel, A., Schieble, T., Davidson, M., Tran, M. C. J., Schoenberg, C., Delphin, E., et al. (2006). Distraction with a hand-held video game reduces pediatric preoperative anxiety [Abstract]. *Pediatric Anesthesia, 16*(10), 1019–1027.

114. Hoffman, H. G., Seibel, E. J., Richards, T. L., Furness, T. A., Patterson, D. R., & Sharar, S. R. (2006). Virtual reality helmet display quality influences the magnitude of virtual reality analgesia [Abstract]. *The Journal of Pain, 7*(11), 843–850.

115. Hoffman, H. G. (2004). Virtual-reality therapy. *Scientific American, 291*, 62.

116. Hoffman, H. G., Richards, T. L., Coda, B., Bills, A. R., Blough, D., Richards, A. L., et al. (2004). Modulation of thermal pain-related brain activity with virtual reality: Evidence from fMRI. *Neuroreport, 15*(8), 1245–1248.

117. Sprenger, C., Eippert, F., Finsterbusch, J., Bingel, U., Rose, M., & Buchel, C. (2012). Attention modulates spinal cord responses to pain. *Current Biology, 22*(11), 1019–1022.

118. Association for Applied Psychophysiology and Biofeedback. (n.d.). About biofeedback. Retrieved from http://www.aapb.org/i4a/pages/index.cfm?pageid=3463

119. Nestoriuc, Y., & Martin, A. (2007). Efficacy of biofeedback for migraine: A meta-analysis. *PAIN, 128*(1), 111–27.

120. Nestoriuc, Y., Martin, A., Rief, W., & Andrasik, F. (2008). Biofeedback treatment for headache disorders: A comprehensive efficacy review. *Applied Psychophysiology and Biofeedback, 33*(3), 125–140.

121. Frank, D. L., Khorshid, L., Kiffer, J. F., Moravec, C. S., & McKee, M. G. (2010). Biofeedback in medicine: Who, when, why and how? *Mental Health in Family Medicine, 7*(2), 85–91.

122. Jensen, M. P., Hakimian, S., Sherlin, L. H., & Fregni, F. (2009). New insights into neuromodulatory approaches for the treatment of pain. *The Journal of Pain, 9*(3), 193–199.

123. DeCharms, R. C., Maeda, F., Glover, G. H., Ludlow, D., Pauly, J. M., Soneji, D., et al. (2005). Control over brain activation and pain learned by using real-time functional MRI. *Proceedings of the National Academy of Sciences, 102*(51), 18626–18631.

124. S. Mackey (personal communication, April 14, 2012).

125. Foreman, J. (2003, April 22). A look at the science behind meditation. *The Boston Globe*, p. F15.

126. Kabat-Zinn, J. (1990). *Full catastrophe living: Using the wisdom of your body and mind to face stress, pain, and illness.* New York: Bantam Dell.

127. Goleman, D. (1988). *The meditative mind: The varieties of meditative experience.* New York: J. P. Tarcher.

128. Goldsmith, J. S. (1990). *The art of meditation.* New York: HarperCollins.

129. Gardner-Nix, J., & Costin-Hall, L. (2009). *The mindfulness solution to pain: Step-by-step techniques for chronic pain management.* Oakland, CA: New Harbinger.

130. Vowles, K. E., McCracken, L. M., & Dahl, J. C. (2010, May 7). *Acceptance and commitment therapy and chronic pain.* PowerPoint slides presented at the American Pain Society's 29th Annual Meeting, Baltimore, MD.

131. Davidson, R. J., Kabat-Zinn, J., Schumacher, J., Rosenkranz, M., Muller, D., Santorelli, S. F., et al. (2003). Alterations in brain and immune function produced by mindfulness meditation. *Psychosomatic Medicine, 65*(4), 564–570.

132. Lazar, S. W., Kerr, C. E., Wasserman, R. H., Gray, J. R., Greve, D. N., Treadway, M. T., et al. (2005). Meditation experience is associated with increased cortical thickness. *Neuroreport, 16*(17), 1893–1897.

133. Grant, J. A., Courtemanche, J., Duerden, E. G., Duncan, G. H., & Rainville, P. (2010). Cortical thickness and pain sensitivity in zen meditators [Abstract]. *Emotion, 10*(1), 43–53.

134. Grant, J. A., Courtemanche, J., & Rainville, P. (2010). A non-elaborative mental stance and decoupling of executive and pain-related cortices predicts low pain sensitivity in Zen meditators [Abstract]. *PAIN, 152*(1), 150–156.

135. Lush, E., Salmon, P., Floyd, A., Studts, J. L., Weissbecker, I., & Sephton, S. E. (2009). Mindfulness meditation for symptom reduction in fibromyalgia: Psychophysiological correlates [Abstract]. *Journal of Clinical Psychology in Medical Settings, 16*(2), 200–207.

136. Grossman, P., Tiefenthaler-Gilmer, U., Raysz, A., & Kesper, U. (2007). Mindfulness training as an intervention for fibromyalgia: Evidence of postintervention and 3-year follow-up benefits in well-being [Abstract]. *Psychotherapy and Psychosomatics, 76*(4), 226–233.

137. Vago, D. R., & Nakamura, Y. (2011). Selective attentional bias towards pain-related threat in fibromyalgia: Preliminary evidence for effects of mindfulness meditation training. *Cognitive Therapy and Research, 35*(6), 581–594.

138. Schmidt, S., Grossman, P., Schwarzer, B., Jena, S., Naumann, J., & Walach, H. (2011). Treating fibromyalgia with mindfulness-based stress reduction: Results from a 3-armed randomized controlled trial [Abstract]. *PAIN, 152*(2), 361–369.

139. Zeidan, F., Martucci, K. T., Kraft, R. A., Gordon, N. S., McHaffie, J. G., & Coghill, R. C. (2011). Brain mechanisms supporting the modulation of pain by mindfulness meditation. *The Journal of Neuroscience, 31*(14), 5540–5548.

140. Zeidan, F., Gordon, N. S., Merchant, J., & Goolkasian, P. (2010). The effects of brief mindfulness meditation training on experimentally induced pain [Abstract]. *The Journal of Pain, 11*(3), 199–209.

141. Rosenzweig, S., Greeson, J. M., Reibel, D. K., Green, J. S., Jasser, S. A., & Beasley, D. (2010). Mindfulness-based stress reduction for chronic pain conditions: Variation in treatment outcomes and role of home meditation practice [Abstract]. *Journal of Psychosomatic Research, 68*(1), 29–36.

142. Brown, C. A., & Jones, A. K. P. (2010). Meditation experience predicts less negative appraisal of pain: Electrophysiological evidence for the

involvement of anticipatory neural responses [Abstract]. *PAIN, 150*(3), 428–438.

143. Hölzel, B. K., Carmody, J., Vangel, M., Congleton, C., Yerramsetti, S. M., Gard, T., et al. (2011). Mindfulness practice leads to increases in regional brain gray matter density. *Psychiatry Research: Neuroimaging, 191*(1), 36–43.

144. Gard, T., Holzel, B. K., Sack, A. T., Hempel, H., Lazar, S. W., Vaitl, D., et al. (2012). Pain attenuation through mindfulness is associated with decreased cognitive control and increased sensory processing in the brain. *Cerebral Cortex, 22*(11), 2692–2702.

145. S. Lazar (personal communication, April 10, 2012).

146. Patterson, D. R., & Jensen, M. P. (2003). Hypnosis and clinical pain. *Psychological Bulletin, 129*(4), 495–521.

147. Barber, J. E. (1996). Hypnosis and suggestion in the treatment of pain: A clinical guide (p. 3). New York: W. W. Norton & Co.

148. Jensen, M. P., Ehde, D. M., Gertz, K. J., Stoelb, B. L., Dillworth, T. M., Hirsh, A. T., et al. (2011). Effects of self-hypnosis training and cognitive restructuring on daily pain intensity and catastrophizing in individuals with multiple sclerosis and chronic pain. *International Journal of Clinical and Experimental Hypnosis, 59*(1), 45–63.

149. Jensen, M. P., Barber, J., Romano, J. M., Hanley, M. A., Raichle, K. A., Molton, I. R., et al. (2009). Effects of self-hypnosis training and EMG biofeedback relaxation training on chronic pain in persons with spinal-cord injury. *International Journal of Clinical and Experimental Hypnosis, 57*(3), 239–268.

150. Zeltzer, L., & LeBaron, S. (1982). Hypnosis and nonhypnotic techniques for reduction of pain and anxiety during painful procedures in children and adolescents with cancer. *The Journal of Pediatrics, 101*(6), 1032–1035.

151. Patterson, D. R., & Jensen, M. P. (2003). Hypnosis and clinical pain. *Psychological Bulletin, 129*(4), 495–521.

152. M. Jensen & D. Patterson (personal communication, February 2, 2010).

153. Jensen, M., McArthur, K., Barber, J., Hanley, M., Engel, J., Romano, J., et al. (2006). Satisfaction with, and the beneficial side effects of, hypnotic analgesia. *International Journal of Clinical and Experimental Hypnosis, 54*(4), 432–447.

154. Prkachin, K. M., Solomon, P. E., & Ross, J. (2007). Underestimation of pain by health-care providers: Towards a model of the process of inferring pain in others [Abstract]. *Canadian Journal of Nursing Research, 39*(2), 88–106.

155. K. Prkachin (personal communication, October 20, 2010).

156. Austin, J. H. (2009). *Selfless insight: Zen and the meditative transformations of consciousness* (p. 213). Cambridge, MA: MIT Press.

157. Jamison, R. N. (2011). Nonspecific treatment effects in pain medicine. *PAIN: Clinical Updates, 19*(2), 1–7.

158. Jackson, P. L., Meltzoff, A. N., & Decety, J. (2005). How do we perceive the pain of others? A window into the neural processes involved in empathy. *NeuroImage, 24*(3), 771–779.

159. M. Loggia (personal communication, February 1, 2011).
160. Iacoboni, M., & Dapretto, M. (2006). The mirror neuron system and the consequences of its dysfunction [Abstract]. *Nature Reviews Neuroscience*, 7(12), 942–951.
161. Dapretto, M., Davies, M. S., Pfeifer, J. H., Scott, A. A., Sigman, M., Bookheimer, S. Y., et al. (2005). Understanding emotions in others: Mirror neuron dysfunction in children with autism spectrum disorders [Abstract]. *Nature Neuroscience*, 9(1), 28–30.
162. Iacoboni, M. (2009). Imitation, empathy, and mirror neurons. *Annual Review of Psychology*, 60, 653–670.
163. Avenanti, A., Paluello, I. M., Bufalari, I., & Aglioti, S. M. (2006). Stimulus-driven modulation of motor-evoked potentials during observation of others' pain [Abstract]. *NeuroImage*, 32(1), 316–324.
164. Avenanti, A., Bueti, D., Galati, G., & Aglioti, S. M. (2005). Transcranial magnetic stimulation highlights the sensorimotor side of empathy for pain [Abstract]. *Nature Neuroscience*, 8(7), 955–960.
165. Fecteau, S., Pascual-Leone, A., & Theoret, H. (2008). Psychopathy and the mirror neuron system: Preliminary findings from a non-psychiatric sample. *Psychiatry Research*, 160, 137–144.
166. Deyo, K. S., Prkachin, K. M., & Mercer, S. R. (2004). Development of sensitivity to facial expression of pain. *PAIN*, 107(1–2), 16–21.
167. Coan, J. A., Schaefer, H. S., & Davidson, R. J. (2006). Lending a hand: Social regulation of the neural response to threat. *Psychological Science*, 17(12), 1032–1039.
168. Loggia, M. L., Mogil, J. S., & Bushnell, M. C. (2008). Empathy hurts: Compassion for another increases both sensory and affective components of pain perception. *PAIN*, 136(1–2), 168–176.
169. Langford, D. J., Crager, S. E., Shehzad, Z., Smith, S. B., Sotocinal, S. G., Levenstadt, J. S., et al. (2006). Social modulation of pain as evidence for empathy in mice [Abstract]. *Science*, 312(5782), 1967–1970.
170. Thomson, H. (2010, March). We feel your pain: Extreme empaths. *The New Scientist*, (2751), 43–45.
171. Jackson, T., Iezzi, T., Chen, H., Ebnet, S., & Eglitis, K. (2005). Gender, interpersonal transactions, and the perception of pain: An experimental analysis [Abstract]. *The Journal of Pain*, 6(4), 228–236.
172. Keefe, F. J., & Somers, T. J. (2010). Psychological approaches to understanding and treating arthritis pain. *Nature Reviews Rheumatology*, 6(4), 210–216.
173. Singer, T., Seymour, B., O'Doherty, J., Kaube, H., Dolan, R. J., & Frith, C. D. (2004). Empathy for pain involves the affective but not sensory components of pain. *Science*, 303(5661), 1157–1162.
174. Botvinick, M., Jha, A. P., Bylsma, L. M., Fabian, S. A., Solomon, P. E., & Prkachin, K. M. (2005). Viewing facial expressions of pain engages cortical areas involved in the direct experience of pain. *NeuroImage*, 25(1), 312–319.
175. Singer, T., Seymour, B., O'Doherty, J. P., Stephan, K. E., Dolan, R. J., & Frith, C. D. (2006). Empathic neural responses are modulated by the perceived fairness of others. *Nature*, 439(7075), 466–469.

CHAPTER 7

1. H. Neizer (personal communication, October 2009).
2. Fishbain, D. A., Cole, B., Lewis, J., Rosomoff, H. L., & Rosomoff, R. S. (2008). What percentage of chronic nonmalignant pain patients exposed to chronic opioid analgesic therapy develop abuse/addiction and/or aberrant drug-related behaviors? A structured evidence-based review. *Pain Medicine, 9*(4), 444–459.
3. L. Webster (personal communication, February 26, 2011).
4. Szalavitz, M. (2011, November 2). Are doctors really to blame for the overdose epidemic? [Blog post]. Retrieved from http://healthland.time.com/2011/11/02/are-doctors-really-to-blame-for-the-overdose-epidemic
5. Institute of Medicine, Committee on Advancing Pain Research, Care, and Education. (2011). *Relieving pain in America: A blueprint for transforming prevention, care, education and research* (p. S-3). Prepublication copy. Washington, DC: National Academies Press.
6. Institute of Medicine, Committee on Advancing Pain Research, Care, and Education. (2011). *Relieving pain in America: A blueprint for transforming prevention, care, education and research* (pp. 3–28). Prepublication copy. Washington, DC: National Academies Press.
7. A. Paolitto (personal communication, October 8, 2012).
8. A. Kolodny (personal communication, October 5, 2012).
9. A. Kolodny (personal communication, March 26, 2013).
10. Orlando Business Journal. (2004, February 27). Orlando Sentinel reporter resigns, two editors reassigned in OxyContin story fallout. Retrieved from http://www.bizjournals.com/orlando/stories/2004/02/23/daily37.html
11. Libby, R. T. (2005, June 16). Treating doctors as drug dealers: The DEA's war on prescription painkillers. *Policy Analysis,* (545), 1–27. Retrieved from http://www.cato.org/pubs/pas/pa545.pdf
12. Centers for Disease Control and Prevention, National Center for Injury Prevention and Control. (2011, November). Prescription painkiller overdoses in the US. Retrieved from http://www.cdc.gov/VitalSigns/pdf/2011-11-vitalsigns.pdf.
13. Centers for Disease Control and Prevention, National Center for Injury Prevention and Control. (2011, November). Policy impact: Prescription painkiller overdoses. Retrieved from http://www.cdc.gov/homeandrecreationalsafety/rxbrief
14. Paulozzi, L., Jones, C. M., Mack, K. A., & Rudd, R. A. (2011). Vital signs: Overdoses of prescription opioid pain relievers—United States, 1999–2008. *Morbidity and Mortality Weekly Report, 60*(43), 1487–1492.
15. Warner, M., Chen, L. H., Makuc, D. M., Anderson, R. N., & Minino, A. M. (2011, December). Drug poisoning deaths in the United States, 1980–2008 [NCHS Data Brief, No. 81]. Retrieved from http://www.cdc.gov/nchs/data/databriefs/db81.pdf
16. M. Von Korff (personal communication, October 5, 2012).
17. Centers for Disease Control and Prevention. (n.d.). Prescription painkiller overdoses in the U.S. Retrieved from http://www.cdc.gov/Features/VitalSigns/PainkillerOverdoses

18. Patrick, S. W., Schumacher, R. E., Benneyworth, B. D., Krans, E. E., McAllister, J. M., & Davis, M. M. (2012). Neonatal abstinence syndrome and associated health care expenditures—United States 2000–2009. *Journal of the American Medical Association, 307*(18), 1934–1040.

19. CNNMoney.com. (2007, July 20). Purdue in $634 million settlement over OxyContin [Press release]. Retrieved from http://money.cnn.com/2007/07/20/news/companies/purdue/index.htm

20. National Institute on Drug Abuse. (2011, April 5). Analysis of opioid prescription practices finds area of concern [Press release]. Retrieved from http://www.drugabuse.gov/news-events/news-releases/2011/04/analysis-opioid-prescription-practices-finds-areas-concern

21. Centers for Disease Control and Prevention, National Center for Injury Prevention and Control. (2011, November). Policy impact: Prescription painkiller overdoses [Issue brief]. Retrieved from http://www.cdc.gov/homeandrecreationalsafety/rxbrief

22. Paulozzi, L., Jones, C. M., Mack, K. A., & Rudd, R. A. (2011). Vital signs: Overdoses of prescription opioid pain relievers—United States, 1999–2008. *Morbidity and Mortality Weekly Report, 60*(43), 1487–1492.

23. Centers for Disease Control and Prevention WONDER. (2013, February). Pharmaceutical overdose deaths, US, 2010. Retrieved from http://wonder.cdc.gov

24. C. Lenard (personal communication, March 27, 2013).

25. Adhikari, B., Kahende, J., Malarcher, A., Pechacek, T., & Tong, V. (2008). Smoking-attributable mortality, years of potential life lost, and productivity losses—United States, 2000–2004. *Morbidity and Mortality Weekly Report, 57*(45), 1226–1228.

26. Centers for Disease Control and Prevention. (2008). Alcohol and public health: Alcohol-Related Disease Impact (ARDI)—Average for United States 2001–2005—Alcohol-attributable deaths due to excessive alcohol use. Retrieved from http://apps.nccd.cdc.gov/DACH_ARDI/default/default.aspx

27. Lanza, F. L., Chan, F. K. L., & Quigley, E. M. M. (2009). Guidelines for prevention of NSAID-related ulcer complications. *American Journal of Gastroenterology, 104*, 728–738.

28. Wiegand, T. J., Wax, P. M., Schwartz, T., Finkelstein, Y., Gorodetsky, R., Brent, J., et al. (2012). The Toxicology Investigators Consortium case registry—the 2011 experience. *Journal of Medical Toxicology, 8*(4), 360–377.

29. Cave, D., & Schmidt, M. S. (2012, July 17). Rise in pill abuse forces new look at U.S. drug fight. *The New York Times*, p. A1.

30. Global Commission on Drug Policy. (2011, June). War on Drugs: Report of the Global Commission on Drug Policy. Retrieved from http://www.globalcommissionondrugs.org/wp-content/themes/gcdp_v1/pdf/Global_Commission_Report_English.pdf

31. Katz, J. M. (2011, June 2). Commission declares drug war failure, urges legalization. *The Boston Globe*, p. A6.

32. Brown, D. (2001, April 2). Nuclear power is safest way to make electricity, according to study. *The Washington Post*. Retrieved from http://www.washingtonpost.com/national/nuclear-power-is-safest-way-to-make-electricity-according-to-2007-study/2011/03/22/AFQUbyQC_story.html

33. Ropeik, D. (2011). *How risky is it, really? Why our fears don't always match the facts* (pp. 26–261). New York: McGraw-Hill.
34. Brooks, D. (2011). *The social animal: The hidden sources of love, character, and achievement* (p. x). New York: Random House.
35. Catan, T., Barrett, D., & Martin, T. W. (2012, October 5). Prescription for addiction [Saturday essay]. *The Wall Street Journal.* Retrieved from http://online.wsj.com/article/SB10000872396390444223104578036933277566700.html
36. Ballantyne, J. C. (2009). U.S. opioid risk management initiatives. *PAIN: Clinical Updates, 17*(6), 1–5.
37. R. Twillman (personal communication, June 1, 2011).
38. Paul, R. (2004, April 19). The federal war on pain relief [Blog post]. Retrieved from http://www.ronpaularchive.com/2004/04/the-federal-war-on-pain-relief/
39. Musto, D. F. (1999). *The American disease: Origins of narcotic control* (3rd ed.). Oxford, UK: Oxford University Press.
40. Ballantyne, J. C. & Shin, N. S. (2008). Efficacy of opioids for chronic pain: A review of the evidence. *The Clinical Journal of Pain, 24*(6), 469–478.
41. Ballantyne, J. C. (2009). U.S. opioid risk management initiatives. *PAIN: Clinical Updates, 17*(6), 1–5.
42. Zogenix. (2012, May 2). NDA submitted for Zohydro [Press release]. Retrieved from http://www.drugs.com/nda/zohydro_120502.html
43. CBC News Canada. (2011, December 26). More powerful painkiller coming: Hydrocodone raises fears of abuse. Retrieved from http://www.cbc.ca/news/health/story/2011/12/26/hydrocodone-painkiller-abuse.html
44. Eban, K. (2011). Painful medicine: What the strange saga of Purdue Pharma—and its $3 billion drug, OxyContin—tells us about our national dependence on painkillers. *Fortune, 164*(8), 144.
45. CBC News Canada. (2012, March 8). OxyContin marketing blamed for addiction epidemic. Retrieved from http://www.cbc.ca/news/canada/story/2012/03/08/oxycontin-marketing.html
46. Meier, B. (2007, May 10). In guilty plea, OxyContin maker to pay $600 million. *The New York Times.* Retrieved from http://www.nytimes.com/2007/05/10/business/11drug-web.html?pagewanted=all
47. Purdue Pharma. (2007, May 10). Statement of Purdue Pharma regarding resolution of the federal investigation in the western district of Virginia [Press release]. Retrieved from http://www.evaluatepharma.com/Universal/View.aspx?type=Story&id=126370
48. CNNMoney.com. (2007, July 20). Purdue in $634 million settlement over OxyContin [Press release]. Retrieved from http://money.cnn.com/2007/07/20/news/companies/purdue/index.htm
49. IMS HEALTH. (n.d.). Top U.S. pharmaceutical products by spending. Retrieved from http://www.imshealth.com/ims/Global/Content/Corporate/Press%20Room/Top-Line%20Market%20Data%20&%20Trends/2011%20Top-line%20Market%20Data/Top_Products_by_Sales.pdf
50. Ornstein, C., & Weber, T. (2012, May 8). American Pain Foundation shuts down as senators launch investigation of

prescription narcotics. Retrieved from http://www.propublica.org/article/senate-panel-investigates-drug-company-ties-to-pain-groups

51. American Pain Foundation. (2010). 2010 Annual Report (p. 16). Retrieved from http://s3.documentcloud.org/documents/277604/apf-2010-annual-report.pdf.

52. Ballantyne, J. (2011). Pain medicine: Repairing a fractured dream. *Anesthesiology, 114*(2), 243–246.

53. IMS Health. (n.d.). Top therapeutic classes by U.S. dispensed prescription. Retrieved from http://www.imshealth.com/deployedfiles/ims/Global/Content/Corporate/Press%20Room/Top-Line%20Market%20Data%20&%20Trends/2011%20Top-line%20Market%20Data/Top_Therapy_Classes_by_RX.pdf

54. Ballantyne, J. C. (2009). U.S. opioid risk management initiatives [Table 1: Summary of U.S. retail drug purchases, 1997–2005]. *PAIN: Clinical Updates, 17*(6), 2.

55. IMS Health. (n.d.). Top therapeutic classes by U.S. dispensed prescription. Retrieved from http://www.imshealth.com/deployedfiles/ims/Global/Content/Corporate/Press%20Room/Top-Line%20Market%20Data%20&%20Trends/2011%20Top-line%20Market%20Data/Top_Therapy_Classes_by_RX.pdf

56. B. Linton (personal communication, March 27, 2013).

57. K. Bush (personal communication, April 25, 2011).

58. R. Twillman (personal communication, June 1, 2011).

59. Department of Defense. (2010, January 5). Department of Defense announces results of 2008 health related behaviors survey [Press release]. Retrieved from http://www.rti.org/newsroom/news.cfm?objectid=9E651A68-5056-B172-B873C3640C367541

60. Office of National Drug Control Policy. (2011, April 19). Obama administration releases action plan to address national prescription drug abuse epidemic; Announces FDA action requiring drug makers to develop education program for prescribers about safe use of opioids [Press release]. Retrieved from http://www.justice.gov/dea/pubs/pressrel/pr041911.html

61. D. E. Hoffmann (personal communication, October 5, 2010).

62. Hoffmann, D. (2008). Treating pain v. reducing drug diversion and abuse: Recalibrating the balance in our drug control laws and policies. *St. Louis University Journal of Health Law and Policy, 1*(2), 256.

63. Executive Office of the President of the United States. (2011). Epidemic: Responding to America's prescription drug abuse crisis (p. 5). Retrieved from http://www.whitehouse.gov/sites/default/files/ondcp/issues-content/prescription-drugs/rx_abuse_plan_0.pdf

64. Valencia, M. J. (2011, March 4). Doctor indicted in 6 drug fatalities. *The Boston Globe*, pp. A1, A9.

65. Van Zeller, M. (2009, October 15). The OxyContin express [Webisode]. *Vanguard*. Retrieved from http://current.com/groups/vanguard-the-oxycontin-express

66. Anderson, C. (2011, April 20). Deadly abuse puts focus on "pill mills." *The Boston Globe*. Retrieved from http://articles.boston.

com/2011-04-20/news/29451932_1_cocaine-deaths-oxycodone-pi
lls-prescription-drugs

67. LaMendola, B., & Campbell, A. (2011, February 23). Feds, police
    raid 11 south Florida pill mills. *The South Florida Sun-Sentinel*.
    Retrieved from http://articles.sun-sentinel.com/2011-02-23/health/
    fl-pill-mill-raids-20110223_1_pain-clinics-pill-mills-pain-pill

68. United States Drug Enforcement Administration. (2011, October 28).
    DEA administrator, attorney general announce enforcement efforts
    against illegal prescription drug distributors in Florida [Press release].
    Retrieved from http://www.justice.gov/dea/pubs/pressrel/pr102811.
    html

69. Hoffmann, D. (2008). Treating pain v. reducing drug diversion and
    abuse: Recalibrating the balance in our drug control laws and policies. *St.
    Louis University Journal of Health Law and Policy, 1*(2), 256.

70. B. L. Carreno (personal communication, April 11, 2011).

71. Richard, J., & Reidenberg, M. M. (2005). The risk of disciplinary action by
    state medical boards against physicians prescribing opioids. *Journal of Medical
    Licensure and Discipline, 91*(2), 14–19.

72. Goldenbaum, D. M., Christopher, M., Gallagher, R. M., Fishman, S.,
    Payne, R., Joranson, D., et al. (2008). Physicians charged with opioid
    analgesic-prescribing offenses. *Pain Medicine, 9*(6), 737–747.

73. Center for Practical Bioethics, National Association of Attorneys General,
    & Federation of State Medical Boards. (2008, September 9). Few physicians
    actually tried or sanctioned for improperly prescribing pain medications
    [Press release]. Retrieved from http://drugcontrol.flgov.com/pdmp/docu-
    ments/Few_physicians_tried_or_sanctioned.pdf

74. Hoffmann, D. (2008). Treating pain v. reducing drug diversion and
    abuse: Recalibrating the balance in our drug control laws and policies. *St.
    Louis University Journal of Health Law and Policy, 1*(2), 231–309.

75. R. Sauber (personal communication, February 23, 2011).

76. L. Webster (personal communication, February 17, 2011).

77. L. Webster (personal communication, May 25, 2011).

78. J. Dahl (personal communication, March 19, 2013).

79. Bates, C., Laciak, R., Southwick, A., & Bishoff, J. (2011). Overprescription
    of postoperative narcotics: A look at postoperative pain medication deliv-
    ery, consumption and disposal in urological practice. *The Journal of Urology,
    185*(2), 551–555.

80. Kehlet, H. (2005). Postoperative opioid sparing to hasten recovery: What are
    the issues? *Anesthesiology, 102*(6), 1083–1085.

81. Kehlet, H., Rung, G. W., & Callesen, T. (1996). Postoperative opioid
    analgesia: Time for a reconsideration? *Journal of Clinical Anesthesia, 8*(6),
    441–445.

82. Von Korff, M. R. (2010, May). *Trends and risks of chronic opioid therapy
    among the elderly. Paper* presented at the 5th Annual NIH Pain Consortium
    Symposium, Washington, DC.

83. M. Von Korff (personal communication, February 23, 2011).

84. C. Stencel (personal communication, March 27, 2012).

85. Portenoy, R. K., Ugarte, C., Fuller, I., & Haas, G. (2004). Population-based survey of pain in the United States: Differences among White, African-American, and Hispanic subjects. *The Journal of Pain, 5*(6), 317–328.

86. The Mayday Fund. (2009). A call to revolutionize chronic pain care in America: An opportunity in health care reform. Retrieved from http://www.maydaypainreport.org/docs/A%20Call%20to%20Revolutionize%20Chronic%20Pain%20Care%20in%20America%2003.04.10.pdf

87. Shi Q., Langer, G., Cohen, J., & Cleeland, C. S. (2007). People in pain: How do they seek relief? *The Journal of Pain, 8*(8), 624–636.

88. Nwokeji, E., Rascati, K., Brown, C., & Eisenberg, A. (2007). Influences of attitudes on family physicians' willingness to prescribe long-acting opioid analgesics for patients with chronic nonmalignant pain. *Clinical Therapeutics, 29*(11), 2589–2602.

89. Quill, T. E., & Meier, D. (2006). The big chill—inserting the DEA into end-of-life care [Perspective]. *New England Journal of Medicine, 354*, 1–3.

90. Cherny, N. I., Baselga, J., de Conno, F., & Radbruch, L. (2010). Formulary availability and regulatory barriers to accessibility of opioids for cancer pain in Europe: A report from the ESMO/EAPC opioid policy initiative. *Annals of Oncology, 21*(3), 615–626.

91. Human Rights Watch. (2009, March). "Please do not make us suffer anymore...": Access to pain treatment as a human right. Retrieved from www.hrw.org/en/node/81079/section/3

92. Human Rights Watch. (2009, October). Unbearable pain: India's obligation to ensure palliative care. Retrieved from http://www.hrw.org/sites/default/files/reports/health1009web.pdf

93. World Health Organization. (2009, February). World Health Organization Briefing Note—February 2009: Access to controlled medications programme. Retrieved from http://www.who.int/medicines/areas/quality_safety/ACMP_BrNoteGenrl_EN_Feb09.pdf

94. Cleary, J. F., Hutson, P., & Joranson, D. (2010). Access to therapeutic opioid medications in Europe by 2011? Fifty years on from the Single Convention on Narcotic Drugs [Editorial]. *Palliative Medicine, 24*(2), 109–110.

95. Human Rights Watch. (2009, March). "Please do not make us suffer anymore...": Access to pain treatment as a human right. Retrieved from www.hrw.org/en/node/81079/section/3

96. Chapman, C. R., Lipschitz, D. L., Angst, M. S., Chou, R., Densico, R. C., Donaldson, G. W., et al. (2010). Opioid pharmacotherapy for chronic non-cancer pain in the United States: A research guideline for developing an evidence-base [Opioid pharmacotherapy research guideline]. *The Journal of Pain, 11*(9), 810.

97. Ross, E. L., Holcomb, C., & Jamison, R. N. (2009). Addressing abuse and misuse of opioid analgesics. *Drug Benefit Trends, 21*(2), 54–63.

98. Institute of Medicine, Committee on Advancing Pain Research, Care, and Education. (2011). *Relieving pain in America: A blueprint for transforming prevention, care, education and research* (p. GL–1). Prepublication copy. Washington, DC: National Academies Press.

99. American Society of Addiction Medicine. (2011, April 12). Public policy statement: Definition of addiction. Retrieved from http://www.asam.org/for-the-public/definition-of-addiction

100. American Society of Addiction Medicine. (2011, August 15). ASAM releases new definition of addiction [Press release]. Retrieved from http://www.eurekalert.org/pub_releases/2011-08/asoa-arn072111.php

101. Szalavitz, M. (2011, August 16). Why the new definition of addiction, as "brain disease," falls short. *Time.* Retrieved from http://healthland.time.com/2011/08/16/why-the-new-definition-of-addiction-as-brain-disease-falls-short

102. J. Dahl (personal communication, March 17, 2013).

103. Ballantyne, J. C., Sullivan, M. D., & Kolodny, A. (2012). Opioid dependence vs addiction: A distinction without a difference? *Archives of Internal Medicine, 172*(17),1342–1343.

104. A. Kolodny (personal communication, October 5, 2012).

105. M. Maglio (personal communication, March 23, 2010)

106. R. Portenoy (personal communication, March 9, 2011).

107. R. Portenoy (personal communication, September 10, 2009).

108. H. Heit (personal communication, March 1, 2011).

109. L. Webster (personal communication, May 17, 2012).

110. Gelernter, J., Panhuysen, C., Wilcox, M., Hesselbrock, V., Rounsaville, B., Poling, J., et al. (2006). Genomewide linkage scan for opioid dependence and related traits. *American Journal of Human Genetics, 78*(5), 759–769.

111. L. Webster (personal communication, March 4, 2011).

112. S. Simson (personal communication, May 24, 2012).

113. Minozzi, S., Amato, L., & Davoli, M. (2013). Development of dependence following treatment with opioid analgesics for pain relief: A systematic review. *Addiction 108*(4), 688–698.

114. Fishbain, D. A., Rosomoff, H. L., & Rosomoff, R. S. (1992). Drug abuse, dependence, and addiction in chronic pain patients. *The Clinical Journal of Pain, 8*(2), 77–85.

115. Fishbain, D. A., Cole, B., Lewis, J., Rosomoff, H. L., & Rosomoff, R. S. (2008). What percentage of chronic nonmalignant pain patients exposed to chronic opioid analgesic therapy develop abuse/addiction and/or aberrant drug-related behaviors? A structured evidence-based review. *Pain Medicine, 9*(4), 444–459.

116. Webster, L. R., & Webster, R. M. (2005). Predicting aberrant behaviors in opioid-treated patients: Preliminary validation of the opioid risk tool. *Pain Medicine, 6*(6), 432–442.

117. Fleming, M. F., Balousek, S. L., Klessig, C. L., Mundt, M. P., & Brown, D. D. (2007). Substance use disorders in a primary care sample receiving daily opioid therapy. *The Journal of Pain, 8*(7), 573–582.

118. Chapman, C. R., Lipschitz, D. L., Angst, M. S., Chou, R., Densico, R. C., Donaldson, G. W., et al. (2010). Opioid pharmacotherapy for chronic non-cancer pain in the United States: A research guideline for developing an

evidence-base [Opioid pharmacotherapy research guideline]. *The Journal of Pain, 11*(9), 810.

119. Noble, M., Treadwell, J. R., Tregear, S. J., Coates, V. H., Wiffen, P. J., Akafomo, C., et al. (2010). Long-term opioid management for chronic noncancer pain [Intervention review]. *Cochrane Database of Systematic Reviews, 2010*(1), CD006605.

120. Banta-Green, C. J., Merrill, J. O., Doyle, S. R., Boudreau, D. M., & Calsyn, D. A. (2009). Opioid use behaviors, mental health and pain—development of a typology of chronic pain patients. *Drug and Alcohol Dependence, 104*(1–2), 34–42.

121. M. Von Korff (personal communication, February 28, 2011).

122. Kauffman, J. F. (2011). Strategies for managing pain & opioid dependence [PowerPoint slides]. Copy in possession of author.

123. J. Kauffman (personal communication, February 23, 2011).

124. Von Korff, M. (2010). Commentary on Boscarino et al. (2010): Understanding the spectrum of opioid abuse, misuse and harms among chronic opioid therapy patients. *Addiction, 105*(10), 1783–1784.

125. Wasan, A., Butler, S. F., Budman, S. H., Benoit, C., Fernandez, K., & Jamison, R. N. (2007). Psychiatric history and psychologic adjustment as risk factors for aberrant drug-related behavior among patients with chronic pain. *The Clinical Journal of Pain, 23*(4), 307–315.

126. Jamison, R. N., Ross, E. L., Michna,E., Chen, L. Q., Holcomb, C., & Wasan A. D. (2010). Substance misuse treatment for high-risk chronic pain patients on opioid therapy: A randomized trial. *PAIN, 150*(3), 390–400.

127. Jamison, R. N., Link, C. L., & Marceau, L. D. (2009). Do pain patients at high risk for substance misuse experience more pain? A longitudinal outcomes study. *Pain Medicine, 10*(6), 1084–1094.

128. Von Korff, M. (2010). Commentary on Boscarino et al. (2010): Understanding the spectrum of opioid abuse, misuse and harms among chronic opioid therapy patients. *Addiction, 105*(10), 1783–1784.

129. World Health Organization. (2009, February). World Health Organization Briefing Note—February 2009: Access to controlled medications programme. Retrieved from http://www.who.int/medicines/areas/quality_safety/ACMP_BrNoteGenrl_EN_Feb09.pdf

130. Foreman, J. (2008, September 15). When pain arrives and help does not. *The Boston Globe.* Retrieved from http://judyforeman.com/columns/when-pain-arrives-and-help-does-not

131. National Institute on Drug Abuse. (2011, April 5). Analysis of opioid prescription practices finds areas of concern [Press release]. Retrieved from http://www.drugabuse.gov/news-events/news-releases/2011/04/analysis-opioid-prescription-practices-finds-areas-concern

132. Centers for Disease Control and Prevention, National Center for Injury Prevention and Control. (2011, November). Policy impact: Prescription painkiller overdoses. Retrieved from http://www.cdc.gov/homeandrecreationalsafety/rxbrief

133. U.S. Department of Justice, National Drug Intelligence Center. (2010, February). National drug threat assessment 2010 [Executive summary]. Retrieved from http://www.justice.gov/ndic/pubs38/38661/execSum.htm

134. Chapman, C. R., Lipschitz, D. L., Angst, M. S., Chou, R., Densico, R. C., Donaldson, G. W., et al. (2010). Opioid pharmacotherapy for chronic non-cancer pain in the United States: A research guideline for developing an evidence-base [Opioid pharmacotherapy research guideline]. *The Journal of Pain, 11*(9), 810.

135. Dunn, K. M., Saunders, K. W., Rutter, C. M., Banta-Green, C. J., Merrill, J. O., Sullivan, M. D., et al. (2010). Opioid prescriptions for chronic pain and overdose. *Annals of Internal Medicine, 152*, 85–92.

136. Bohnert, A. S. B., Valenstein, M., Bair, M. J., Ganoczy, D., McCarthy, J. F., Ilgen, M. A., et al. (2011). Association between opioid prescribing patterns and opioid overdose-related deaths. *Journal of the American Medical Association, 305*(13), 1315–1321.

137. Gomes, T., Mamdani, M. M., Dhalla, I. A., Paterson, J. M., & Juurlink, D. N. (2011). Opioid dose and drug-related mortality in patients with nonmalignant pain. *Archives of Internal Medicine, 171*(7), 686–691.

138. Hall, A. J., Logan, J. E., Toblin, R. L., Kaplan, J. A., Kraner, J. C., Bixler, D., et al. (2008). Patterns of abuse among unintentional pharmaceutical overdose fatalities. *Journal of the American Medical Association, 300*(22), 2613–2620.

139. Arria, A. M., Garnier-Dykstra, L. M., Caldeira, K. M., Vincent, K. B., & O'Grady, K. E. (2001). Prescription analgesic use among young adults: Adherence to physician instructions and diversion. *Pain Medicine, 12*(6), 898–903.

140. Cruciani, R., Fine, P., & January, C. (2010, May 8). *Methadone prescribing: Everything you wanted to know but were afraid to ask.* Paper presented at the 29th Annual Scientific Meeting of the American Pain Society Meeting, Baltimore, MD.

141. J. Dahl (personal communication, May 24, 2011).

142. H. Heit (personal communication, May 18, 2012).

143. D. Carr (personal communication, April 23, 2012).

144. L. Webster (personal communication, May 17, 2012).

145. U.S. Food and Drug Administration. (2006, November 27). Public health advisory: Methadone use for pain control may result in death and life-threatening changes in breathing and heart beat [Press release]. Retrieved from http://www.fda.gov/Drugs/DrugSafety/PostmarketDrugSafetyInformationforPatientsandProviders/DrugSafetyInformationforHeathcareProfessionals/PublicH

146. J. Kauffman (personal communication, February 23, 2011).

147. Seattle Times staff. (2012, April 16). Seattle Times methadone investigation wins Pulitzer Prize. *The Seattle Times.* Retrieved from http://seattletimes.nwsource.com/html/localnews/2017994882_pulitzer17m.html

148. Chapman, C. R., Lipschitz, D. L., Angst, M. S., Chou, R., Densico, R. C., Donaldson, G. W., et al. (2010). Opioid pharmacotherapy for chronic

non-cancer pain in the United States: A research guideline for developing an evidence-base [Opioid pharmacotherapy research guideline]. *The Journal of Pain, 11*(9), 807–829.

149. J. Dahl (personal communication, March 17, 2013).

150. Saunders, K. W., Dunn, K. M., Merrill, J. O., Sullivan, M., Weisner, C., Braden, J. B., et al. (2010). Relationship of opioid use and dosage levels to fractures in older chronic pain patients. *Journal of General Internal Medicine, 25*(4), 310–315.

151. National Osteoporosis Foundation. (2011). Fast facts. Retrieved from http://www.nof.org/node/40

152. Rajagopal, A., Vassilopoulou-Sellin, R., Palmer, J. L., Kaur, G., & Bruera, E. (2003). Hypogonadism and sexual dysfunction in male cancer survivors receiving chronic opioid therapy. *Journal of Pain Symptom Management, 26*(5), 1055–1061.

153. Rubinstein, A., Carpenter, D. M., & Minkoff, J. (2013). Hypogonadism in men with chronic pain linked to the use of long-acting rather than short-acting opioids. *The Clinical Journal of Pain*. Advance online publication. Retrieved from http://journals.lww.com/clinicalpain/Abstract/publisha-head/Hypogonadism_in_Men_With_Chronic_Pain_Linked_to.99660.aspx

154. J. Dahl (personal communication, March 17, 2013).

155. Katz, M. H. (2010). Long-term opioid treatment of nonmalignant pain: A believer loses his faith [Editorial]. *Archives of General Medicine, 170*(16), 1422–1423.

156. Von Korff, M. (2010). Commentary on Boscarino et al. (2010): Understanding the spectrum of opioid abuse, misuse and harms among chronic opioid therapy patients. *Addiction, 105*(10), 1783–1784.

157. Chapman, C. R., Lipschitz, D. L., Angst, M. S., Chou, R., Densico, R. C., Donaldson, G. W., et al. (2010). Opioid pharmacotherapy for chronic non-cancer pain in the United States: A research guideline for developing an evidence-base [Opioid pharmacotherapy research guideline]. *The Journal of Pain, 11*(9), 807–829.

158. Chu, L. F., Angst, M. S., & Clark, D. (2008). Opioid-induced hyperalgesia in humans: Molecular mechanisms and clinical considerations [Special topic series]. *The Clinical Journal of Pain, 24*(6), 479–496.

159. L. Watkins (personal communication, October 28, 2009).

160. Chu, L. F., Angst, M. S., & Clark, D. (2008). Opioid-induced hyperalgesia in humans: Molecular mechanisms and clinical considerations [Special topic series]. *The Clinical Journal of Pain, 24*(6), 479–496.

161. US Department of Health and Human Services, Substance Abuse and Mental Health Services Administration. (2010, September). *Results from the 2009 National Survey on Drug Use and Health: Volume I. Summary of national findings* (HHS Publication No. SMA 10-4586 Findings). Retrieved from http://oas.samhsa.gov/NSDUH/2k9NSDUH/2k9ResultsP.pdf

162. United States Drug Enforcement Administration. (2012, September 25). DEA holds its fifth prescription drug take-back day September 29 as public

participation continues to rise [Press release]. Retrieved from http://www. justice.gov/dea/divisions/hq/2012/hq092512.shtml

163. Smarxt Disposal. (n.d.). Smarxt disposal: A prescription for a healthy planet. Retrieved from www.smarxtdisposal.net/index.html

164. Inciardi, J. A., Surratt, H. L., Kurtz, S. P., & Cicero, T. J. (2007). Mechanisms of prescription drug diversion among drug-involved club- and street-based populations. *Pain Medicine, 8*(2), 171–183.

165. Institute of Medicine, Committee on Advancing Pain Research, Care, and Education. (2011). *Relieving pain in America: A blueprint for transforming prevention, care, education and research* (pp. 2–26). Prepublication copy. Washington, DC: National Academies Press.

166. Fisch, M. J., Lee, J-W., Weiss, M., Wagner, L. I., Chang, V. T., Cella, D., et al. (2012). Prospective, observational study of pain and analgesic prescribing in medical oncology outpatients with breast, colorectal, lung, or prostate cancer. *Journal of Clinical Oncology, 30*(16), 1980–1988.

167. Ackerman, T. (2012, April 19). Pain treatment lacking for a third of cancer patients, study says. *Houston Chronicle*. Retrieved from http://www.chron.com/news/houston-texas/article/A-third-of-cancer-patients-pain-3496068.php

168. T. Fersch (personal communication, March 9, 2011).

169. R. Jamison (personal communication, February 14, 2011).

170. Chou, R., Fanciullo, G. J., Fine, P. G., Adler, J. A., Ballantyne, J. C., Davies, P., et al. (2009). Clinical guidelines for the use of chronic opioid therapy in chronic noncancer pain. *The Journal of Pain, 10*(2), 113–130.

171. Ballantyne, J. C., & Shin, N. S. (2008). Efficacy of opioids for chronic pain: A review of the evidence. *The Clinical Journal of Pain, 24*(6), 469–478.

172. Tennant, F. (2010, January 1). Opioid treatment 10-year longevity survey final report. *Practical Pain Management*. Retrieved from http://www. practicalpainmanagement.com/treatments/pharmacological/opioids/opioid-treatment-10-year-longevity-survey-final-report

173. Hamza, M., Doleys, D., Wells, M., Weisbein, J., Hoff, J., Martin, M., et al. (2012). Prospective study of 3-year follow-up of low-dose intrathecal opioids in the management of chronic nonmalignant pain. *Pain Medicine, 13*(10), 1304–1313.

174. Chapman, C. R., Lipschitz, D. L., Angst, M. S., Chou, R., Densico, R. C., Donaldson, G. W., et al. (2010). Opioid pharmacotherapy for chronic non-cancer pain in the United States: A research guideline for developing an evidence-base [Opioid pharmacotherapy research guideline]. *The Journal of Pain, 11*(9), 807–829.

175. Manchikanti, L., Ailinani, H., Koyyalagunta, D., Datta, S., Singh, V., Eriator, I., et al. (2011). A systematic review of randomized trials of long-term opioid management for chronic non-cancer pain. *Pain Physician, 14*, 91–121.

176. Andrews, N. (2012, July 9). Moving pain treatments forward: An FDA public scientific workshop. Retrieved from http://www.painresearchforum.org/news/17889-moving-pain-treatments-forward-fda-public-scientific-workshop

177. Noble, M., Tregear, S. J., Treadwell, J. R., & Schoelles, K. (2008). Long-term opioid management for chronic noncancer pain: A systematic review and meta-analysis of efficacy and safety. *Journal of Pain and Symptom Management, 35*(2), 214–228.

178. Physicians for Responsible Opioid Prescribing. (n.d.). Cautious, evidence-based opioid prescribing. Retrieved from http://www.support-prop.org/educational/PROP_OpioidPrescribing.pdf

179. Von Korff, M., Kolodny, A., Deyo, R. A., & Chou, R. (2011). Long-term opioid therapy reconsidered. *Annals of Internal Medicine, 155*(5), 325–328.

180. Noble, M., Tregear, S. J., Treadwell, J. R., & Schoelles, K. (2008). Long-term opioid management for chronic noncancer pain: A systematic review and meta-analysis of efficacy and safety. *Journal of Pain and Symptom Management, 35*(2), 214–228.

181. Noble, M., Treadwell, J. R., Tregear, S. J., Coates, V. H., Wiffen, P. J., Akafomo, C., et al. (2010). Long-term opioid management for chronic non-cancer pain [Intervention review]. *Cochrane Database of Systematic Reviews, 2010*(1), CD006605.

182. Chapman, C. R., Lipschitz, D. L., Angst, M. S., Chou, R., Densico, R. C., Donaldson, G. W., et al. (2010). Opioid pharmacotherapy for chronic non-cancer pain in the United States: A research guideline for developing an evidence-base [Opioid pharmacotherapy research guideline]. *The Journal of Pain, 11*(9), 807–829.

183. Eriksen, J., Sjogren, P., Bruera, E., Ekhold, O., & Rasmussen, N. K. (2006). Critical issues on opioids in chronic non-cancer pain: An epidemiological study. *PAIN, 125,* 172–179.

184. Joranson, D. E. (2004). Improving availability of opioid pain medications: Testing the principle of balance in Latin America. *Journal of Palliative Medicine, 7*(1), 105–114.

185. Sjogren, P., Gronbaek, M., Peuckmann, V., & Ekholm, O. (2010) A population-based cohort study on chronic pain: The role of opioids. *The Clinical Journal of Pain, 26*(9), 763–769.

186. Ballantyne, J. C., & Shin, N. S. (2008). Efficacy of opioids for chronic pain: A review of the evidence. *The Clinical Journal of Pain, 24*(6), 469–478.

187. Katz, M. H. (2010). Long-term opioid treatment of nonmalignant pain: A believer loses his faith [Editorial]. *Archives of General Medicine, 170*(16), 1422–1423.

188. Foley, K. M., Fins, J. J., & Inturrisi, C. E. (2011). A true believer's flawed analysis. *Archives of Internal Medicine, 171*(9), 867–868.

189. US Drug Enforcement Administration. (2012, April 17). Controlled substances by CSA schedule. Retrieved from http://www.deadiversion.usdoj.gov/schedules/orangebook/e_cs_sched.pdf

190. Office of Diversion Control, U.S. Department of Justice. (2013, May). List of controlled substances. Retrieved from http://www.deadiversion.usdoj.gov/schedules/#define

CHAPTER 8

1. Leavitt, S. B. (2010). Intranasal naloxone for at-home opioid rescue. *Practical Pain Management*. Retrieved from http://www.practicalpainmanagement.com/treatments/pharmacological/opioids/intranasal-naloxone-home-opioid-rescue

2. Szalavitz, M. (2011, September 27). Drugs, risk and the myth of the "evil" addict [Blog post]. Retrieved from http://opinionator.blogs.nytimes.com/2011/09/27/drugs-risk-and-the-myth-of-the-evil-addict

3. Project Lazarus. (n.d.). Project Lazarus results for Wilkes County. Retrieved from http://www.projectlazarus.org/project-lazarus-results-wilkes-county

4. Albert, S., Brason, F. W., II, Sanford, C. K., Dasgupta, N., Graham, J., & Lovette, B. (2011). Project Lazarus: Community-based overdose prevention in rural North Carolina. *Pain Medicine, 12*(Supplement 2), S77–S85.

5. J. Dahl (personal communication, March 27, 2013).

6. Lazar, K. (2011, August 31). Progress seen in fight on heroin. *The Boston Globe*. Retrieved from http://articles.boston.com/2011-08-31/news/29949874_1_narcan-overdose-deaths-addicts

7. The Massachusetts Department of Public Health. (2012, April 25). The Massachusetts Department of Public Health opioid overdose prevention and reversal information sheet. Retrieved from http://www.mass.gov/eohhs/docs/dph/substance-abuse/naloxone-info.pdf

8. Centers for Disease Control and Prevention. (2012). Community-based opioid overdose prevention programs providing naloxone—United States, 2010. *Morbidity and Mortality Weekly Report, 61*(6), 101–105.

9. US Food and Drug Administration. (2011, November 22). Role of naloxone in opioid overdose fatality prevention; Public workshop, preliminary agenda. Retrieved from http://pain-topics.org/docs/FDA-NaloxoneMeeting-April2012.pdf

10. D. Carr (personal communication, April 23, 2012).

11. D. Carr (personal communication, April 23, 2012).

12. Johnson, K. (2012, April 12). Taking it to feel normal: My Oxycodone experience [Blog post]. Retrieved from http://commonhealth.wbur.org/2012/04/painkiller-addiction

13. D. Carr (personal communication, October 4, 2012).

14. J. Dahl (personal communication, March 27, 2013).

15. C. Garner (personal communication, March 16, 2011).

16. L. Webster (personal communication, May 25, 2011).

17. J. Kauffman (personal communication, February 23, 2011).

18. J. Kauffman (personal communication, May 13, 2012).

19. J. Dahl (personal communication, May 25, 2011).

20. J. Kauffman (personal communication, May 13, 2012).

21. MacArthur, G. J., Minozzi, S., Martin, N., Vickerman, P., Deren, S., Bruneau, J., et al. (2012). Opiate substitution treatment and HIV transmission in people who inject drugs: Systematic review and meta-analysis. *British Medical Journal, 345*, e5945.

22. Arbuck, D. M. (2011, April 6). Is buprenorphine effective for chronic pain? Retrieved from http://updates.pain-topics.org/2011/04/is-buprenorphine-effective-for-chronic.html
23. D. Carr (personal communication, April 23, 2012).
24. Arbuck, D. M. (2011, April 6). Is buprenorphine effective for chronic pain? Retrieved from http://updates.pain-topics.org/2011/04/is-buprenorphine-effective-for-chronic.html
25. L. Webster (personal communication, May 25, 2011).
26. S. B. Leavitt (personal communication, May 10, 2011).
27. Weiss, R. D., Potter, J. S., Fiellin, D. A., Byrne, M., Connery, H. S., Dickinson, W., et al. (2011). Adjunctive counseling during brief and extended buprenorphine-naloxone treatment for prescription opioid dependence. *Archives of General Psychiatry, 68*(12), 1238–1246.
28. Drugs.com. (n.d.). Butrans approval history. Retrieved from http://www.drugs.com/history/butrans.html
29. Ling, W., Casadonte, P., Bigelow, G., Kampman, K. M., Patkar, A., Bailey, G. L., et al. (2010). Buprenorphine implants for treatment of opioid dependence: A randomized clinical trial. *Journal of the American Medical Association, 304*(14), 1576–1583.
30. O'Connor, P. G. (2010). Advances in the treatment of opioid dependence: Continued progress and ongoing challenges [Editorial]. *Journal of the American Medical Association, 304*(14), 1612–1614.
31. Steiner, D., Munera, C., Hale, M., Ripa, S., & Landau, C. (2011). Efficacy and safety of buprenorphine transdermal system (BTDS) for chronic moderate to severe low back pain: A randomized, double-blind study. *The Journal of Pain, 12*(11), 1163–1172.
32. Arbuck, D. M. (2011, April 6). Is buprenorphine effective for chronic pain? Retrieved from http://updates.pain-topics.org/2011/04/is-buprenorphine-effective-for-chronic.html
33. Hitt, E. (2010, October 14). Once-monthly naltrexone approved for treatment of opioid addiction. Retrieved from http://www.medscape.com/viewarticle/730457?src=rss
34. P. Fine (personal communication, October, 2009).
35. Knotkova, H., Fine, P. G., & Portenoy, R. K. (2009). Opioid rotation: The science and the limitations of the equianalgesic dose table. *Journal of Pain and Symptom Management, 38*(3), 426–439.
36. Chou, R., Fanciullo, G. J., Fine, P. G., Adler, J. A., Ballantyne, J. C., Davies, P., et al. (2009). Clinical guidelines for the use of chronic opioid therapy in chronic noncancer pain. *The Journal of Pain, 10*(2), 113–130.
37. Leavitt, S. B. (2009, November 21). Opioid rotation: Benefits, challenges, hazards. Retrieved from http://updates.pain-topics.org/2009/11/opioid-rotation-benefits-challenges.html
38. Arbuck, D. M. (2012, February 8). New views of opioid equivalency. Retrieved from http://updates.pain-topics.org/2012/02/new-views-on-opioid-equivalency.html
39. Webster, L. R., & Fine, P. G. (2012). Overdose deaths demand a new paradigm for opioid rotation. *Pain Medicine, 13*(4), 571–574.

40. Webster, L. R., & Fine, P. G. (2012). Review and critique of opioid rotation practices and associated risks of toxicity. *Pain Medicine, 13*(4), 562–570.
41. Leavitt, S. B. (2012, April 5). New perspectives on safer opioid rotation. Retrieved from http://updates.pain-topics.org/2012/04/new-perspectives-on-safer-opioid.html
42. R. Twillman (personal communication, June 2, 2011).
43. Katz, N. (2008). Abuse-deterrent opioid formulations: Are they a pipe dream? *Current Rheumatology Reports, 10*(1), 11–18.
44. L. Webster (personal communication, February 17, 2011).
45. J. Heins (personal communication, May 15, 2012).
46. Eban, K. (2011, November 21). OxyContin: Purdue Pharma's painful medicine. Retrieved from http://features.blogs.fortune.cnn.com/2011/11/09/oxycontin-purdue-pharma/
47. Purdue Pharma. (2002, June 27). Purdue Pharma implements national surveillance system to track diversion and abuse of controlled pain medications [Press release]. Retrieved from http://headaches.about.com/bl-radars.htm
48. Dart, R. (2011). RADARS system abuse/tamper deterrent formulations: 2011 update and analysis. Retrieved from http://www.radars.org/Portals/1/04_DartR_ADF_Update_distribution_20120502.pdf
49. Burke, J. (2011, May 16). The OxyContin reformulation: Is it working? Retrieved from http://www.pharmacytimes.com/publications/issue/2011/May2011/DrugDiversion-0511
50. Cicero, T. J., Ellis, M. S., & Surratt, H. L. (2012). Effect of abuse-deterrent formulation of OxyContin [Letter to the editor]. *New England Journal of Medicine, 367,* 187–198.
51. Leavitt, S. B. (2012, July 13). Abuse-deterrent opioids spawn upsurge in heroin. Retrieved from http://updates.pain-topics.org/2012/07/abuse-deterrent-opioids-spawn-upsurge.html
52. Leger, D. L. (2012, July 10). Opana abuse in USA overtakes OxyContin. Retrieved from http://www.usatoday.com/news/nation/story/2012-07-10/opana-painkiller-addiction/56137086/1#
53. EMBEDA. (n.d.). Important information for patients and prescribers. Retrieved from http://www.embeda.com
54. L. Webster (personal communication, February 17, 2011).
55. Drugs.com. (n.d.). Remoxy approval status. Retrieved from http://www.drugs.com/history/remoxy.html
56. Leavitt, S. B. (2011, August 12). Abuse-deterrent opioids; A better mousetrap? Retrieved from http://updates.pain-topics.org/2011/08/abuse-deterrent-opioids-better.html
57. National Institute of Drug Abuse. (2012, July 25). NIDA supports development of combined anti-heroin and HIV vaccine [Press release]. Retrieved from http://www.drugabuse.gov/news-events/news-releases/2012/07/nida-supports-development-combined-anti-heroin-hiv-vaccine-0
58. Payne, R., Anderson, E., Arnold, R., Duensing, L., Gilson, A. Green, C., et al. (2010). A rose by any other name: Pain contracts/agreements. *American Journal of Bioethics, 10*(11), 5–12.

59. Andrews, M. (2011, April 4). Some doctors require patients to sign contracts get opioid painkillers. *The Washington Post*. Retrieved from http://www.washingtonpost.com/national/health/some-doctors-require-patients-to-sign-contracts-get-opioid-painkillers/2011/03/29/AF7D31dC_story.html

60. Payne, R., Anderson, E., Arnold, R., Duensing, L., Gilson, A. Green, C., et al. (2010). A rose by any other name: Pain contracts/agreements. *American Journal of Bioethics*, 10(11), 5–12.

61. Hariharan, J., Lamb, G. C., & Neuner, J. M. (2007). Long-term opioid contract use for chronic pain management in primary care practice: A five year experience. *Journal of General Internal Medicine*, 22(4), 485–490.

62. Starrels, J. L., Becker, W. C., Alford, D. P., Kapoor, A., Williams, A. R., & Turner, B. J. (2010). Systematic review: Treatment agreements and urine drug testing to reduce opioid misuse in patients with chronic pain. *Annals of Internal Medicine*, 152(11), 712–720.

63. R. Jamison (personal communication, February 14, 2011).

64. Katz, M. H. (2010). Long-term opioid treatment of nonmalignant pain: A believer loses his faith [Editorial]. *Archives of General Medicine*, 170(16), 1422–1423.

65. Collen, M. (2009). Opioid contracts and random drug testing for people with chronic pain—think twice. *Journal of Law, Medicine & Ethics*, 37(4), 841–845.

66. Centers for Disease Control and Prevention. (2010, July). Unintentional drug poisoning in the United States. Retrieved from http://www.cdc.gov/HomeandRecreationalSafety/pdf/poison-issue-brief.pdf

67. Federation of State Medical Boards of the United States. (2004). Model policy for the use of controlled substances for the treatment of pain. Retrieved from http://www.fsmb.org/pdf/2004_grpol_Controlled_Substances.pdf

68. Chou, R., Fanciullo, G. J., Fine, P. G., Adler, J. A., Ballantyne, J. C., Davies, P., et al. (2009). Clinical guidelines for the use of chronic opioid therapy in chronic noncancer pain. *The Journal of Pain*, 10(2), 113–130.

69. R. Twillman (personal communication, June 2, 2011).

70. Collen, M. (2011). The Fourth Amendment and random drug testing of people with chronic pain. *Journal of Pain & Palliative Care Pharmacology*, 25, 42–48.

71. Becker, W. C., Starrels, J. L., Heo, M., Li, X., Weiner, M. G., & Turner, B. J. (2011). Racial differences in primary care opioid risk reduction strategies. *Annals of Family Medicine*, 9(3), 219–225.

72. Michna, E., Jamison, R. N., Pham, L-D., Ross, E. L., Janfaza, D., Nedeljkovic, S. S., et al. (2007). Urine toxicology screening among chronic pain patients on opioid therapy: Frequency and predictability of abnormal findings. *Clinical Journal of Pain*, 23(2), 173–179.

73. Quest Diagnostics. (2012, April 27). Three in five Americans misuse their prescription drugs, finds national study of prescription medication lab testing [Press release]. Retrieved from http://markets.on.nytimes.com/research/stocks/news/press_release.asp?docTag=201204271507PR_NEWS_USPRX____NY95661&feedID=600&press_symbol=89411

74. Quest Diagnostics. (2012). Prescription drug monitoring report 2012. Prescription drug misuse in America—laboratory insights into the

new drug epidemic. Retrieved from http://www.questdiagnostics.com/dms/Documents/health-trends/PDF-MI3040_PDM-Report_24638_FIN_Digital_4-20-12/PDF%20MI3040_PDM%20Report_24638_FIN_Digital_4-20-12.pdf

75. West, R., Pesce, A., West, C., Crews, B., Mikel, C., Rosenthal, M., et al. (2010). Observations of medication compliance by measurement of urinary drug concentrations in a pain management population. *Journal of Opioid Management, 6*(4), 253–257.

76. Heit, H. (2010). Tackling the difficult problem of prescription opioid misuse [Editorial]. *Annals of Internal Medicine, 152*(11), 747–748.

77. Collen, M. (2009). Opioid contracts and random drug testing for people with chronic pain—think twice. *Journal of Law, Medicine & Ethics, 37*(4), 841–845.

78. S. B. Leavitt (personal communication, May 19, 2012).

79. Leavitt, S. B. (2011, March 3). Biased UDT research distorts opioid misuse, again. Retrieved from http://updates.pain-topics.org/2011/03/biased-udt-research-distorts-opioid.html

80. Leavitt, S. B. (2010, September 11). Another UDT study distorts opioid noncompliance. Retrieved from http://updates.pain-topics.org/2010/09/another-udt-study-distorts-opioid.html

81. Anson, P. (2012, April 30). Industry funded study promotes more drug testing. Retrieved from http://americannewsreport.com/industry-funded-study-promotes-more-drug-testing-8814015.html

82. Cuoto, J. E., Peppin, J. F., Fine, P. G., Passik, S. D., & Goldfarb, N. I. (2012, February). *Developing recommendations for urine drug monitoring for patients on long-term opioid therapy.* Paper presented at the 2012 American Academy of Pain Medicine Annual meeting, Palm Springs, CA. Abstract retrieved from http://www.painmed.org/2012posters/abstract-215/

83. United States ex rel. Maul v. Ameritox, LLC, No. 8:07-cv-953-T- 26EAJ (M.D. Fla. 2010).

84. Collen, M. (2012). Profit-driven drug testing. *Journal of Pain and Palliative Care Pharmacology, 26*, 13–17.

85. Department of Justice. (2010, November 16). Ameritox, Ltd. Agrees to pay $16.3 million to resolve kickback claims associated with laboratory testing services. Retrieved from http://pharmacychoice.us/News/article.cfm?Article_ID=653009

86. Millennium Laboratories. (2012, June 13). Millennium laboratories wins lawsuit; federal jury finds Ameritox repeatedly lied to physicians regarding Rx Guardian and Rx Guardian CD [Press release]. Retrieved from http://www.bizjournals.com/sanfrancisco/prnewswire/press_releases/California/2012/06/13/LA24201

87. Ameritox. (2012, June 15). Science behind Ameritox pain medication monitoring products emerges from trial unscathed [Press release]. Retrieved from http://www.ameritox.com/science-behind-ameritox-pain-medication-monitoring-products-emerges-from-trial-unscathed/

88. R. Twillman (personal communication, June 2, 2011).

89. S. B. Leavitt (personal communication, May 19, 2012).

90. Meadway, C., George, S., & Braithwaite, R. (1998). Opiate concentrations following the ingestion of poppy products—evidence for "the poppy seed defence." *Forensic Science International, 96*(1), 29–38.

91. AllianceofStateswithPrescriptionMonitoringPrograms.(n.d.).Prescription monitoring frequently asked questions (FAQ). Retrieved from http://www.pmpalliance.org/content/prescription-monitoring-frequently-asked-questions-faq

92. Leavitt, S. B. (2011, February 24). Rx monitoring doesn't stem opioid overdose deaths. Retrieved from http://updates.pain-topics.org/2011/02/rx-monitoring-doesnt-stem-opioid.html

93. Simeone, R., & Holland, L. (2006, September 1). An evaluation of prescription drug monitoring programs [Executive summary]. Retrieved from https://www.bja.gov/publications/pdmpexecsumm.pdf

94. Executive Office of the President of the United States. (2011). Epidemic: Responding to America's prescription drug abuse crisis (p. 5). Retrieved from http://www.whitehouse.gov/sites/default/files/ondcp/issues-content/prescription-drugs/rx_abuse_plan_0.pdf

95. R. Twillman (personal communication, October 8, 2012).

96. Wang, J., & Christo, P. J. (2009). The influence of prescription monitoring programs on chronic pain management. *Pain Physician, 12,* 507–515.

97. Pain & Policy Studies Group. (n.d.). Prescription monitoring programs (PMPs). Retrieved from http://www.painpolicy.wisc.edu/domestic/pmp.htm

98. Simeone, R., & Holland, L. (2006, September 1). An evaluation of prescription drug monitoring programs [Executive summary]. Retrieved from https://www.bja.gov/publications/pdmpexecsumm.pdf

99. Leavitt, S. B. (2011, February 24). Rx monitoring doesn't stem opioid overdose deaths. Retrieved from http://updates.pain-topics.org/2011/02/rx-monitoring-doesnt-stem-opioid.html

100. Gilson, A., Twillman, R., Dahl, J., & Fishman, S. (2010, May 7). Prescription Monitoring *Programs' impact on medication diversion and availability: What do we know and where should we go?* Paper presented at the 29th Annual Scientific Meeting of the American Pain Society Meeting, Baltimore, MD.

101. Katz, N., Houle, B., Fernandez, K. C., Kreiner, P., Thomas, C. P., Kim, M., et al. (2008). Update on prescription monitoring in clinical practice: A survey study of prescription monitoring program administrators. *Pain Medicine, 9*(5), 587–594.

102. United States General Accounting Office. (2002, May 17). Prescription drugs: State monitoring programs provide useful tool to reduce diversion (Report No. GAO-02-634). Retrieved from http://www.gao.gov/assets/240/234687.pdf

103. Simeone, R., & Holland, L. (2006, September 1). An evaluation of prescription drug monitoring programs [Executive summary]. Retrieved from https://www.bja.gov/publications/pdmpexecsumm.pdf

104. Katz, N., Panas, L., Kim, M., Audet, A. D., Bilansky, A., Eadie, J., et al. (2010). Usefulness of prescription monitoring programs for surveillance—analysis of Schedule II opioid prescription data in Massachusetts, 1996–2006. *Pharmacoepidemiology and Drug Safety, 19*(2), 115–123.

105. Gilson, A., Twillman, R., & Dahl, J. (2010, May 7). *Prescription Monitoring Programs' impact on medication diversion and availability: What do we know and where should we go?* Paper presented at the 29th Annual Scientific Meeting of the American Pain Society Meeting, Baltimore, MD.

106. Walter, S. (2012, April 7). Meager participation hobbles drug oversight. *The New York Times.* Retrieved from http://www.nytimes.com/2012/04/08/us/poor-participation-hobbles-californias-drug-oversight.html?pagewanted=all

107. Twillman, R. K. (2003). Report from the 10th World Congress on Pain. *Journal of Pain and Palliative Care Pharmacotherapy, 17*(2), 83–88.

108. Twillman, R. K. (2006). Impact of prescription monitoring programs on prescription patterns and indicators of opioid abuse. *The Journal of Pain, 7*(4), S6.

109. R. Twillman (personal communication, June 2, 2011).

110. Kerlikowske, G., Jones, C. M., LaBelle, R. M., & Condon, T. P. (2011). Prescription drug monitoring programs—lack of effectiveness or a call to action? [Editorial]. *Pain Medicine, 12,* 687–689.

111. Paulozzi L. J., Kilbourne E. M., & Desai, H. A. (2011). Prescription drug monitoring programs and death rates from drug overdose. *Pain Medicine, 12*(5), 747–754.

112. Reifler, L. M., Droz, D., Bailey, J. E., Schnoll, S. H., Fant, R., Dart, R. C., et al. (2012). Do prescription monitoring programs impact state trends in opioid abuse/misuse? *Pain Medicine, 13*(3), 434–442.

113. C. Steinberg. (2012, July 20). Massachusetts Pain Initiative testimony on proposed regulations to enhance the Prescription Monitoring Program (105CMR 700.000 & 105 CMR 701.000) [Personal communication].

114. US Food and Drug Administration. (n.d.). Approved risk evaluation and mitigation strategies (REMS): Currently approved individual REMS. Retrieved from http://www.fda.gov/Drugs/DrugSafety/PostmarketDrugSafetyInformationforPatientsandProviders/ucm111350.htm

115. US Food and Drug Administration. (n.d.). List of long-acting and extended-release opioid products required to have an opioid REMS. Retrieved from http://www.fda.gov/Drugs/DrugSafety/InformationbyDrugClass/ucm251735.htm

116. J. Dahl (personal communication, July 27, 2012).

117. The White House, Office of National Drug Control Policy. (2011, April 19). Obama administration releases action plan to address national prescription drug abuse epidemic; announces FDA action requiring drug makers to develop education program for prescribers about safe use of opioids [Press release]. Retrieved from http://www.whitehouse.gov/ondcp/news-releases-remarks/obama-administration-releases-action-plan

118. Executive Office of the President of the United States. (2011). Epidemic: Responding to America's prescription drug abuse crisis (p. 5). Retrieved from http://www.whitehouse.gov/sites/default/files/ondcp/ issues-content/prescription-drugs/rx_abuse_plan_0.pdf

119. Leavitt, S. B. (2011, April 20). U.S. FDA releases long-awaited opioid-REMS. Retrieved from http://updates.pain-topics.org/2011/04/us-fda-releases-l ong-awaited-opioid.html

120. Department of Health and Human Services, Food and Drug Administration. (2009). Risk evaluation and mitigation strategies for certain opioid drugs; notice of public meeting. *Federal Register, 74*(74), 17967–17970. Retrieved from http://www.gpo.gov/fdsys/pkg/FR-2009-04-20/pdf/E9-8903.pdf

121. US Food and Drug Administration. (2012, July 9). FDA introduces new safety measures for extended-release and long-acting opioid medications [Press release]. Retrieved from http://www.fda.gov/NewsEvents/ Newsroom/PressAnnouncements/ucm310870.htm

122. J. Dahl (personal communication, July 27, 2012).

123. Nelson, L. S., & Perrone, J. (2012). Curbing the opioid epidemic in the United States—the risk evaluation and mitigation strategy (REMS). *Journal of the American Medical Association, 308*(5), 457–458.

124. US Food and Drug Administration Consumer Health Information. (2009, February 23). A guide to safe use of pain medicine. Retrieved from http://www.fda.gov/downloads/ForConsumers/ConsumerUpdates/ ucm095742.pdf

125. US Food and Drug Administration. (n.d.). Approved risk evaluation and mitigation strategies (REMS): Currently approved individual REMS. Retrieved from http://www.fda.gov/Drugs/DrugSafety/ PostmarketDrugSafetyInformationforPatientsandProviders/ucm111350. htm

126. US Food and Drug Administration. (2012, July 9). FDA introduces new safety measures for extended-release and long-acting opioid medications [Press release]. Retrieved from http://www.fda.gov/NewsEvents/ Newsroom/PressAnnouncements/ucm310870.htm

127. Leavitt, S. B. (2012, July 10). U.S. FDA launches the long-awaited opioid REMS. Retrieved from http://updates.pain-topics.org/2012/07/ us-fda-launches-long-awaited-opioid.html

128. US Food and Drug Administration. (2012, July 9). FDA introduces new safety measures for extended-release and long-acting opioid medications [Press release]. Retrieved from http://www.fda.gov/NewsEvents/ Newsroom/PressAnnouncements/ucm310870.htm

129. S. B. Leavitt (personal communication, May 19, 2012).

130. J. Dahl (personal communication, July 27, 2012).

131. H. Neuman (personal communication, April 5, 2011).

132. L. Webster (personal communication, May 13, 2012).

133. Michna, E., Ross, E. L., Hynes, W. L., Nedeljkovic, S. S., Soumekh, S., Janfaza, D., et al. (2004). Predicting aberrant drug behavior in patients

treated for chronic pain: Importance of abuse history. *Journal of Pain and Symptom Management, 28*(3), 250–258.

134. Chou, R., Fanciullo, G. J., Fine, P. G., Adler, J. A., Ballantyne, J. C., Davies, P., et al. (2009). Clinical guidelines for the use of chronic opioid therapy in chronic noncancer pain. *The Journal of Pain, 10*(2), 113–130.

135. American Pain Society. (2009, February 10). New guidelines for prescribing opioid pain drugs published [Press release]. Retrieved from http://www.ampainsoc.org/press/2009/downloads/20090210.pdf

136. Federation of State Medical Boards of the United States. (2004). Model policy for the use of controlled substances for the treatment of pain. Retrieved from http://www.fsmb.org/pdf/2004_grpol_Controlled_Substances.pdf

137. Schiff, G. D., Galanter, W. L., Duhig, J., Lodolce, A. E., Koronowski, M. J., & Lambert, B. L. (2011). Principles of conservative prescribing [Review article]. *Archives of Internal Medicine, 171*(16), 1433–1440.

138. Physicians for Responsible Opioid Prescribing. (n.d.). Cautious, evidence-based opioid prescribing. Retrieved from http://www.support-prop.org/educational/PROP_OpioidPrescribing.pdf

139. Leavitt, S. B. (2010, September). Common opioid pain relievers. Retrieved from http://opioids911.org/opioidproducts.php

140. L. Webster (personal communication, May 14, 2012).

141. Utah Department of Health. (2011). Utah's winnable health battles: Prescription drug misuse, abuse and overdose deaths. Retrieved from https://health.utah.gov/phi/getfile.php?id=236

142. Katz, M. H. (2010). Long-term opioid treatment of nonmalignant pain: A believer loses his faith [Editorial]. *Archives of General Medicine, 170*(16), 1422–1423.

143. Foley, K. M., Fins, J. J., & Inturrisi, C. E. (2011). A true believer's flawed analysis. *Archives of Internal Medicine, 171*(9), 867–868.

144. Physicians for Responsible Opioid Prescribing. (2012, July 25). Citizen petition (Document ID: FDA-2012-P-0818-0001). Retrieved from http://www.regulations.gov/#!documentDetail;D=FDA-2012-P-0818-0001

145. Bono Mack, M. (2012, July 26). [Letter to Margaret Hamburg, M.D., Commissioner, Food and Drug Administration]. Retrieved from http://bono.house.gov/uploadedfiles/fda_opioid_labels_letter7_26_12.pdf

146. Public Citizen. (2012, July 25). Doctors, researchers and health officials call on FDA to change labels on opioid painkillers to deter misprescribing [Press release]. Retrieved from http://www.citizen.org/pressroom/pressroomredirect.cfm?ID=3674

147. Physicians for Responsible Opioid Prescribing. (2012, July 25). Citizen petition (Document ID: FDA-2012-P-0818-0001). Retrieved from http://www.regulations.gov/#!documentDetail;D=FDA-2012-P-0818-0001

148. Twillman, R. (2012, August 2). Group petitions FDA to change opioid label. Retrieved from http://updates.pain-topics.org/2012/08/group-petitions-fda-to-change-opioid.html

CHAPTER 9

1. Fields, R. D. (2009). New culprits in chronic pain. *Scientific American*, *301*(5), 50–57.
2. Fields, R. D. (2011). *The other brain: The scientific and medical break-throughs that will heal our brains and revolutionize our health* (pp. 234–244). New York: Simon & Schuster.
3. Fields, R. D. (2011). The hidden brain. *Scientific American Mind*, *22*(2), 52–59.
4. Miller, G. (2005). The dark side of glia. *Science*, *308*(5723), 778–781.
5. Milligan, E. D., & Watkins, L. R. (2009). Pathological and protective roles of glia in chronic pain. *Nature Reviews Neuroscience*, *10*(1), 23–36.
6. Watkins, L. R., Wieseler-Frank, J., Milligan, E. D., Johnston, I., & Maier, S. F. (2006). Contribution of glia to pain processing in health and disease. In J. Cervero, & T. S. Jensen (Eds.), *Handbook of clinical neurology: Pain* (3rd ed., pp. 309–323). New York: Elsevier.
7. Watkins, L. R., & Maier, S. F. (2003). When good pain turns bad. *Current Directions in Psychological Science*, *12*(6), 232–236.
8. Halassa, M. M., Florian, C., Fellin, T., Munoz, J. R., Lee, S. Y., Abel, T., et al. (2009). Astrocytic modulation of sleep homeostasis and cognitive consequences of sleep loss. *Neuron*, *61*(2), 213–219.
9. Watkins, L. R., & Maier, S. F. (2003). Glia: A novel drug discovery target for clinical pain [Abstract]. *Nature Reviews Drug Discovery*, *2*(12), 973–985.
10. Watkins, L. R., Milligan, E. D., & Maier, S. F. (2001). Glial activation: A driving force for pathological pain. *Trends in Neurosciences*, *24*(8), 450–455.
11. Fields, R. D. (2011). The hidden brain. *Scientific American Mind*, *22*(2), 52–59.
12. Scholz, J., & Woolf, C. J. (2007). The neuropathic pain triad: Neurons, immune cells and glia. *Nature Neuroscience*, *10*(11), 1361.
13. Ji, R. R., Kawasaki, Y., Zhuang, Z. Y., Wen, Y. R., & Decosterd, I. (2006). Possible role of spinal astrocytes in maintaining chronic pain sensitization: Review of current evidence with focus on bFGF/JNK pathway. *Neuron Glia Biology*, *2*(4), 259–269.
14. Meller, S. T., Dykstra, C., Grzybycki, D., Murphy, S., & Gebhart, G. F. (1994). The possible role of glia in nociceptive processing and hyperalgesia in the spinal cord of the rat [Abstract]. *Neuropharmacology*, *33*(11), 1471–1478.
15. Zhang, J. H., & Huang, Y. G. (2006). The immune system: A new look at pain. *Chinese Medical Journal*, *119*(11), 930–938.
16. Watkins, L. R., Hutchinson, M. R., Ledeboer, A., Wieseler-Frank, J., Milligan, E. D., & Maier, S. F. (2007). Glia as the "bad guys": Implications for improving clinical pain control and the clinical utility of opioids. *Brain, Behavior, and Immunity*, *21*(2), 131–146.
17. L. R. Watkins (personal communication, October 28, 2009).
18. Watkins, L. R., Milligan, E. D., & Maier, S. F. (2003). Glial proinflammatory cytokines mediate exaggerated pain states: Implications for clinical pain [Abstract]. *Advances in Experimental Medicine and Biology*, *521*, 1–21.
19. L. R. Watkins (personal communication, November 9, 2009).

20. Younger, J., & Mackey, S. (2009). Fibromyalgia symptoms are reduced by low-dose naltrexone: A pilot study. *Pain Medicine, 10*(4), 663–672.
21. Younger, J., McCue, R., Noor, N., & Mackey, S. (2012). *Low-dose naltrexone reduces the symptoms of fibromyalgia: A double-blind and placebo-controlled crossover study.* Paper presented at the 2012 American Academy of Pain Medicine Annual Meeting, Palm Springs, FL. Abstract retrieved from http://www.painmed.org/2012posters/abstract-251
22. L. R. Watkins (personal communication, November 9, 2009).
23. R. Chavez (personal communication, May 13, 2011).
24. Sloane, E. M., Soderquist, R.G., Maier, S. F., Mahoney, M. J., Watkins, L. R., & Milligan, E. D. (2009). Long-term control of neuropathic pain in a non-viral gene therapy paradigm. *Gene Therapy, 16*(4), 470–475.
25. Milligan, E. D., Soderquist, R. G., Malone, S. M., Mahoney, J. H., Hughes, T. S., Langer, S. J., et al. (2006). Intrathecal polymer-based interleukin-10 gene delivery for neuropathic pain [Abstract]. *Neuron Glia Biology, 2*(4), 293–308.
26. Soderquist, R. G., Sloane, E. M., Loram, L. C., Harrison, J. A., Dengler, E. C., Johnson, S. M., et al. (2010). Release of plasmid DNA-encoding IL-10 from PLGA microparticles facilitates long-term reversal of neuropathic pain following a single intrathecal administration. *Pharmaceutical Research, 27*(5), 841–854.
27. Fink, D. J., Wechuck, J., Mata, M., Glorioso, J. C., Goss, J., Krisky, D., & Wolfe, D. (2011). Gene therapy for pain: Results of a phase I clinical trial. *Annals of Neurology, 70*(2), 207–212.
28. TedTalks (Producer). (2011). Elliot Krane: The mystery of chronic pain [Video file]. Retrieved from http://www.ted.com/talks/elliot_krane_the_mystery_of_chronic_pain.html
29. L. R. Watkins (personal communication, March 1, 2012).
30. Watkins, L. R., Hutchinson, M. R., Rice, K. C., & Maier, S. F. (2009). The "toll" of opioid-induced glial activation: Improving the clinical efficacy of opioids by targeting glia. *Trends in Pharmacological Sciences, 30*(11), 581–591.
31. L. R. Watkins (personal communication, October 28, 2009).
32. K. Johnson (personal communication, May 13, 2011).
33. Rolan, P., Hutchinson, M. R., & Johnson, K. W. (2009). Ibudilast: A review of its pharmacology, efficacy and safety in respiratory and neurological disease. *Expert Opinion on Pharmacotherapy, 10*(17), 2897–2904.
34. Ledeboer, A., Liu, T., Shumilla, J. A., Mahoney, J. H., Vijay, S., Gross, M. I., et al. (2006). The glial modulatory drug AV411 attenuates mechanical allodynia in rat models of neuropathic pain. *Neuron Glia Biology, 2*(04), 279–291.
35. Ledeboer, A., Hutchinson, M. R., Watkins, L. R., & Johnson, K. W. (2007). Ibudilast (AV-411): A new class therapeutic candidate for neuropathic pain and opioid withdrawal syndromes. *Expert Opinion on Investigational Drugs, 16*(7), 935–950.
36. K. Johnson (personal communication, March 5, 2012).
37. Tanga, F. Y., Nutile-McMenemy, N., & DeLeo, J. A. (2005). The CNS role of toll-like receptor 4 in innate neuroimmunity and painful

neuropathy. *Proceedings of the National Academy of Sciences, 102*(16), 5856–5861.

38. DeLeo, J. A., Tanga, F. Y., & Tawfik, V. L. (2004). Neuroimmune activation and neuroinflammation in chronic pain and opioid tolerance/hyperalgesia. *The Neuroscientist, 10*(1), 40–52.

39. DeLeo, J., Schubert, P., & Kreutzberg, G. W. (1988). Protection against ischemic brain damage using propentofylline in gerbils [Abstract]. *Stroke, 19*(12), 1535–1539.

40. Sweitzer, S. M., Schubert, P., & DeLeo, J. A. (2001). Propentofylline, a glial modulating agent, exhibits antiallodynic properties in a rat model of neuropathic pain. *Journal of Pharmacology and Experimental Therapeutics, 297*(3), 1210–1217.

41. Sweitzer, S. M., Pahl, J. L., & DeLeo, J. A. (2006). Propentofylline attenuates vincristine-induced peripheral neuropathy in the rat. *Neuroscience Letters, 400*(3), 258–261.

42. Ledeboer, A., Sloane, E. M., Milligan, E. D., Frank, M. G., Mahony, J. H., Maier, S. F., et al. (2005). Minocycline attenuates mechanical allodynia and proinflammatory cytokine expression in rat models of pain facilitation [Abstract]. *PAIN, 115*(1–2), 71–83.

43. Raghavendra, V., Tanga, F., & DeLeo, J. A. (2003). Inhibition of microglial activation attenuates the development but not existing hypersensitivity in a rat model of neuropathy [Abstract]. *Journal of Pharmacology and Experimental Therapeutics, 306*(2), 624–630.

44. J. DeLeo (personal communication, May 11, 2011).

45. Sun, X. C., Chen, W. N., Li, S. Q., Cai, J. S., Li, W. B., Xian, X. H., et al. (2009). Fluorocitrate, an inhibitor of glial metabolism, inhibits the up-regulation of NOS expression, activity and NO production in the spinal cord induced by formalin test in rats. *Neurochemical Research, 34*(2), 351–359.

46. Meller, S. T., Dykstra, C., Grzybycki, D., Murphy, S., & Gebhart, G. F. (1994). The possible role of glia in nociceptive processing and hyperalgesia in the spinal cord of the rat [Abstract]. *Neuropharmacology, 33*(11), 1471–1478.

47. Raghavendra, V., Tanga, F. Y., & DeLeo, J. A. (2004). Attenuation of morphine tolerance, withdrawal-induced hyperalgesia, and associated spinal inflammatory immune responses by propentofylline in rats. *Neuropsychopharmacology, 29*(2), 327–334.

48. Solace Pharmaceuticals. (2009). Solace Pharmaceuticals initiates phase IIa trial of glial cell modulator SLC022 in post-herpetic neuralgia. Retrieved from http://www.reuters.com/article/2009/01/12/idUS89208+12-Jan-2009+PRN20090112

49. J. DeLeo (personal communication, May 11, 2011).

50. Talkington, M. (2011, June 9). Where are glia going? Retrieved from http://www.painresearchforum.org/news/6905-where-are-glia-going?search_term=ere%20glia%20going

51. Stovall, S. (2011, March 27). R&D cuts curb brain-drug pipeline. *The Wall Street Journal*. Retrieved from http://online.wsj.com/article/SB10001424052748704474804576222463927753954.html

52. J. DeLeo (personal communication, May 11, 2011).
53. Fields, R. D. (2011). *The other brain: The scientific and medical breakthroughs that will heal our brains and revolutionize our health* (p. 197). New York: Simon & Schuster.
54. Fields, R. D., & Burnstock, G. (2006). Purinergic signalling in neuron–glia interactions [Abstract]. *Nature Reviews Neuroscience, 7*(6), 423–436.
55. Tsuda, M., Shigemoto-Mogami, Y., Koizumi, S., Mizokoshi, A., Kohsaka, S., Salter, M. W., et al. (2003). P2X4 receptors induced in spinal microglia gate tactile allodynia after nerve injury [Abstract]. *Nature, 424*(6950), 778–783.
56. K. Inoue (personal communication, May 26, 2011).
57. Fields, R. D. (2011). *The other brain: The scientific and medical breakthroughs that will heal our brains and revolutionize our health* (p. 195). New York: Simon & Schuster.
58. M. Costigan (personal communication, March 3, 2012).
59. Costigan, M., Moss, A., Latremoliere, A., Johnston, C., Verma-Gandhu, M., Herbert, T. A., et al. (2009). T-cell infiltration and signaling in the adult dorsal spinal cord is a major contributor to neuropathic pain-like hypersensitivity. *Journal of Neuroscience, 29*(46), pp. 14, 415–14, 422.
60. M. Costigan (personal communication, March 3, 2012).
61. Klein, C. J., Lennon, V. A., Aston, P. A., McKeon, A., & Pittock, S. J. (2012). Chronic pain as a manifestation of potassium channel-complex autoimmunity. *Neurology, 79*(11), 1136–1144.
62. Talkington, M. (2012, September 4). An autoimmune basis for chronic pain? Retrieved from http://www.painresearchforum.org/news/19697-autoimmune-basis-chronic-pain
63. Bennett, D. L., & Vincent, A. (2012). Autoimmune pain: An emerging concept. *Neurology, 79*, 1080–1081.
64. Paterniti, M. (2001). *Driving Mr. Albert: A trip across America with Einstein's brain*. New York: Dial Press Trade Paperback.
65. Fields, R. D. (2004). The other half of the brain. *Scientific American, 290*(4), 54–61.
66. Fields, R. D. (2011). *The other brain: The scientific and medical breakthroughs that will heal our brains and revolutionize our health* (pp. 3–7). New York: Simon & Schuster.

CHAPTER 10

1. B. McCauley (personal communication, June 13, 2011).
2. M. Duda (personal communication, June 22, 2009).
3. Pierre, J. M. (2011). Cannabis, synthetic cannabinoids, and psychosis risk: What the evidence says. *Current Psychiatry, 10*(9), 49–57.
4. Goodnough, A., & Zezima, K. (2011, July 16). An alarming new stimulant, legal in many states. *The New York Times.* Retrieved from http://www.nytimes.com/2011/07/17/us/17salts.html?pagewanted=all

5. United States Drug Enforcement Administration. (2011). Chemicals used in "Spice" and "K2" type products now under federal control and regulation [Press release]. Retrieved from http://www.justice.gov/dea/pubs/pressrel/pr030111.html
6. United States Drug Enforcement Administration. (2010). DEA moves to emergency control synthetic marijuana [Press release]. Retrieved from http://www.justice.gov/dea/pubs/pressrel/pr112410.html
7. MontanaPBS (Producer). (2011). Clearing the smoke: The science of cannabis [Documentary series]. Retrieved from http://video.pbs.org/video/1825223761#
8. Substance Abuse and Mental Health Service Administration. (2011). National survey shows a rise in illicit drug use from 2008 to 2010 [Press release]. Retrieved from http://www.samhsa.gov/newsroom/advisories/1109075503.aspx
9. K. Hunter (personal communication, March 22, 2012).
10. Sidney, S. (2003). Comparing cannabis with tobacco-again [Editorial]. British Medical Journal, 327(7416), 635.
11. Centers for Disease Control and Prevention. (2008). Smoking-attributable mortality, years of potential life lost and productivity losses—United States, 2000–2004. Morbidity and Mortality Weekly Report, 57(45), 1226–1228.
12. Centers for Disease Control and Prevention. (2008). Alcohol-Related Disease Impact (ARDI): Average for United States 2001–2005, alcohol-attributable deaths due to excessive alcohol use. Retrieved from http://apps.nccd.cdc.gov/DACH_ARDI/Default/Report.aspx?T=AAM&P=de9de51e-d51b-4690-a9a4-358859b692bc&R=804296a0-ac47-41d3-a939-9df26a176186&M=E2769A53-0BFC-453F-9FD7-63C5AA6CE5D7&F=AAMCauseGenderNew&D=H
13. Lanza, F. L., Chan, F. K. L., Quigley, E. M. M., & the Practice Parameters Committee of the American College of Gastroenterology. (2009). Guidelines for prevention of NSAID-related ulcer complications. The American Journal of Gastroenterology, 104, 728–738.
14. Ware, M. A., & Tawfik, V. L. (2005). Safety issues concerning the medical use of cannabis and cannabinoids. Pain Research & Management: The Journal of the Canadian Pain Society, 10(Supplement A), 33A.
15. Sidney, S. (2003). Comparing cannabis with tobacco-again [Editorial]. British Medical Journal, 327(7416), 635.
16. S. Gust (personal communication, March 22, 2012).
17. Young, F. L. (1988, September 6). In the matter of marijuana rescheduling petition—opinion and recommended ruling, findings of fact, conclusions of law and decision of administrative law judge (Docket No. 86-22, Part VIII). Retrieved from http://iowamedicalmarijuana.org/pdfs/young.pdf
18. National Institute on Drug Abuse. (n.d.). DrugFacts: Marijuana. Retrieved from http://www.drugabuse.gov/publications/drugfacts/marijuana
19. Substance Abuse and Mental Health Services Administration. (2011). National survey shows a rise in illicit drug use from 2008 to 2010 [Press

release]. Retrieved from http://www.samhsa.gov/newsroom/advisories/1109075503.aspx

20. Abrams, D. I. (2010). Cannabis in pain and palliative care. *The Pain Practitioner*, 20(4), 35–45.

21. Russo, E. B. (2007). History of cannabis and its preparations in saga, science, and sobriquet. *Chemistry & Biodiversity*, 4(8), 1614–1648.

22. Eadie, M. J. (2007). The neurological legacy of John Russell Reynolds (1828–1896). *Journal of Clinical Neuroscience*, 14(4), 309–316.

23. Russo, E. (2001). Hemp for headache: An in-depth historical and scientific review of cannabis in migraine treatment. *Journal of Cannabis Therapeutics*, 1(2), 21–92.

24. Russo, E. (1998). Cannabis for migraine treatment: The once and future prescription? An historical and scientific review. *PAIN*, 76(1–2), 3–8.

25. Abrams, D. I. (2010). Cannabis in pain and palliative care. *The Pain Practitioner*, 20(4), 35–45.

26. Musto, D. (n.d.). Transcript from Busted: America's War on Marijuana. Retrieved from http://www.pbs.org/wgbh/pages/frontline/shows/dope/etc/script.html. (Original work broadcast April 28, 1998).

27. U.S Pharmacopeia. (n.d.). About USP. Retrieved from http://www.usp.org.

28. Ferguson, A. (2010). Don't call it pot; it's "medicine" now. Dealers are caregivers, and buyers are patients…how marijuana got mainstreamed. *Time*, 176(21), 30–32, 34, 36–37.

29. PatentStorm. (n.d.). Cannabinoids as antioxidants and neuroprotectants. Retrieved from http://www.patentstorm.us/patents/6630507/fulltext.html

30. M. Cutler (personal communication, July 12, 2011).

31. Shaffer Library of Drug Policy. (n.d.). The report of the National Commission on Marihuana and Drug Abuse. Retrieved from http://www.druglibrary.org/schaffer/Library/studies/nc/ncmenu.htm

32. M. Cutler (personal communication, July 12, 2011).

33. Schlosser, E. (n.d.). Transcript from Busted: America's War on Marijuana. Retrieved from http://www.pbs.org/wgbh/pages/frontline/shows/dope/etc/script.html (Original work broadcast April 28, 1998).

34. S. Gust (personal communication, March 23, 2012).

35. R. Doblin (personal communication, July 14, 2011).

36. Griffiths, R. R., Richards, W. A., McCann, U., & Jesse, R. (2006). Psilocybin can occasion mystical-type experiences having substantial and sustained personal meaning and spiritual significance. *Psychopharmacology*, 187(3), 268–283.

37. Multidisciplinary Association for Psychedelic Studies. (n.d.). [Food and Drug Administration approval letter to Rick Doblin], (IND 101, 825). Retrieved from http://www.maps.org/research/cluster/psilo-lsd/maps.lsd.research-fda_removes_hold.pdf

38. Multidisciplinary Association for Psychedelic Studies. (n.d.). [Food and Drug Administration approval letter to Rick Doblin] (IND 63384). Retrieved from http://www.maps.org/mdma/mt1_docs/ind_63384_may_proceed_ltr.pdf

39. Winter, J. (2006, May 28). Weed control. *The Boston Globe*. Retrieved from http://www.boston.com/news/globe/ideas/articles/2006/05/28/weed_control/?page=full
40. S. Gust (personal communication, March 22, 2012).
41. American Botanical Council. (2010). The state of clinical cannabis research in the United States. *HerbalGram, 85,* 64–68.
42. Bittner, M. E. (2007, February 12). In the matter of Lyle E. Craker—opinion and recommended ruling, findings of fact, conclusions of law, and decision of the administrative law judge (Docket No. 05-16). Retrieved from http://www.maps.org/ALJfindings.PDF
43. S. Gust (personal communication, March 22, 2012).
44. National Advisory Council on Drug Abuse, NIDA. (1998, January). Provision of Marijuana and Other Compounds for Scientific Research—Recommendations of the National Institute on Drug Abuse National Advisory Council. Retrieved June 20, 2013, from http://archives.drugabuse.gov/about/organization/nacda/MarijuanaStatement.html
45. Bittner, M. E. (2007, February 12). In the matter of Lyle E. Craker—opinion and recommended ruling, findings of fact, conclusions of law, and decision of the administrative law judge (Docket No. 05-16). Retrieved from http://www.maps.org/ALJfindings.PDF
46. L. Craker (personal communication, July 13, 2011).
47. R. Doblin (personal communication, July 14, 2011).
48. American Society of Addiction Medicine. (2011, March 23). American Society of Addiction Medicine rejects use of "medical marijuana," citing dangers and failure to meet standards of patient care [Press release]. Retrieved from http://www.prnewswire.com/news-releases/american-society-of-addiction-medicine-rejects-use-of-medical-marijuana-citing-dangers-and-failure-to-meet-standards-of-patient-care-118534464.html
49. American College of Physicians. (2008). Supporting research into the therapeutic role of marijuana: A position paper. Retrieved from http://www.acponline.org/fcgi/search?q=therapeutic+role+of+marijuana&site=ACP_Online&x=23&y=10
50. O'Reilly, K. B. (2009, November 23). AMA meeting: Delegates support review of marijuana's schedule I status. *American Medical News*. Retrieved from http://www.ama-assn.org/amednews/2009/11/23/prse1123.htm
51. R. Doblin (personal communication, July 14, 2011).
52. Laughren, T. (2011, April 28). [Advice/Information request to Multidisciplinary Association for Psychedelic Studies, attention: Rick Doblin] (IND110513). Retrieved from http://www.maps.org/mmj/110513_Advice_Ltr_4_28_11.pdf
53. American Botanical Council. (2010). The state of clinical cannabis research in the United States. *HerbalGram, 85,* 64–68.
54. Bittner, M. E. (2007, February 12). In the matter of Lyle E. Craker—opinion and recommended ruling, findings of fact, conclusions of law, and decision of the administrative law judge (Docket No. 05-16). Retrieved from http://www.maps.org/ALJfindings.PDF

55. Marijuana Policy Project. [MPP]. (2008, March 22). Barack Obama and medical marijuana (interview Q&A) [Video file]. Retrieved from http://www.youtube.com/watch?v=LvUziSfMwAw&feature=player_embedded

56. Marijuana Policy Project. (2011, December). Federal enforcement policy de-prioritizing medical marijuana: Statements from Pres. Obama, his spokesman, and the Justice Department. Retrieved from http://www.mpp.org/assets/pdfs/library/Federal-Enforcement-Policy-De-Prioritizing-Medical-Marijuana.pdf

57. Ogden, D. W. (2009, October 19). Memorandum for selected United States attorneys on investigations and prosecutions in states authorizing the medical use of marijuana. Retrieved from http://blogs.usdoj.gov/blog/archives/192

58. Kampia, R. (2011, July 4). Obama needs to honor his medical marijuana campaign promise [Blog post]. Retrieved from http://www.theweedblog.com/obama-needs-to-honor-his-medical-marijuana-campaign-promise/

59. Fox, M. (2011, July 7). DOJ clarification of medical marijuana policy still unclear [Blog post]. Retrieved from http://blog.mpp.org/medical-marijuana/doj-clarification-of-medical-marijuana-policy-still-unclear/07072011/

60. Riggs, M. (2011, June 30). Obama administration overrides 2009 Ogden memo, declares open season on pot shops in states where medical marijuana is legal [Blog post]. Retrieved from http://reason.com/blog/2011/06/30/white-house-overrides-2009-memo

61. Cole, J. M. (2011, June 29). Guidance regarding the Ogden memo in jurisdictions seeking to authorize marijuana for medical use. Retrieved from http://proxychi.baremetal.com/www.drugsense.org/temp/guidance_regarding_medical_mariju.pdf

62. Multidisciplinary Association for Psychedelic Studies. (2012, May 8). DEA goes to court for blocking medical marijuana research [Email newsletter]. Retrieved from B. Burge (personal communication, May 8, 2012).

63. Multidisciplinary Association for Psychedelic Studies. (2012, May 11). U.S. First Circuit Court hears oral arguments in Lyle Craker v. Drug Enforcement Administration [Press release]. Retrieved from http://www.maps.org/media/view/u.s._first_circuit_court_hears_oral_arguments_in_lyle_e._craker_v._dru/

64. E. Russo (personal communication, August 16, 2011).

65. Institute of Medicine. (1999). The medical value of marijuana and related substances. In J. E. Joy, S. J. Watson, & J. A. Benson (Eds.), *Marijuana and medicine: Assessing the science base* (pp. 137–192). Washington, DC: National Academies Press.

66. Russo, E. B. (2011). Taming THC: Potential cannabis synergy and phytocannabinoid-terpenoid entourage effects. *British Journal of Pharmacology, 163*(7), 1344–1364.

67. J. H. Atkinson (personal communication, June 30, 2011).

68. Hoeffel, J. (2010, February 9). UC studies find promise in medical marijuana. *LA Times.* Retrieved from http://articles.latimes.com/2010/feb/18/local/la-me-medical-marijuana18-2010feb18

69. Center for Medicinal Cannabis Research, University of California (2010, February 11). Report to the legislature and governor of the state of California presenting findings pursuant to SB847 which created the CMCR and provided state funding (p. 2). Retrieved from http://www.cmcr.ucsd.edu/images/pdfs/CMCR_REPORT_FEB17.pdf

70. Coalition for Rescheduling Cannabis: Members. (n.d.). Retrieved from http://www.drugscience.org/coalition_members.html

71. Arguments supporting the Cannabis Rescheduling Petition. (n.d.). Retrieved from http://www.drugscience.org/intro/arguments.html

72. The Global Commission on Drug Policy. (2011, June). War on drugs: Report of the Global Commission on Drug Policy (p. 3). Retrieved from http://www.globalcommissionondrugs.org/wp-content/themes/gcdp_v1/pdf/Global_Commission_Report_English.pdf

73. Denial of Petition to Initiate Proceedings to Reschedule Marijuana, 76 Fed. Reg. 40552 (proposed July 8, 2011) (to be codified at 21 C.F.R. Chapter II). Retrieved from http://www.gpo.gov/fdsys/pkg/FR-2011-07-08/pdf/2011-16994.pdf

74. Arguments supporting the Cannabis Rescheduling Petition. (n.d.). Retrieved from http://www.drugscience.org/intro/arguments.html

75. M. Cutler (personal communication, July 12, 2011).

76. Denial of Petition to Initiate Proceedings to Reschedule Marijuana, 76 Fed. Reg. 40552 (proposed July 8, 2011) (to be codified at 21 C.F.R. Chapter II). Retrieved from http://www.gpo.gov/fdsys/pkg/FR-2011-07-08/pdf/2011-16994.pdf

77. Americans for Safe Access. (2011, July 8). Patients' lawsuit forces federal gov't to answer 9-year-old medical marijuana rescheduling petition [Press release]. Retrieved from http://www.safeaccessnow.org/article.php?id=6703

78. R. Merchoulam (personal communication, April 16, 2010).

79. E. A. Romero-Sandoval (personal communication, August 29, 2011).

80. Riachlen, D. A., Foster, A. D., Gerdeman, G. L., Seillier, A., & Giuffrida, A. (2012). Wired to run: Exercise-induced endocannabinoid signaling in humans and cursorial mammals with implications for the "runner's high." The Journal of Experimental Biology, 215(Pt. 8), 1331–136.

81. Reynolds, G. (2012, April 25). Like it or not, our brains are enticing us to run. The New York Times. Retrieved from http://well.blogs.nytimes.com/2012/04/25/the-evolution-of-the-runners-high/

82. Abrams, D. I. (2010). Cannabis in pain and palliative care. The Pain Practitioner, 20(4), 35–45.

83. Di Marzo, V., Melck, D., Bisogno, T., & De Petrocellis, L. (1998). Endocannabinoids: Endogenous cannabinoid receptor ligands with neuromodulatory action. Trends in Neuroscience, 21(12), 521–528.

84. Russo, E. B., & Hohmann, A. (2013). Role of cannabinoids in pain management. In T. R. Deer et al. (Eds.), Comprehensive treatment of chronic pain by medical, interventional, and behavioral approaches: The American Academy of Pain Medicine textbook on patient management (pp. 181–198). New York: Springer.

85. Rossi, C., Pini, L. A., Cupini, M. L., Calabresi, P., & Sarchielli, P. (2008). Endocannabinoids in platelets of chronic migraine patients and medication-overuse headache patients: Relation with serotonin levels. *European Journal of Clinical Pharmacology, 64*(1), 1–8.

86. Russo, E. B. (2004). Clinical endocannabinoid deficiency (CECD): Can this concept explain therapeutic benefits of cannabis in migraine, fibromyalgia, irritable bowel syndrome and other treatment-resistant conditions? *Neuroendocrinology Letters, 25*(1/2), 31–39.

87. Juhasz, G., Lazary, J., Chase, D., Pegg, E., Downey, D., Toth, Z. G., et al. (2009). Variations in the cannabinoid receptor 1 gene predispose to migraine. *Neuroscience Letters, 461*(2), 116–120.

88. Talkington, M. (2011, December 1). FLAT-tening pain: Blocking transporter boosts endocannabinoid levels in mice. Retrieved from http://www.painresearchforum.org/news/11548-flat-tening-pain?search_term=FLAT-tening%20Pain

89. Duggan, K. C., Hermanson, D. J., Musee, L., Prusakiewicz, J. J., Scheib, J. L., Carter, B. D., et al. (2011). R-Profens are substrate-selective inhibitors of endocannabinoid oxygenation by COX-2. *Nature Chemical Biology, 7*(11), 803–809.

90. E. A. Romero-Sandoval (personal communication, June 20, 2011).

91. Abrams, D. I. (2010). Cannabis in pain and palliative care. *The Pain Practitioner, 20*(4), 35–45.

92. Martin, M., Ledent, C., Parmentier, M., Maldonado, R., & Valverde, O. (2002). Involvement of CB1 cannabinoid receptors in emotional behaviour. *Psychopharmacology, 159*(4), 379–387.

93. Poncelet, M., Maruani, J., Calassi, R., & Soubrie, P. (2003). Overeating, alcohol and sucrose consumption decrease in CB1 receptor deleted mice. *Neuroscience Letters, 343*(3), 216–218.

94. Cota, D., Marsicano, G., Tschop, M., Grubler, Y., Flachskamm, C., Schubert, M., et al. (2003). The endogenous cannabinoid system affects energy balance via central orexigenic drive and peripheral lipogenesis. *The Journal of Clinical Investigation, 112*(3), 423–431.

95. Benedetti, F., Amanzio, M., Rosato, R., & Blanchard, C. (2011). Nonopioid placebo analgesia is mediated by CB1 cannabinoid receptors. *Nature Medicine, 17*(10), 1228–1230.

96. Society for Nuclear Medicine. (2011, June 6). Molecular imaging shows chronic marijuana smoking affects brain chemistry [Press release]. Retrieved from http://www.eurekalert.org/pub_releases/2011-06/sonm-mis060211.php

97. E. Russo (personal communication, August 16, 2011).

98. Beltramo, M. (2009). Cannabinoid type 2 receptor as a target for chronic pain. *Mini-Reviews in Medicinal Chemistry, 9*(1), 11–25.

99. Abrams, D. I. (2010). Cannabis in pain and palliative care. *The Pain Practitioner, 20*(4), 35–45.

100. Russo, E. B. (2011). Taming THC: Potential cannabis synergy and phytocannabinoid-terpenoid entourage effects. *British Journal of Pharmacology, 163*(7), 1344–1364.

101. Lee, M. C., Ploner, M., Wiech, K., Bingel, U., Wanigasekera, V., Brooks, J., et al. (2013). Amygdala activity contributes to the dissociative effect of cannabis on pain perception. *PAIN, 154*(1), 124–134.

102. Ware, M. A., & Tawfik, V. L. (2005). Safety issues concerning the medical use of cannabis and cannabinoids. *Pain Research & Management: The Journal of the Canadian Pain Society, 10*(Supplement A), 32A.

103. Mehmedic, Z., Chandra, S., Slade, D., Denham, H., Foster, S., Patel, A. S., et al. (2010). Potency trends of Delta-9 THC and other cannabinoids in confiscated cannabis preparations from 1993 to 2008. *Journal of Forensic Sciences, 55*(5), 1209–1217.

104. E. Russo (personal communication, August 16, 2011).

105. Russo, E., & Guy, G. W. (2006). A tale of two cannabinoids: The therapeutic rationale for combining tetrahydrocannabinol and cannabidiol. *Medical Hypotheses, 66*, 234–246.

106. E. A. Romero-Sandoval (personal communication, June 20, 2011).

107. Beltramo, M. (2009). Cannabinoid type 2 receptor as a target for chronic pain. *Mini-Reviews in Medicinal Chemistry, 9*(1), 11–25.

108. Vann, R. E., Cook, C. D., Martin, B. R., & Wiley, J. L. (2007). Cannabimimetic properties of ajulemic acid. *Journal of Pharmacology and Experimental Therapeutics, 320*(2), 678–686.

109. Burstein, S. H., Karst, M., Schneider, U., & Zurier, R. B. (2004). Ajulemic acid: A novel cannabinoid produces analgesia without a "high." *Life Sciences, 75*(12), 1513–1522.

110. Ware, M., Fitzcharles, M-A., Joseph, L., & Shir, Y. (2010). The effects of nabilone on sleep in fibromyalgia: Results of a randomized controlled trial. *Anesthesia & Analgesia, 110*(2), 604–610.

111. Frank, B., Serpell, M. G., Hughes, J., Matthews, J. N. S., & Kapur, D. (2008). Comparison of analgesic effects and patient tolerability of nabilone and dihydrocodeine for chronic neuropathic pain: Randomised, crossover, double blind study. *British Medical Journal, 336*(7637), 199.

112. Berlach, D. M., Shir, Y., & Ware, M. (2006). Experience with the synthetic cannabinoid nabilone in chronic noncancer pain. *Pain Medicine, 7*(1), 25–29.

113. Ware, M., & St. Arnaud-Trempe, E. (2010). The abuse potential of the synthetic cannabinoid nabilone. *Addiction, 105*(3), 494–503.

114. Narang, S., Gibson, D., Wasan, A.D., Ross, E. L., Michna, E., Nedeljkovic, S. S., et al. (2008). Efficacy of dronabinol as an adjuvant treatment for chronic pain patients on opioid therapy. *The Journal of Pain, 9*(3), 254–264.

115. Grant, I. (2010, October 22). Medical marijuana: The science behind the smoke and fears. *San Diego Union Tribune*. Retrieved from http://www.utsandiego.com/news/2010/oct/22/medical-marijuana-science-behind-smoke-and-fears/

116. E. Russo (personal communication, August 16, 2011).

117. Russo, E. B. (2008). Cannabinoids in the management of difficult to treat pain. *Therapeutics and Clinical Risk Management, 4*(1), 245–259.

118. Johnson, J. R., Burnell-Nugent, M., Lossignol, D., Ganae-Motan, E. D., Potts, R., & Fallon, M. T. (2010). Multicenter, double-blind, randomized,

placebo-controlled, parallel-group study of the efficacy, safety, and tolerability of THC:CBD extract and THC extract in patients with intractable
cancer-related pain. *Journal of Pain and Symptom Management, 39*(2),
167–179.

119. Nurmikko, T. J., Serpell, M. G., Hoggart, B., Toomey, P. J., Morlion, B. J., &
Haines, D. (2007). Sativex successfully treats neuropathic pain characterized by allodynia: A randomized, double-blind, placebo-controlled clinical
trial. *PAIN, 133,* 210–220.

120. Rog, D. J., Nurmikko, T. J., Friede, T., & Young, C. A. (2005). Randomized,
controlled trial of cannabis-based medicine in central pain in multiple sclerosis. *Neurology, 65*(6), 812–819.

121. Drug and Therapeutics Bulletin. (2012). What place for cannabis extract in
MS? *Drug and Therapeutics Bulletin, 50*(12), 141–144.

122. Blake, D. R., Robson, P., Ho, M., Jubb, R. W., & McCabe, C. S. (2006).
Preliminary assessment of the efficacy, tolerability and safety of a
cannabis-based medicine (Sativex) in the treatment of pain caused by rheumatoid arthritis. *Rheumatology, 45*(1), 50–52.

123. Portenoy, R. K., Ganae-Motan, E. D., Allende, S., Yanagihara, R., Shaiova, L.,
Weinstein, S., et al. (2012). Nabiximols for opioid-treated cancer patients
with poorly-controlled chronic pain: Randomized, placebo-controlled,
graded-dose trial. *The Journal of Pain, 13*(5), 438–449.

124. Hazekamp, A. (2010). Review on clinical studies with cannabis and cannabinoids 2005–2009. *Cannabinoids, 5*(Special issue), 1–21.

125. Ben Amar, M. (2006). Cannabinoids in medicine: A review of their therapeutic potential. *Journal of Ethnopharmacology, 105*(1–2), 1–25.

126. Amtmann, D., Weydt, P., Johnson, K. L., Jensen, M. P., & Carter, G. T.
(2004). Survey of cannabis use in patients with amyotrophic lateral sclerosis. *American Journal of Hospice and Palliative Medicine, 21*(2), 95–104.

127. Lago, E. D., & Fernandez-Ruiz, J. (2007). Cannabinoids and neuropro-
tection in motor-related disorders. *CNS & Neurological Disorders—Drug
Targets, 6*(6), 377–387.

128. Carter, G. T. (2001). Marijuana in the management of amyotrophic lateral
sclerosis. *American Journal of Hospice and Palliative Care, 18*(4), 264–270.

129. Marijuana Policy Project. (n.d.). Medical marijuana research. Retrieved
from http://www.mpp.org/assets/pdfs/library/MedConditionsHandout.
pdf

130. International Association for Cannabinoid Medicines. (n.d.).
General remarks. Retrieved from http://www.cannabis-med.org/index.
php?tpl=page&id=21&lng=en

131. Guzman, M. (2003). Cannabinoids: Potential anticancer agents. *Nature
Reviews/Cancer, 3,* 745–755.

132. Sarfaraz, S., Adhami, V. M., Syed, D. N., Afaq, F., & Mukhtar, H. (2008).
Cannabinoids for cancer treatment: Progress and promise. *Cancer Research,
68*(2), 339–342.

133. Marcu, J. P., Christian, R. T., Lau, D., Zielinski, A. J., Horowitz, M. P.,
Lee, J., et al. (2010). Cannabidiol enhances the inhibitory effects of

delta-9-tetrahydrocanabinol on human glioblastoma cell proliferation and survival. *Molecular Cancer Therapeutics, 9*(1), 180–189.

134. University of South Carolina, Department of Pathology, Microbiology and Immunology. (n.d.). Dr. Prakash Nagarkatti, research interests: Cannabinoid-induced immunosuppression and use of cannabinoids in cancer therapy: (Supported by NIH grants R01 DA016545 and R21 DA014885). Retrieved from http://pathmicro.med.sc.edu/2004-fac/nagarkattip.htm

135. Abrams, D., Jay, C. A., Shade, S. B., Vizoso, H., Reda, H., Press, S., et al. (2007). Cannabis in painful HIV-associated sensory neuropathy: A randomized placebo-controlled trial. *Neurology, 68*(7), 515–521.

136. Russo, E. B. (2008). Cannabinoids in the management of difficult to treat pain. *Therapeutics and Clinical Risk Management, 4*(1), 245–259.

137. Turcotte, D., Le Dorze, J-A., Esfahani, F., Frost, E., Gomori, A., & Namaka, M. (2010). Examining the roles of cannabinoids in pain and other therapeutic indications: A review. *Expert Opinion on Pharmacotherapy, 11*(1), 17–31.

138. Lynch, M. E., & Campbell, F. (2011). Cannabinoids for treatment of chronic non-cancer pain: A systematic review of randomized trials. *British Journal of Clinical Pharmacology, 72*(5), 735–744.

139. Abrams, D. I. (2010). Cannabis in pain and palliative care. *The Pain Practitioner, 20*(4), 35–45.

140. Narang, S., Gibson, D., Wasan, A. D., Ross, E. L., Michna, E., Nedeljkov, S., et al. (2008). Efficacy of dronabinol as an adjuvant treatment for chronic pain patients on opioid therapy. *The Journal of Pain, 9*(3), 254–264.

141. Cichewicz, D. L. (2004). Synergistic interactions between cannabinoid and opioid analgesics. *Life Sciences, 74*(11), 1317–1324.

142. Hazekamp, A. (2010). Review on clinical studies with cannabis and cannabinoids 2005–2009. *Cannabinoids, 5*(Special issue), 1–21.

143. Holdcroft, A., Maze, M., Tebbs, S., & Thompson, S. (2006). A multicenter dose-escalation study of analgesic and adverse effects of an oral cannabis extract (cannador) for postoperative pain management. *Anesthesiology, 104*(5), 1040–1046.

144. Wallace, M., Schulteis, G., Atkinson, J. H., Wolfson, T., Lazzaretto, D., Bentley, H., et al. (2007). Dose-dependent effects of smoked cannabis on capsaicin-induced pain and hyperalgesia in healthy volunteers. *Anesthesiology, 107*(5), 785–796.

145. Center for Medicinal Cannabis Research, University of California. (2010, February 11). Report to the legislature and governor of the state of California presenting findings pursuant to SB847 which created the CMCR and provided state funding (p. 4). Retrieved from http://www.cmcr.ucsd.edu/images/pdfs/CMCR_REPORT_FEB17.pdf

146. Canadian Consortium for the Investigation of Cannabinoids. (n.d.). Completed clinical research on cannabinoids. Retrieved from http://www.ccic.net/index.php?id=212,685,0,0,1,0

147. Abrams, D., Jay, C. A., Shade, S. B., Vizoso, H., Reda, H., Press, S., et al. (2007). Cannabis in painful HIV-associated sensory neuropathy: A randomized placebo-controlled trial. *Neurology, 68*(7), 515–521.

148. Wilsey, B., Marcotte, T., Tsodikov, A., Millman, J., Bentley, H., Gouaux, B., et al. (2008). A randomized, placebo-controlled, crossover trial of cannabis cigarettes in neuropathic pain. *The Journal of Pain, 9*(6), 506–521.

149. Ellis, R. J., Toperoff, W., Vaida, F., van den Brande, G., Gonzales, J., Gouaux, B., et al. (2009). Smoked medicinal cannabis for neuropathic pain in HIV: A randomized, crossover clinical trial. *Neuropsychopharmacology, 34,* 672–680.

150. Ware, M. A., Wang, T., Shapiro, S., Robinson, A., Ducruet, T., Huynh, T., et al. (2010). Smoked cannabis for chronic neuropathic pain: A randomized controlled trial. *Canadian Medical Association Journal, 182,* 1489.

151. Leavitt, S. B. (2010, September 4). Is smoking "pot" helpful for neuro-pathic pain? Retrieved from http://updates.pain-topics.org/2010/09/is-smoking-pot-helpful-for-neuropathic.html

152. M.Ware (personal communication, November 11, 2009).

153. Skrabek, R. Q., Galimova, L., Ethans, K., & Perry, K. (2008). Nabilone for the treatment of pain in fibromyalgia. *The Journal of Pain, 9*(2), 164–178.

154. Fiz, J., Duran, M., Capella, D., Carbonell, J., & Farre, M. (2011). Cannabis use in patients with fibromyalgia: Effect on symptoms relief and health-related quality of life. *PLoSOne, 6*(4), e18440.

155. Rog, D. J., Nurmikko, T. J., Friede, T., & Young, C. A. (2005). Randomized, controlled trial of cannabis-based medicine in central pain in multiple scle-rosis. *Neurology, 65*(6), 812–819.

156. Russo, E. (1998). Cannabis for migraine treatment: The once and future prescription? An historical and scientific review. *PAIN, 76*(1–2), 3–8.

157. Akerman, S., Holland, P. R., & Goadsby, P. J. (2007). Cannabinoid (CB1) receptor activation inhibits trigeminovascular neurons. *Journal of Pharmacology and Experimental Therapeutics, 320*(1), 64–77.

158. Juhasz, G., Lazary, J., Chase, D., Pegg, E., Downey, D., Toth, Z. G., et al. (2009). Variations in the cannabinoid receptor 1 gene predispose to migraine. *Neuroscience Letters, 461*(2), 116–120.

159. Joy, J. E., & Benson, J. A. (Eds.). (1999). *Marijuana and medicine: Assessing the science base* (p. 6). Washington, DC: National Academies Press.

160. Degenhardt, L., & Hall, W. D. (2008). The adverse effects of cannabi-noids: Implications for use of medicinal marijuana. *Journal of the Canadian Medical Association, 178*(13), 1685–1686.

161. Wang, T., Collet, J-P., Shapiro, S., & Ware, M. A. (2008). Adverse effects of medical cannabinoids: A systematic review. *Journal of the Canadian Medical Association, 178*(13), 1669–1678.

162. Degenhardt, L., & Hall, W. D. (2008). The adverse effects of cannabi-noids: Implications for use of medicinal marijuana. *Journal of the Canadian Medical Association, 178*(13), 1685–1686.

163. Vandrey, R., Budney, A. J., Kamon, J. L., & Stanger, C. (2005). Cannabis withdrawal in adolescent treatment seekers. *Drug and Alcohol Dependence, 78*(2), 205–210.

164. Grant, I. (2010, October 22). Medical marijuana: The science behind the smoke and fears. *San Diego Union Tribune.* Retrieved from http://www.

utsandiego.com/news/2010/oct/22/medical-marijuana-science-behind-smoke-and-fears/

165. National Institute on Drug Abuse. (n.d.). Research reports: Marijuana abuse: Is marijuana addictive? Retrieved from http://www.drugabuse.gov/publications/research-reports/marijuana-abuse/marijuana-addictive

166. National Institute on Drug Abuse. (2011). Topics in brief: Marijuana. Marijuana and addiction. Retrieved from http://www.drugabuse.gov/publications/topics-in-brief/marijuana

167. S. Weiss (personal communication, March 22, 2012).

168. Ware, M. A., & Tawfik, V. L. (2005). Safety issues concerning the medical use of cannabis and cannabinoids. *Pain Research & Management: The Journal of the Canadian Pain Society, 10*(Supplement A), 33A.

169. S. Weiss (personal communication, March 22, 2012).

170. Anthony, J. C., Warner, L. A., & Kessler, R. C. (1994). Comparative epidemiology of dependence on tobacco, alcohol, controlled substances, and inhalants: Basic findings from the national comorbidity study. *Experimental and Clinical Psychopharmacology, 2*(3), 244–268.

171. Singh, R., Sandhu, J., Kaur, B., Juren, T., Steward, W. P., Segerback, D., et al. (2009). Evaluation of the DNA damaging potential of cannabis cigarette smoke by the determination of acetaldehyde derived N2-ethyl-2-deoxyguanosine adducts. *Chemical Research in Toxicology, 22*(6), 1181–1188.

172. Guzman, M. (2003). Cannabinoids: Potential anticancer agents. *Nature Reviews/Cancer, 3*, 745–755.

173. Hashibe, M., Morgenstern, H., Cui, Y., Tashkin, D. P., Zhang, Z-F., Cozen, W., et al. (2006). Marijuana use and the risk of lung and upper aerodigestive tract cancers: Results of a population-based case-control study. *Cancer Epidemiology, Biomarkers and Prevention, 15*(10), 1829–1834.

174. Foreman, J. (2009, July 13). Evil weed or useful drug? *The Boston Globe.* Retrieved from http://articles.boston.com/2009-07-13/news/29262455_1_medical-marijuana-marinol-marijuana-policy-project

175. Berthiller, J., Yuan-chin, A. L., Boffetta, P., Wei, Q., Sturgis, E. M., Greenland, S., et al. (2009). Marijuana smoking and the risk of head and neck cancer: Pooled analysis in the INHANCE consortium. *Cancer Epidemiology, Biomarkers and Prevention, 18*(5), 1544–1551

176. National Institute on Drug Abuse. (n.d.). Marijuana: Facts parents need to know. Does smoking marijuana cause lung cancer? Retrieved from http://www.drugabuse.gov/publications/marijuana-facts-parents-need-to-know/want-to-know-more-some-faqs-about-marijuana

177. Zammit, S., Allebeck, P., Andreasson, S., Lundberg, I., & Lewis, G. (2002). Self-reported cannabis use as a risk factor for schizophrenia in Swedish conscripts of 1969: Historical cohort. *British Medical Journal, 325*, 1199, 1212.

178. Arseneault, L., Cannon, M., Poulton, R., Murray, R., Caspi, A., & Moffitt, T. E. (2002). Cannabis use in adolescence and risk for adult psychosis: Longitudinal prospective study. *British Medical Journal, 325*(7374), 1195, 1199.

179. van Os, J., Bak, M., Hanssen, M., Bijl, R.V., de Graaf, R., & Verdoux, H. (2002). Cannabis use and psychosis: A longitudinal population-based study. *American Journal of Epidemiology, 156*, 319–327.

180. Smit, F., Bolier, L., & Cuijpers, P. (2004). Cannabis use and the risk of later schizophrenia: A review. *Addiction, 99*, 425–430.

181. Moore, T. H. M., Zammit, S., Lingford-Hughes, A., Barnes, T. R. E., Jones, P. B., Burke, M., et al. (2007). Cannabis use and risk of psychotic or affective mental health outcomes: A systematic review. *The Lancet, 370*(9584), 319–328.

182. McGrath, J., Welham, J., Scott, J., Varghese, D., Degenhardt, L., Hayatbakhsh, M. R., et al. (2010). Association between cannabis use and psychosis-related outcomes using sibling pair analysis in a cohort of young adults. *Archives of General Psychiatry, 67*(5), 440–447.

183. Large, M., Sharma, S., Compton, M. T., Slade, T., & Nielssen, O. (2011). Cannabis use and earlier onset of psychosis. *Archives of General Psychiatry, 68*(6), 555–561.

184. Frisher, M., Crome, I., Martino, O., & Croft, P. (2009). Assessing the impact of cannabis use on trends in diagnosed schizophrenia in the United Kingdom from 1996 to 2005. *Schizophrenia Research, 113*(2–3), 123–128.

185. van Winkel, R. (2011). Family-based analysis of genetic variation underlying psychosis-inducing effects of cannabis. *Archives of General Psychiatry, 68*(2), 148–157.

186. Stokes, P. R., Mehta, M. A., Curran, H. V., Breen, G., & Grasby, P. M. (2009). Can recreational doses of THC produce significant dopamine release in the human striatum? *Neuroimage, 48*(1), 186–190.

187. Leweke, F. M., Koethe, D., Gerth, C. W., Nolden, B. M., Schreibe, D., Hansel, A., et al. (2005, September). *Cannabidiol as an antipsychotic. A double-blind, controlled clinical trial on cannabidiol vs. amisulpride in acute schizophrenia.* Paper presented at the IACM 3rd Conference on Cannabinoids in Medicine, Leiden, the Netherlands. Abstract retrieved from http://www.cannabis-med.org/studies/ww_en_db_study_show.php?s_id=171

188. Pierre, J. M. (2011). Cannabis, synthetic cannabinoids, and psychosis risk: What the evidence says. *Current Psychiatry, 10*(9), 49–57.

189. Ware, M. A., & Tawfik, V. L. (2005). Safety issues concerning the medical use of cannabis and cannabinoids. *Pain Research & Management: The Journal of the Canadian Pain Society, 10*(Supplement A), 34A.

190. Patton, G. C., Coffey, C., Carlin, J. B., Degenhardt, L., Lynskey, M., & Hall, W. (2002). Cannabis use and mental health in young people: Cohort study. *British Medical Journal, 325*(7374), 1195.

191. Ware, M. A., & Tawfik, V. L. (2005). Safety issues concerning the medical use of cannabis and cannabinoids. *Pain Research & Management: The Journal of the Canadian Pain Society, 10*(Supplement A), 34A.

192. Pope, H. G., Gruber, A. J., Hudson, J. I., Cohane, G., Huestis, M. A., & Yurgelun-Todd, D. (2003). Early-onset cannabis use and cognitive

deficits: What is the nature of the association? *Drug and Alcohol Dependence, 69,* 303–310.

193. Gruber, A. J., Pope, H. G., Hudson, J. I., & Yurgelun-Todd, D. (2003). Attributes of long-term heavy cannabis users: A case-control study. *Psychological Medicine, 33,* 1415–1422.

194. Yucel, M., Solowij, N., Respondek, C., Whittle, S., Fornito, A., Pantelis, C., et al. (2008). Regional brain abnormalities associated with long-term heavy cannabis use. *Archives of General Psychiatry, 65*(6), 694–701.

195. Hester, R., Nestor, L., & Garavan, H. (2009). Impaired error awareness and anterior cingulate cortex hypoactivity in chronic cannabis users. *Neuropsychopharmacology, 34,* 2450–2458.

196. McLean Hospital. (2010, November 15). McLean Hospital study shows greater cognitive deficits in marijuana users who start young [Press release]. Retrieved from http://www.mclean.harvard.edu/news/press/current. php?kw=mclean-study-shows-greater-cognitive-deficits-in-marijuana-users-who-start-&id=162

197. Meier, M. H., Caspi, A., Ambler, A., Harrington, H., Houts, R., Keefe, R. S. E., et al. (2012). Persistent cannabis users show neuropsychological decline from childhood to midlife. *Proceedings of the National Academy of Sciences, 109*(40), E2657–E2664.

198. Ware, M. A., & Tawfik, V. L. (2005). Safety issues concerning the medical use of cannabis and cannabinoids. *Pain Research & Management: The Journal of the Canadian Pain Society, 10*(Supplement A), 32A.

199. Pope, H. G., Gruber, A. J., Hudson, J. I., Huestis, M. A., & Yurgelun-Todd, D. (2001). Neuropsychological performance in long-term cannabis users. *Archives of General Psychiatry, 58,* 909–915.

200. Grant, I., Gonzalez, R., Carey, C. L., Natarajan, L., & Wolfson, T. (2003). Non-acute (residual) neurocognitive effects of cannabis use: A meta-analytic study. *Journal of the International Neuropsychological Society, 9*(5), 679–689.

201. Aldington, S., Williams, M., Nowitz, M., Weatherall, M., Pritchard, A., McNaughton, A., et al. (2007). Effects of cannabis on pulmonary structure, function and symptoms. *Thorax, 62,* 1058–1063.

202. R. Doblin (personal communication, August 9, 2011).

203. Pletcher, M. J., Vittinghoff, E., Kalhan, R., Richman, J., Safford, M., Sidney, S., et al. (2012). Association between marijuana exposure and pulmonary function over 20 years. *Journal of the American Medical Association, 307*(2), 173–181

204. Moir, D., Rickert, W. S., Levasseur, G., Larose, Y., Maertens, R., White, P., et al. (2008). A comparison of mainstream and sidestream marijuana and tobacco cigarette smoke produced under two machine smoking conditions. *Chemical Research in Toxicology, 21*(2), 494–502.

205. Ware, M. A., & Tawfik, V. L. (2005). Safety issues concerning the medical use of cannabis and cannabinoids. *Pain Research & Management: The Journal of the Canadian Pain Society, 10*(Supplement A), 32A.

206. Abrams, D. I., Vizoso, H. P., Shade, S. B., Jay, C., Kelly, M. E., & Benowitz, N. L. (2007). Vaporization as a smokeless cannabis delivery system: A pilot study. *Clinical Pharmacology & Therapeutics, 82,* 572–578.

207. Van Dam, N. T., & Earleywine, M. (2010). Pulmonary function in cannabis users: Support for a clinical trial of the vaporizer. *The International Journal of Drug Policy, 21*(6), 511–513.

208. Ware, M. A., & Tawfik, V. L. (2005). Safety issues concerning the medical use of cannabis and cannabinoids. *Pain Research & Management: The Journal of the Canadian Pain Society, 10*(Supplement A), 34A.

209. Clark, A. J., Lynch, M. E., Beaulieu, P., McGilveray, I. J., & Gourlay, D. (2005). Guidelines for the use of cannabinoid compounds for chronic pain. *Pain Research Management, 10*(Supplement A), 44A–46A.

210. Sidney, S. (2002). Cardiovascular consequences of marijuana use. *Journal of Clinical Pharmacology, 42*(11 Supplement), 64S–70S.

211. Reisfield, G. M. (2010). Medical cannabis and chronic opioid therapy. *Journal of Pain and Palliative Care Pharmacotherapy, 24*(4), 356–361.

212. Ware, M. A. (2007). Rebuttal: Is there a role for marijuana in medical practice? *Canadian Family Physician, 53*, 22.

213. McKinley, J. (2012, March 7). Pat Robertson says marijuana should be legal. *The New York Times*. Retrieved from http://www.nytimes.com/2012/03/08/us/pat-robertson-backs-legalizing-marijuana.html

214. Johnson, C. (2011, July 12). Obama cracks down on medical marijuana. Retrieved from http://www.npr.org/2011/07/12/137791944/obama-cracks-down-on-medical-marijuana

215. Hutchison, C. (2011, July 12). Marijuana advocates sue feds after DEA rejects weed as medicine. Retrieved from http://abcnews.go.com/Health/PainNews/marijuana-advocates-sue-feds-dea-rejects-weed-medicine/story?id=14046823#.T8V8uI6HpBI

216. Newport, F. (2011, October 17). Record-high 50% of Americans favor legalizing marijuana use. Retrieved from http://www.gallup.com/poll/150149/record-high-americans-favor-legalizing-marijuana.aspx

217. Nagourney, A. (2012, December 20). Marijuana, not yet legal for Californians, might as well be. *The New York Times*. Retrieved from http://www.nytimes.com/2012/12/21/us/politics/stigma-fading-marijuana-common-in-california.html?pagewanted=1

218. Mendoza, M. (2012, March 3). VP Biden goes to Latin America amid drug debate. Retrieved from http://abcnews.go.com/International/wireStory/vp-biden-latin-american-amid-drug-debate-15839428#.T1kkuc1WDld

219. FRONTLINE, The Center for Investigative Reporting & KQED (Producers). (2011). The Pot Republic: One sheriff's quietly radical experiment. Available from http://www.pbs.org/wgbh/pages/frontline/the-pot-republic/

220. Cave, D. (2012, July 30). South America sees drug path to legalization. *The New York Times*, pp. A1, A7.

221. Ferguson, A. (2010). Don't call it pot; it's "medicine" now. Dealers are caregivers, and buyers are patients…how marijuana got mainstreamed. *Time, 176*(21), 30–32, 34, 36–37.

222. Coffman, K., & Neroulias, N. (2012, November 7). Colorado, Washington first states to legalize recreational pot. Retrieved from

http://www.reuters.com/article/2012/11/07/us-usa-marijuana-legalization-idUSBRE8A602D20121107

223. Voth, E. (n.d.). [Transcript of *Doctors, patients assess effectiveness of medical marijuana*]. Retrieved from http://www.pbs.org/newshour/bb/health/july-dec11/marijuana_08-23.html (Original work broadcast August 23, 2011).
224. Kerlikowske, G. (n.d.). Official White House response to "legalize and regulate marijuana in a manner similar to alcohol": What we have to say about legalizing marijuana. Retrieved from https://wwws.whitehouse.gov/petitions#!/petition/legalize-and-regulate-marijuana-manner-similar-alcohol/y8l45gb1
225. H. Gural (personal communication, March 12, 2012).
226. Johnson, G. (2012, February 4). The big story, APNewsBreak: Effort building to change US pot laws. Retrieved from http://bigstory.ap.org/article/apnewsbreak-effort-building-change-us-pot-laws
227. Dwyer, D. (2012, December 14). Marijuana not high Obama priority. Retrieved from http://abcnews.go.com/Politics/OTUS/president-obama-marijuana-users-high-priority-drug-war/story?id=17946783#.UVBU6qUZfQM
228. Miron, J. A. (2005). The budgetary implications of marijuana prohibition. Retrieved from http://www.prohibitioncosts.org/wp-content/uploads/2012/04/MironReport.pdf
229. McKim, J. B. (2012, August 5). Maine a case study in medical marijuana. *The Boston Globe*, pp. A1, A8.
230. M. Blumenthal (personal communication, June 22, 2011).
231. E. Russo (personal communication, July 30, 2011).
232. Center for Drug Evaluation and Research, Food and Drug Administration, U.S. Department of Health and Human Services. (2004, June). Guidance for industry: Botanical drug products. Retrieved from http://www.fda.gov/downloads/Drugs/GuidanceComplianceRegulatoryInformation/Guidances/ucm070491.pdf
233. Reichbach, G. L. (2012, May 16). A judge's plea for pot. *The New York Times*. Retrieved from http://www.nytimes.com/2012/05/17/opinion/a-judges-plea-for-medical-marijuana.html?_r=2&smid=tw-share
234. Dwyer, J. (2012, July). Gustin Reichbach, judge with a radical history, dies at 65. *The New York Times*. Retrieved from http://www.nytimes.com/2012/07/19/nyregion/gustin-reichbach-judge-with-a-radical-history-dies-at-65.html?_r=0

CHAPTER 11

1. Institute of Medicine, Committee on Advancing Pain Research, Care, and Education. (2011). *Relieving pain in America: A blueprint for transforming prevention, care, education and research* (pp. 2–6). Prepublication copy. Washington, DC: National Academies Press.

2. S. Parazin (personal communication, December 21, 2011).
3. Haldeman, S., & Dagenais, S. (2008). What have we learned about the evidence-informed management of chronic low back pain? *The Spine Journal*, *8*(1), 277.
4. R. Chou (personal communication, April 3, 2012).
5. Chou, R., Loeser, J. D., Owens, D. K., Rosenquist, R. W., Atlas, S. J., Baisden, J., et al. (2009). Interventional therapies, surgery, and interdisciplinary rehabilitation for low back pain: An evidence-based clinical practice guideline from the American Pain Society. *Spine*, *34*(10), 1066–1077.
6. J. Loeser (personal communication, October 24, 2011).
7. Melzack, R., & Wall, P. D. (1965). Pain mechanisms: A new theory. *Science*, *150*(699), 971–979.
8. S. Fishman (personal communication, October 10, 2011).
9. S. Parazin (personal communication, December 21, 2011).
10. The Burton Report. (n.d.) The history of neurostimulation: Part I. Retrieved from http://www.burtonreport.com/infspine/NSHistNeurostimPartI.htm
11. Johnson, M., & Martinson, M. (2007). Efficacy of electrical nerve stimulation for chronic musculoskeletal pain: A meta-analysis of randomized controlled trials [Abstract]. *PAIN*, *130*(1), 157–165.
12. Haldeman, S., Carroll, L., Cassidy, J. D., Schubert, J., & Nygren, Å, (2008). The bone and joint decade 2000–2010 task force on neck pain and its associated disorders: Executive summary. *Spine*, *33*(4S), S5–S7.
13. Haldeman, S., & Dagenais, S. (2008). What have we learned about the evidence-informed management of chronic low back pain? *The Spine Journal*, *8*(1), 266–277.
14. Poitras, S., & Brosseau, L. (2008). Evidence-informed management of chronic low back pain with transcutaneous electrical nerve stimulation, interferential current, electrical muscle stimulation, ultrasound, and thermotherapy. *The Spine Journal*, *8*(1), 226–233.
15. Dubinsky, R. M., & Miyasaki, J. (2010). Assessment: Efficacy of transcutaneous electric nerve stimulation in the treatment of pain in neurologic disorders (an evidence-based review) [Abstract]. *Neurology*, *74*(2), 173–176.
16. Mulvey, M. R., Bagnall, A. M., Johnson, M. I., & Marchant, P. R. (2010). Transcutaneous electrical nerve stimulation (TENS) for phantom pain and stump pain following amputation in adults. *Cochrane Database of Systematic Reviews*, *2010*(5), CD007264.
17. Centers for Medicare & Medicaid Services. (n.d.). Proposed decision memo for transcutaneous electrical nerve stimulation for chronic low back pain (CAG-00429N). Retrieved from http://www.cms.gov/medicare-coverage-database/details/nca-proposed-decision-memo.aspx?NCAId=256&ver=9&NcaName=Tran
18. J. Loeser (personal communication, October 24, 2011).
19. Columbia University Medical Center. (n.d.). Peripheral nerve stimulation. Retrieved from http://www.cumc.columbia.edu/dept/peripheral-nerve/problems/pns.html

20. Raphael, J. H., Raheem, T. A., Southall, J. L., Bennett, A., Ashford, R. L., & Williams, S. (2011). Randomized double-blind sham-controlled crossover study of short-term effect of percutaneous electrical nerve stimulation in neuropathic pain [Abstract]. *Pain Medicine, 12*(10), 1515–1522.

21. Deyo, R. A., Mirza, S. K., Turner, J. A., & Martin, B. I. (2009). Overtreating chronic back pain: Time to back off? *The Journal of the American Board of Family Medicine, 22*(1), 62–68.

22. Guyer, R. D., Patterson, M., & Ohnmeiss, D. D. (2006). Failed back surgery syndrome: Diagnostic evaluation [Abstract]. *Journal of the American Academy of Orthopaedic Surgeons, 14*(9), 534–543.

23. Bederman, S. S., Mahomed, N. N., Kreder, H. J., McIsaac, W. J., Coyte, P. C., & Wright, J. G. (2010). In the eye of the beholder: Preferences of patients, family physicians, and surgeons for lumbar spinal surgery [Abstract]. *Spine, 35*(1), 108–115.

24. R. Chou (personal communication, April 3, 2012).

25. Kumar, K., Taylor, R. S., Jacques, L., Eldabe, S., Meglio, M., Molet, J., et al. (2008). The effects of spinal cord stimulation in neuropathic pain are sustained: A 24-month follow-up of the prospective randomized controlled multicenter trial of the effectiveness of spinal cord stimulation. *Neurosurgery, 63*(4), 762.

26. Mailis-Gagnon, A., Furlan, A., Sandoval, J., & Taylor, R. (2004). Spinal cord stimulation for chronic pain [Abstract]. *Cochrane Database of Systematic Reviews, 2004*(3), CD003783.

27. Kunnumpurath, S., Srinivasagopalan, R., & Vadivelu, N. (2009). Spinal cord stimulation: Principles of past, present and future practice: A review. *Journal of Clinical Monitoring and Computing, 23*(5), 333–339.

28. WebMD. (n.d). Spinal cord stimulation for chronic pain. Retrieved October 30, 2011, from http://www.webmd.com/back-pain/spinal-cord-stimulation-for-low-back-pain

29. Bittar, R. G., Kar-Purkayastha, I., Owen, S. L., Bear, R. E., Green, A., Wang, S. Y., & Aziz, T. Z. (2005). Deep brain stimulation for pain relief: A meta-analysis [Abstract]. *Journal of Clinical Neuroscience, 12*(5), 515–519.

30. J. Loeser (personal communication, October 24, 2011).

31. A. Pascual-Leone (personal communication, December 28, 2011).

32. Lefaucheur, J. P., Drouot, X., Keravel, Y., & Nguyen, J. P. (2001). Pain relief induced by repetitive transcranial magnetic stimulation of precentral cortex [Abstract]. *Neuroreport, 12*(13), 2963–2065.

33. Lefaucheur, J., Drouot, X., Menard-Lefaucheur, I., Zerah, F., Bendib, B., Cesaro, P., et al. (2004). Neurogenic pain relief by repetitive transcranial magnetic cortical stimulation depends on the origin and the site of pain. *Journal of Neurology, Neurosurgery & Psychiatry, 75*(4), 612–616.

34. Rosen, A. C., Ramkumar, M., Nguyen, T., & Hoeft, F. (2009). Noninvasive transcranial brain stimulation and pain. *Current Pain and Headache Reports, 13*(1), 12–17.

35. Leung, A., Donohue, M., Xu, R., Lee, R., Lefaucheur, J. P., Khedr, E. M., et al. (2009). rTMS for suppressing neuropathic pain: A meta-analysis [Abstract]. *The Journal of Pain, 10*(12), 1205–1216.

36. Lipton, R. B., Dodick, D. W., Silberstein, S. D., Saper, J. R., Aurora, S. K., Pearlman, S. H., et al. (2010). Single-pulse transcranial magnetic stimulation for acute treatment of migraine with aura: A randomised, double-blind, parallel-group, sham-controlled trial. *The Lancet Neurology, 9*(4), 373–380.

37. Soler, M. D., Kumru, H., Pelayo, R., Vidal, J., Tormos, J. M., Fregni, F., et al. (2010). Effectiveness of transcranial direct current stimulation and visual illusion on neuropathic pain in spinal cord injury [Abstract]. *Brain, 133*(9), 2565–2577.

38. Mhalla, A., Baudic, S., De Andrade, D. C., Gautron, M., Perrot, S., Teixeira, M. J., et al. (2011). Long-term maintenance of the analgesic effects of transcranial magnetic stimulation in fibromyalgia [Abstract]. *PAIN, 152*(7), 1478–1485.

39. Fregni, F., Freedman, S., & Pascual-Leone, A. (2007). Recent advances in the treatment of chronic pain with non-invasive brain stimulation techniques. *The Lancet Neurology, 6*(2), 188–191.

40. O'Connell, N. E., Wand, B. M., Marston, L., Spencer, S., & DeSouza, L. H. (2010). Non-invasive brain stimulation techniques for chronic pain [Abstract]. *Cochrane Database of Systematic Reviews, 2010*(9), CD008208.

41. Cohen, S. P. (2011). Epidural steroid injections for low back pain: Editorial. *British Medical Journal, 343*, d5301.

42. Iversen, T., Solberg, T. K., Romner, B., Wilsgaard, T., Twisk, J., Anke, A., et al. (2011). Effect of caudal epidural steroid or saline injection in chronic lumbar radiculopathy: Multicentre, blinded, randomised controlled trial. *British Medical Journal, 343*, d5278.

43. Carette, S., Marcoux, S., Truchon, R., Grondin, C., Gagnon, J., Allard, Y., & Latulippe, M. (1991). A controlled trial of corticosteroid injections into facet joints for chronic low back pain [Abstract]. *New England Journal of Medicine, 325*(14), 1002–1007.

44. Carette, S., Leclaire, R., Marcoux, S., Morin, F., Blaise, G. A., St.-Pierre, A., et al. (1997). Epidural corticosteroid injections for sciatica due to herniated nucleus pulposus [Abstract]. *New England Journal of Medicine, 336*(23), 1634–1640.

45. Peloso, P., Gross, A., Haines, T., Trinh, K., Goldsmith, C. H., Aker, P., et al. (2005). Medicinal and injection therapies for mechanical neck disorders. *Cochrane Database of Systematic Reviews, 2005*(3), CD000319.

46. Luijsterburg, P. A. J., Verhagen, A. P., Ostelo, R. W. J. G., Van Os, T. A. G., Peul, W. C., & Koes, B. W. (2007). Effectiveness of conservative treatments for the lumbosacral radicular syndrome: A systematic review. *European Spine Journal, 16*(7), 881–899.

47. Haldeman, S., & Dagenais, S. (2008). What have we learned about the evidence-informed management of chronic low back pain? *The Spine Journal, 8*(1), 266–277.

48. DePalma, M. J., & Slipman, C. W. (2008). Evidence-informed management of chronic low back pain with epidural steroid injections. *The Spine Journal, 8*(1), 45–55.

49. Ghahreman, A., Ferch, R., & Bogduk, N. (2010). The efficacy of transforaminal injection of steroids for the treatment of lumbar radicular pain. *Pain Medicine, 11*(8), 1149–1168.

50. Staal, J., De Bie, R., De Vet, H., Hildebrandt, J., & Nelemans, P. (2008). Injection therapy for subacute and chronic low-back pain [Abstract]. *Cochrane Database of Systematic Reviews, 2008*(3), CD001824.
51. Cohen, S. P., White, R. L., Kurihara, C., Larkin, T. M., Chang, A., Griffith, S. R., et al. (2012). Epidural steroids, etanercept, or saline in subacute sciatica. *Annals of Internal Medicine, 156*(8), 551–559.
52. Radcliff, K., Kepler, C., Hilibrand, A., Rihn, J., Zhao, W., Lurie, J., et al. (2013). Epidural steroid injections are associated with less improvement in patients with lumbar spinal stenosis: A subgroup analysis of the Spine Patient Outcomes Research Trial [Abstract]. *Spine, 38*(4), 279–291.
53. Chou, R., Loeser, J. D., Owens, D. K., Rosenquist, R. W., Atlas, S. J., Baisden, J., et al. (2009). Interventional therapies, surgery, and interdisciplinary rehabilitation for low back pain: An evidence-based clinical practice guideline from the American Pain Society. *Spine, 34*(10), 1066–1077.
54. Johnson, C. Y. (2012, October 10). Doctors split on value of low-back injections. *The Boston Globe*, pp. A1, A4.
55. WebMD. (n.d). Pain management and nerve blocks. Retrieved November 15, 2011, from http://www.webmd.com/pain-management/guide/nerve-blocks
56. Ilfeld, B. M. (2011). Continuous peripheral nerve blocks: A review of the published evidence [Abstract]. *Anesthesia & Analgesia, 113*(4), 904–925.
57. The U.S. Food and Drug Administration. (2010, October 15). FDA approves Botox to treat chronic migraine [Press release]. Retrieved from http://www.fda.gov/NewsEvents/Newsroom/PressAnnouncements/ucm229782.htm
58. Dagenais, S., Yelland, M. J., Del Mar, C., & Schoene, M. L. (2007). Prolotherapy injections for chronic low back pain. *Cochrane Database of Systematic Reviews, 2007*(2), CD00409.
59. Dagenais, S., Mayer, J., Haldeman, S., & Borg-Stein, J. (2008). Evidence-informed management of low back pain with prolotherapy. *The Spine Journal, 8(1)*, 203–212.
60. Chou, R., Loeser, J. D., Owens, D. K., Rosenquist, R. W., Atlas, S. J., Baisden, J., et al. (2009). Interventional therapies, surgery, and interdisciplinary rehabilitation for low back pain: An evidence-based clinical practice guideline from the American Pain Society. *Spine, 34*(10), 1066–1077.
61. Distel, L. M., & Best, T. M. (2011). Prolotherapy: A critical review of its role in treating chronic musculoskeletal pain. *PM&R, 3*(6 Supplement 1), S78–S81.
62. Malanga, G., & Wolff, E. (2008). Evidence-informed management of chronic low back pain with trigger point injections. *The Spine Journal, 8(1)*, 243–252.
63. Cheng, O. T., Souzdalnitski, D., Vrooman, B., & Cheng, J. (2012). Evidence-based knee injections for the management of arthritis. *Pain Medicine, 13*(6), 740–753.
64. Rutjes, A. W. S., Juni, P., da Costa, B. R., Trelle, S., Nuesch, E., & Reichenbach, S. (2012). Viscosupplementation for osteoarthritis of the knee: A systematic review and meta-analysis. *Annals of Internal Medicine, 157*(3), 180–191.

65. Coombes, B. K., Bisset, L., Brooks, P., Khan, A., & Vicenzino, B. (2013). Effect of corticosteroid injection, physiotherapy, or both on clinical outcome in patients with unilateral lateral epicondylalgia: A randomized controlled trial [Abstract]. *Journal of the American Medical Association, 309*(5), 461–469.

66. Rutjes, A. W. S., Juni, P., da Costa, B. R., Trelle, S., Nuesch, E., & Reichenbach, S. (2012). Viscosupplementation for osteoarthritis of the knee: A systematic review and meta-analysis. *Annals of Internal Medicine, 157*(3), 180–191.

67. Doheny, K. (2012, June 12). Knee injections for arthritis? Save your money, study says. Retrieved from http://news.yahoo.com/ knee-injections-arthritis-save-money-study-says- 231207566.html

68. Dumais, R., Benoit, C., Dumais, A., Babin, L., Bordage, R., de Arcos, C., et al. (2012). Effect of regenerative injection therapy on function and pain in patients with knee osteoarthritis: A randomized crossover study. *Pain Medicine, 13*(8), 990–999.

69. Nuensch, E., Trelle, S., Reichenbach, S., Rutjes, A. W. S., Tschannen, B., & Altman, D. G. (2012). Small study effects in meta-analyses of osteoarthritis trials: Meta-epidemiological study. *British Medical Journal, 341*, c3515.

70. Straube, S., Derry, S., Moore, R. A., & McQuay, H. J. (2010). Cervico-thoracic or lumbar sympathectomy for neuropathic pain and complex regional pain syndrome [Abstract]. *Cochrane Database of Systematic Reviews, 2010*(7), CD002918.

71. J. Loeser (personal communication, October 24, 2011).

72. S. P. Cohen (personal communication, November 21, 2011).

73. S. P. Cohen (personal communication, November 17, 2011).

74. J. Loeser (personal communication, November 22, 2011).

75. S. P. Cohen (personal communication, November 17, 2011).

76. J. Loeser (personal communication, November 22, 2011).

77. Cohen, S. P., Williams, K. A., Kurihara, C., Nguyen, C., Shields, C., Kim, P., et al. (2010). Multicenter, randomized, comparative cost-effectiveness study comparing 0, 1 and 2 diagnostic medial branch (facet joint nerve) block treatment paradigms before lumbar facet radiofrequency denervation. *Anesthesiology, 113*(2), 395–405.

78. Gupta, A. (2010). Evidence-based review of radiofrequency ablation techniques for chronic sacroiliac joint pain. *Pain Medicine News, 8*(12), 69–77.

79. Niemisto, L., Kalso, E. A., Malmivaara, A., Seitsalo, S., & Hurri, H. (2003). Radiofrequency denervation for neck and back pain. *Cochrane Database of Systematic Reviews, 2003*(1), CD004058.

80. R. Chou (personal communication, April 3, 2012).

81. Chou, R., Atlas, S. J., Stanos, S. P., & Rosenquist, R. (2009). Nonsurgical interventional therapies for low back pain: A review of the evidence for an American Pain Society clinical practice guideline. *Spine, 34*(10), 1078–1093.

82. R. Chou (personal communication, April 3, 2012).

83. Don, A. S., & Carragee, E. (2008). A brief review of evidence-informed management of chronic low back pain with surgery. *The Spine Journal, 8*(1), 258–265.

84. Weinstein, J. N., Lurie, J. D., Olson, P., Bronner, K. K., Fisher, E. S., Morgan, T. S. (2006). United States trends and regional variations in lumbar spine surgery: 1992–2003. *Spine, 31*(23), 2707–2714.
85. S. Parazin (personal communication, December 21, 2011).
86. Weinstein, J. N., Tosteson, T. D., Lurie, J. D., Tosteson, A. N. A, Hanscom, B., Skinner, J. S., et al. (2006). Surgical vs. nonoperative treatment for lumbar disk herniation: The Spine Patient Outcomes Research Trial (SPORT): A randomized trial [Abstract]. *Journal of the American Medical Association, 296*(20), 2441–1450.
87. Chou, R., Loeser, J. D., Owens, D. K., Rosenquist, R. W., Atlas, S. J., Baisden, J., et al. (2009). Interventional therapies, surgery, and interdisciplinary rehabilitation for low back pain: An evidence-based clinical practice guideline from the American Pain Society. *Spine, 34*(10), 1066–1077.
88. R. Chou (personal communication, April 3, 2012).
89. Don, A. S., & Carragee, E. (2008). A brief review of evidence-informed management of chronic low back pain with surgery. *The Spine Journal, 8*(1), 258–265.
90. R. Chou (personal communication, April 3, 2012).
91. S. Parazin (personal communication, April 4, 2012).
92. S. Parazin (personal communication, December 21, 2011).
93. R. Chou (personal communication, April 3, 2012).
94. Haldeman, S., & Dagenais, S. (2008). What have we learned about the evidence-informed management of chronic low back pain? *The Spine Journal, 8*(1), 266–277.
95. Don, A. S., & Carragee, E. (2008). A brief review of evidence-informed management of chronic low back pain with surgery. *The Spine Journal, 8*(1), 258–265.
96. Derby, R., Baker, R. M., & Lee, C. H. (2008). Evidence-informed management of chronic low back pain with minimally invasive nuclear decompression. *The Spine Journal, 8*(1), 150–159.
97. R. Chou (personal communication, April 3, 2012).
98. G. Bennett (personal communication, September 12, 2009).
99. G. Bennett (personal communication, September 12, 2009).
100. Zheng, H., Xiao, W. H., & Bennett, G. J. (2011). Functional deficits in peripheral nerve mitochondria in rats with paclitaxel- and oxaliplatin-evoked painful peripheral neuropathy. *Experimental Neurology, 232*(2), 154–161.
101. Wilson, A. D. H., Hart, A., Brannstrom, T., Wiberg, M., & Terenghi, G. (2007). Delayed acetyl-l-carnitine administration and its effect on sensory neuronal rescue after peripheral nerve injury. *Journal of Plastic, Reconstructive and Aesthetic Surgery, 60*(2), 114–118.
102. U.S. National Institutes of Health. (2013, March 20). Safety and efficacy of Olesoxime (TRO19622) in 3–25 years SMA patients. Retrieved from http://clinicaltrials.gov/show/NCT01302600
103. Ward, S. J., Ramirez, M. D., Neelakantan, M. S., & Walker, E. A. (2011). Cannabidiol prevents the development of cold and mechanical allodynia

in paclitaxel-treated female C57Bl6 mice. *Anesthesia & Analgesia, 113*(4), 947–950.

104. C. Serhan (personal communication, October 25, 2011).
105. Goldman, N., Chen, M., Fujita, T., Xu, Q., Peng, W., Liu, W., et al. (2010). Adenosine A1 receptors mediate local anti-nociceptive effects of acupuncture. *Nature Neuroscience, 13*, 883–888.
106. M. Zylka (personal communication, November 2, 2011).
107. Zylka, M. J., Sowa, N. A., Taylor-Blake, B., Twomey, M. A., Herrala, A., Voikar, V., et al. (2008). Prostatic acid phosphatase is an ectonucleotidase and suppresses pain by generating adenosine. *Neuron, 60*(1), 111–122.
108. Street, S. E., & Zylka, M. J. (2011). Emerging roles for ectonucleotidases in pain-sensing neurons. *Neuropsychopharmacology, 36*(1), 358.
109. Zylka, M. J. (2011). Pain-relieving properties for adenosine receptors and ectonucleotidases [Abstract]. *Trends in Molecular Medicine, 17*(4), 188–196.
110. Sowa, N. A., Street, S. E., Vihko, P., & Zylka, M. J. (2010). Prostatic acid phosphatase reduces thermal sensitivity and chronic pain sensitization by depleting phosphatidylinositol 4,5-bisphosphate [Abstract]. *Journal of Neuroscience, 30*(31), 10282–10293.
111. Sowa, N. A., Taylor-Blake, B., & Zylka, M. J. (2010). Ecto-5' nucleotidase (CD73) inhibits nociception by hydrolyzing AMP to adenosine in nociceptive circuits [Abstract]. *Journal of Neuroscience, 30*(6), 2235–2244.
112. Hurt, J. K., & Zylka, M. J. (2012). PAPupuncture has localized and long-lasting antinociceptive effects in mouse models of acute and chronic pain. *Molecular Pain, 8*(1), 28.
113. Schnabel, J. (2011, January 14). Drug for chronic pain shows promise in pre-clinical tests. Retrieved from http://www.dana.org/news/features/detail.aspx?id=29760
114. Sharif-Naeini, R., & Basbaum, A. I. (2011). Targeting pain where it resides…in the brain. *Science Translational Medicine, 3*(65), 65ps1.
115. Wang, H., Xu, H., Wu, L. J., Kim, S. S., Chen, T., Koga, K., et al. (2011). Identification of an adenylyl cyclase inhibitor for treating neuropathic and inflammatory pain [Abstract]. *Science Translational Medicine, 3*(65), 65ra3.
116. Jimenez-Andrade, J. M., Martin, C. D., Koewler, N. J., Freeman, K. T., Sullivan, L. J., Halvorson, K. G., et al. (2001). Nerve growth factor sequestering therapy attenuates non-malignant skeletal pain following fracture [Abstract]. *PAIN, 133*(1–3), 183–196.
117. Watson, J. J., Allen, S. J., & Dawbarn, D. (2008). Targeting nerve growth factor in pain: What is the therapeutic potential? [Abstract]. *BioDrugs, 22*(6), 349–359.
118. Woolf, C. J. (1996). Phenotypic modification of primary sensory neurons: The role of nerve growth factor in the production of persistent pain. *Philosophical Transactions: Biological Sciences, 351*(1338), 441–448.
119. U.S. National Institutes of Health. (2008, August 11). Tanezumab in osteoarthritis of the knee. Retrieved from http://www.clinicaltrials.gov/show/NCT00733902

120. U.S. National Institutes of Health. (2008, August 29). Tanezumab in osteo-arthritis of the hip. Retrieved from http://www.clinicaltrials.gov/show/NCT00744471

121. Ko, J. (2011, May 19). *Efficacy and safety of IV tanezumab in osteoarthritis hip and knee pain.* Results presented at the American Pain Society's 30th Annual Scientific Meeting, Austin, Texas. Retrieved from http://www.empr.com/efficacy-and-safety-of-iv-tanezumab-in-osteoarthritis-hip-and-knee-pain/article/203193/

122. Lane, N. E., Schnitzer, T. J., Birbara, C. A., Mokhtarani, M., Shelton, D. L., Smith, M. D., et al. (2010). Tanezumab for the treatment of pain from osteo-arthritis of the knee. *New England Journal of Medicine, 363,* 1521–1531.

123. Wood, J. N. (2010). Nerve growth factor and pain [Editorial]. *New England Journal of Medicine, 363,* 1572–1573.

124. Allen, J. E. (2010, September 30). "Game-changing" arthritis drug blocks pain too well in some. *ABC News.* Retrieved from http://abc-news.go.com/Health/PainArthritis/pfizer-arthritis-drug-blocks-pain/story?id=11758493

125. McCaffrey, P. (2012, October 2). NGF update: Antibodies get a second chance and small molecules zero in on TrkA. Retrieved from http://www.painresearchforum.org/news/20470-ngf-update-antibodies-get-second-chance-and-small-molecules-zero-trka?search_term=antibodies%20get%20second%20chance

126. Pfizer. (2010, June 23). Pfizer suspends chronic pain studies in tan-ezumab clinical trial [Press release]. Retrieved from http://www.pfizer.com/news/press_releases/pfizer_press_release_archive.jsp#guid=tanezumab_clinical_hold_062310&source=RSS_2010&page=6

127. M. Brown (personal communication, October 11, 2012).

128. Hucho, T. B., Dina, O. A., & Levine, J. D. (2005). Epac mediates a cAMP-to-PKC signaling in inflammatory pain: An isolectin B4(+) neuron-specific mechanism. *The Journal of Neuroscience, 25*(26), 6119–6126.

129. Yamamoto, T., Nair, P., Davis, P., Ma, S., Navratilova, E., Moye, S., et al. (2007). Design, synthesis, and biological evaluation of novel bifunc-tional c-terminal-modified peptides for δ/µ opioid receptor agonists and neurokinin-1 receptor antagonists. *Journal of Medicinal Chemistry, 50*(12), 2779–2786.

130. Andrews, N. (2012, July 9). Moving pain treatments forward: NIH Pain Consortium Symposium. Retrieved from http://www.painresearchforum.org/news/17877-moving-pain-treatments-forward-nih-pain-consor-tium-symposium

131. Andrews, N. (2012, July 9). Moving pain treatments forward: NIH Pain Consortium Symposium. Retrieved from http://www.painresearchforum.org/news/17877-moving-pain-treatments-forward-nih-pain-consor-tium-symposium

132. Wolfe, D., Mata, M., & Fink, D. J. (2009). A human trial of HSV-mediated gene transfer for the treatment of chronic pain HSV-mediate gene transfer. *Gene Therapy, 16,* 455–460.

133. Fink, D. J., & Wolfe, D. (2011). Gene therapy for pain: A perspective. *Pain Management, 1*(5), 379–381.

134. U.S. National Library of Medicine. (n.d.). Gabapentin. Retrieved from http://www.ncbi.nlm.nih.gov/pubmedhealth/PMH0000940

135. U.S. National Library of Medicine. (n.d.). Pregabalin. Retrieved from http://www.ncbi.nlm.nih.gov/pubmedhealth/PMH0000327/

136. G. Bennett (personal communication, November 1, 2011).

137. Moore, R. A., Straube, S., Wiffen, P. J., Derry, S., & McQuay, H. J. (2009). Pregabalin for acute and chronic pain in adults. *Cochrane Database of Systematic Reviews, 2009*(3), CD007076.

138. Backonja, M., Beydoun, A., Edwards, K. R., Schwartz, S. L., Fonseca, V., Hes, M., et al. (1998). Gabapentin for the symptomatic treatment of painful neuropathy in patients with diabetes mellitus: A randomized controlled trial. *Journal of the American Medical Association, 280*(21), 1831–1836.

139. Moore, R. A., Straube, S., Wiffen, P. J., Derry, S., & McQuay, H. J. (2009). Pregabalin for acute and chronic pain in adults. *Cochrane Database of Systematic Reviews, 2009*(3), CD007076.

140. Urquhart, D. M., Hoving, J. L., Assendelft, W. J. J., Roland, M., & van Tulder, M. W. (2008). Antidepressants for non-specific low back pain. *Cochrane Database of Systematic Reviews, 2008*(1), CD001703.

141. U.S. National Library of Medicine. (n.d.). Duloxetine. Retrieved from http://www.ncbi.nlm.nih.gov/pubmedhealth/PMH0000274/

142. U.S. Food and Drug Administration. (2010, November 4). FDA clears Cymbalta to treat chronic musculoskeletal pain [Press release]. Retrieved from http://www.fda.gov/NewsEvents/Newsroom/PressAnnouncements/ucm232708.htm

143. U.S. National Library of Medicine. (n.d.). Venlaxafine. Retrieved from http://www.ncbi.nlm.nih.gov/pubmedhealth/PMH0000947/

144. U.S. National Library of Medicine. (n.d.). Milnacipran. Retrieved from http://www.ncbi.nlm.nih.gov/pubmedhealth/PMH0000495/

145. U.S. National Library of Medicine. (n.d.). Nortriptyline. Retrieved from http://www.ncbi.nlm.nih.gov/pubmedhealth/PMH0000732/

146. U.S. National Library of Medicine. (n.d.). Amitriptyline. Retrieved from http://www.ncbi.nlm.nih.gov/pubmedhealth/PMH0000732/

147. U.S. National Library of Medicine. (n.d.). Desipramine. Retrieved from http://www.ncbi.nlm.nih.gov/pubmedhealth/PMH0000665/

148. U.S. National Library of Medicine. (n.d.). Olanzapine. Retrieved from http://www.ncbi.nlm.nih.gov/pubmedhealth/PMH0000161/

149. U.S. National Library of Medicine. (n.d.). Carisoprodol. Retrieved from http://www.ncbi.nlm.nih.gov/pubmedhealth/PMH0000717/

150. U.S. National Library of Medicine. (n.d.). Cyclobenzaprine. Retrieved from http://www.ncbi.nlm.nih.gov/pubmedhealth/PMH0000699/

151. U.S. National Library of Medicine. (n.d.). Diazepam. Retrieved from http://www.ncbi.nlm.nih.gov/pubmedhealth/PMH0000556/

152. Schofferman, J., & Mazanec, D. (2008). Evidence-informed management of chronic low back pain with opioid analgesics. *The Spine Journal, 8*(1), 185–194.

153. P. Fine (personal communication, October 27, 2011).

154. Woodcock, J. (2009). A difficult balance—pain management, drug safety and the FDA. *New England Journal of Medicine, 361*(22), 2105–2107.

155. U.S. Food and Drug Administration. (2011, January 13). FDA drug safety communication: Prescription acetaminophen products to be limited to 325 mg per dosage unit; boxed warning will highlight potential for severe liver failure. Retrieved from http://www.fda.gov/Drugs/DrugSafety/ucm239821.htm

156. U.S. National Library of Medicine. (n.d.). Ibuprofen—important warning. Retrieved from http://www.ncbi.nlm.nih.gov/pubmedhealth/PMH0000598

157. Lanza, F. L., Chan, F. K. L., Quigley, E. M. M., & the Practice Parameters Committee of the American College of Gastroenterology. (2009). Guidelines for prevention of NSAID-related ulcer complications. *American Journal of Gastroenterology, 104*, 728–738.

158. American Geriatrics Society Panel on the Pharmacological Management of Persistent Pain in Older Persons. (2009). Pharmacological management of persistent pain in older persons. *Journal of the American Geriatrics Society, 57*(8), 1331–1346.

159. Agency for Healthcare Research and Quality, John M. Eisenberg Center at Oregon Health and Science University. (2009, March). Choosing non-opioid analgesics for osteoarthritis [Clinician's Guide]. Retrieved from http://effectivehealthcare.ahrq.gov/index.cfm/search-for-guides-reviews-and-reports/?pageaction=displayproduct&productID=5&returnpage=

160. Fauber, J., & Gabler, E. (2012, May 29). Experts linked to drug firms tout benefits but downplay chance of addiction, other risks. *The Milwaukee-Wisconsin Journal Sentinel.* Retrieved from http://search.jsonline.com/Search.aspx?k=John%20Fauber,%20experts%20linked

161. Schmidt, M., Christiansen, C. F., Mehnert, F., Rothman, K. J., & Sorensen, H. T. (2011). Non-steroidal anti-inflammatory drug use and risk of atrial fibrillation or flutter: Population based case-control study. *British Medical Journal, 343*, d3450.

162. Fosbel, E. L., Folke, F., Jacobsen, S., Rasmussen, J. N., Sorensen, R., Schramm T. K., et al. (2010). Cause-specific cardiovascular risk associated with nonsteroidal anti-inflammatory drugs among healthy individuals. *Circulation: Cardiovascular Quality and Outcomes, 3*, 395–405.

163. Trelle, S., Reichenbach, S., Wandel, S., Hildebrand, P., Tschannen, B., Villiger, P. M., et al. (2011). Cardiovascular safety of non-steroidal anti-inflammatory drugs: Network meta-analysis. *British Medical Journal, 342*, c7086.

164. McGettigan, P., & Henry, D. (2011). Cardiovascular risk with non-steroidal anti-inflammatory drugs: Systematic review of population-based controlled observational studies. *PLoS Medicine, 8*(9), e1001098.

165. Coxib and traditional NSAID Trialists' (CNT) Collaboration. (2013). Vascular and upper gastrointestinal effects of non-steroidal anti-inflammatory drugs: Meta-analyses of individual participant data from randomised trials. *The Lancet.* Early online publication.

166. S. Parazin (personal communication, December 21, 2011).
167. Mayo Clinic. (2010, November 13). Arthritis pain: Creams and gels for aching joints. Retrieved from http://www.mayoclinic.com/health/pain-medications/PN00041
168. Hayman, M., & Kam, P. C. A. (2008). Capsaicin: A review of its pharmacology and clinical applications [Abstract]. *Current Anaesthesia & Critical Care*, *19*(5), 338–343.
169. Caterina, M. J., Schumacher, M. A., Tominaga, M., Rosen, T. A., Levine, J. D., & Julius, D. (1997). The capsaicin receptor: A heat-activated ion channel in the pain pathway. *Nature*, *389*(6653), 816–824.
170. Patwardhan, A. M., Akopian, A. N., Ruparel, N. B., Diogenes, A., Weintraub, S. T., Uhlson, C., et al. (2010). Heat generates oxidized linoleic acid metabolites that activate TRPV1 and produce pain in rodents. *The Journal of Clinical Investigation*, *120*(5), 1617–1626.
171. Agency for Healthcare Research and Quality, John M. Eisenberg Center at Oregon Health and Science University. (2009, March). Choosing non-opioid analgesics for osteoarthritis [Clinician's Guide]. Retrieved from http://effectivehealthcare.ahrq.gov/index.cfm/search-for-guides-reviews-and-reports/?pageaction=displayproduct&productID=5&return page=
172. De Silva, V., El-Metwally, A., Ernst, E., Lewith, G., & Macfarlane, G. J. (2011). Evidence for the efficacy of complementary and alternative medicines in the management of osteoarthritis: A systematic review. *Rheumatology*, *50*(5), 911–920.
173. Medline Plus. (n.d.). Lidocaine transdermal patches. Retrieved from http://www.nlm.nih.gov/medlineplus/druginfo/meds/a603026.html
174. Agency for Healthcare Research and Quality, John M. Eisenberg Center at Oregon Health and Science University. (2009, March). Choosing non-opioid analgesics for osteoarthritis [Clinician's Guide]. Retrieved from http://effectivehealthcare.ahrq.gov/index.cfm/search-for-guides-reviews-and-reports/?pageaction=displayproduct&productID=5&returnpage=http://www.sciencedirect.com/science/article/pii/S0965229911001063, accessed 12/13/11. have
175. J. Loeser (personal communication, October 24, 2011).
176. Mayfield Clinic for Brain and Spine. (n.d.). Intrathecal drug pump. Retrieved from http://www.mayfieldclinic.com/PE-Pump.htm
177. Smith, H., Deer, T., Staats, P., Singh, V., Sehgal, N., & Cordner, H. (2008). Intrathecal drug delivery [Abstract]. *Pain Physician*, *11*(2 Supplement), S89–S104.
178. Jazz Pharmaceuticals. (n.d.). The Prialt difference. Retrieved from http://www.prialt.com
179. Braz, J. M., Sharif-Naeini, R., Vogt, D., Kriegstein, A., Alvarez-Buylla, A., Rubenstein, J. L., et al. (2012). Forebrain GABAergic neuron precursors integrate into adult spinal cord and reduce injury-induced neuropathic pain. *Neuron*, *74*(4), 663–675.

CHAPTER 12

1. National Center for Complementary and Alternative Medicine. (2008). Health conditions prompting CAM use. Retrieved from http://nccam.nih.gov/news/camstats/2007/camsurvey_fs1.htm

2. Barnes, P. M., Bloom, B., & Nahin, R. L. (2008). Complementary and alternative medicine use among adults and children: United States, 2007 (National Health Statistics Reports No. 12). Retrieved from http://www.cdc.gov/nchs/data/nhsr/nhsr012.pdf

3. Cohen, S. P., Argoff, C. E., & Carragee, E. J. (2009). Management of low back pain [Clinical review]. *British Journal of Medicine, 338,* 100–106.

4. National Center for Complementary and Alternative Medicine. (n.d.). Statistics on complementary and alternative medicine national health interview survey. Retrieved from http://nccam.nih.gov/news/camstats/NHIS.htm

5. National Center for Complementary and Alternative Medicine. (2009). The use of complementary and alternative medicine in the United States: Cost data. Retrieved from http://nccam.nih.gov/news/camstats/costs/cost-datafs.htm

6. Barnes, P. M., Bloom, B., & Nahin, R. L. (2008). Complementary and alternative medicine use among adults and children: United States, 2007 (National Health Statistics Reports No. 12). Retrieved from http://www.cdc.gov/nchs/data/nhsr/nhsr012.pdf

7. National Center for Complementary and Alternative Medicine. (n.d.). NCCAM facts-at-a-glance and mission. Retrieved from http://nccam.nih.gov/about/ataglance

8. Mielczarek, E. V., & Engler, B. D. (2012). Measuring mythology: Startling concepts in NCCAM grants. *Skeptical Inquirer, 36*(1), 35–43.

9. Barnes, P. M., Bloom, B., & Nahin, R. L. (2008). Complementary and alternative medicine use among adults and children: United States, 2007 (National Health Statistics Reports No. 12). Retrieved from http://www.cdc.gov/nchs/data/nhsr/nhsr012.pdf

10. Consumer Reports. (2011). Natural health: Alternative treatments. Retrieved from http://www.consumerreports.org/health/natural-health/alternative-treatments/overview/index.htm

11. National Center for Complementary and Alternative Medicine. (2005). Herbs at a glance: Echinacea. Retrieved from http://nccam.nih.gov/health/echinacea/ataglance.htm

12. Barnes, P. M., Bloom, B., & Nahin, R. L. (2008). Complementary and alternative medicine use among adults and children: United States, 2007 (National Health Statistics Reports No. 12). Retrieved from http://www.cdc.gov/nchs/data/nhsr/nhsr012.pdf

13. Foreman, J. (2006, February 6). Trick or treatment? *The Boston Globe.* Retrieved from http://www.boston.com/yourlife/health/diseases/articles/2006/02/06/trick_or_treatment/

14. Barnes, P. M., Bloom, B., & Nahin, R. L. (2008). Complementary and alternative medicine use among adults and children: United States, 2007 (National

Health Statistics Reports No. 12). Retrieved from http://www.cdc.gov/nchs/data/nhsr/nhsr012.pdf

15. MacPherson, H., & Asghar, A. (2006). Acupuncture needle sensations associated with De Qi: A classification based on experts' ratings. *Journal of Alternative and Complementary Medicine, 12*(7), 633–637.

16. Hui, K. K. S., Liu, J., Marina, O., Napadow, V., Haselgrove, C., Kwong, K. K., et al. (2005). The integrated response of the human cerebro-cerebellar and limbic systems to acupuncture stimulation at ST 36 as evidenced by fMRI. *NeuroImage, 27*(3), 479–496.

17. Kong, J., Gollub, R., Huang, T., Polich, G., Napadow, V., Hui, K., et al. (2007). Acupuncture De Qi, from qualitative history to quantitative measurement. *Journal of Alternative and Complementary Medicine, 13*(10), 1059–1070.

18. Langevin, H. M., Wayne, P. M., MacPherson, H., Schnyer, R., Milley, R. M., Napadow, V., et al. (2011). Paradoxes in acupuncture research: Strategies for moving forward [Review article]. *Evidence-Based Complementary and Alternative Medicine (eCAM),* 2011(180805), 1–11.

19. Derry, C. J., Derry, S., McQuay, H. J., & Moore, R. A. (2006). Systematic review of systematic reviews of acupuncture published 1996–2005. *Clinical Medicine, 6*(4), 381–386.

20. Johnson, M. I. (2006). The clinical effectiveness of acupuncture for pain relief—you can be certain of uncertainty. *Acupuncture in Medicine,* 24, 71–79.

21. Cherkin, D. C., Sherman, K. J., Deyo, R. A., & Shekelle, P. G. (2003). A review of the evidence for the effectiveness, safety, and cost of acupuncture, massage therapy, and spinal manipulation for back pain. *Annals of Internal Medicine, 138*(11), 898–906.

22. Vickers, A. J., Cronin, A. M., Maschino, A. C., Lewith, G., MacPherson, H., Foster, N. E., et al. (2012). Acupuncture for chronic pain. *Archives of Internal Medicine, 172*(19), 1444–1453.

23. Cho, Z. H., Chung, S. C., Jones, J. P., Park, H. J., Lee, H. J., Wong, E. K., & Min, B. I. (1998). New findings of the correlation between acupoints and corresponding brain cortices using functional MRI. *Proceedings of the National Academy of Sciences, 95*(5), 2670–2673.

24. P. Wayne (personal communication, November 28, 2011).

25. V. Napadow (personal communication, November 29, 2011).

26. Cho, Z. H., Chung, S. C., Jones, J. P., Park, H. J., Lee, H. J., Wong, E. K., & Min, B. I. (1998). New findings of the correlation between acupoints and corresponding brain cortices using functional MRI. *Proceedings of the National Academy of Sciences USA, 95*(5), 2670–2673.

27. Singh, S., & Ernst, E. (2008). *Trick or treatment: The undeniable facts about alternative medicine* (p. 77). New York: Norton.

28. Ernst, E. (2006). Acupuncture—a critical analysis. *Journal of Internal Medicine, 259*(2), 125–137.

29. Singh, S., & Ernst, E. (2008). *Trick or treatment: The undeniable facts about alternative medicine* (p. 79). New York: Norton.

30. Ernst, E., Soo Lee, M., & Choi, T-Y. (2011). Acupuncture: Does it alleviate pain and are there serious risks? A review of reviews. *PAIN, 152*(4), 755–764.
31. Ernst, E. (2012). Acupuncture: What does the most reliable evidence tell us? An update. *Journal of Pain and Symptom Management, 43*(2), e11–e13.
32. V. Napadow (personal communication, November 29, 2011).
33. Sun, Y., Gan, T. J., Dubose, J. W., & Habib, A. S. (2008). Acupuncture and related techniques for postoperative pain: A systematic review of randomized clinical trials. *British Journal of Anesthesia, 101*(2), 151–160.
34. Berman, B. M., Lao, L., Langenberg, P., Lee, W. L., Gilpin, A. M. K., & Hochberg, M. C. (2004). Effectiveness of acupuncture as adjunctive therapy in osteoarthritis of the knee: A randomized, controlled trial. *Annals of Internal Medicine, 141*(12), 901–910.
35. Jubb, R. W., Tukmachi, E. S., Jones, P. W., Dempsey, E., Waterhouse, L., & Brailsford, S. (2008). A blinded randomised trial of acupuncture (manual and electroacupuncture) compared with a non-penetrating sham for the symptoms of osteoarthritis of the knee. *Acupuncture in Medicine, 26,* 69–78.
36. P. Wayne (personal communication, November 28, 2011).
37. Manheimer, E., White, A., Berman, B., Forys, K., & Ernst, E. (2005). Meta-analysis: Acupuncture for low back pain. *Annals of Internal Medicine, 142*(8), 651–663.
38. Shen, Y. F., Younger, J., Goddard, G., & Mackey, S. (2009). Randomized clinical trial of acupuncture for myofascial pain of the jaw muscles. *Journal of Orofacial Pain, 23*(4), 353–359.
39. Berman, B. M., Langevin, H. M., Witt, C. M., & Dubner, R. (2010). Acupuncture for chronic low back pain. *New England Journal of Medicine, 363*(5), 454–461.
40. Ammendolia, C., Furlan, A. D., Imamura, M., Irvin, E., & van Tulder, M. (2008). Evidence-informed management of chronic low back pain with needle acupuncture. *The Spine Journal, 8*(1), 160–172.
41. Cherkin, D. C., Sherman, K. J., Avins, A. L., Erro, J. H., Ichikawa, L., Barlow, W. E., et al. (2009). A randomized trial comparing acupuncture, simulated acupuncture and usual care for chronic low back pain. *Archives of Internal Medicine, 169*(9), 858–866.
42. Singh, S., & Ernst, E. (2008). *Trick or treatment: The undeniable facts about alternative medicine* (p. 87). New York: Norton.
43. The National Institutes of Health Consensus Development Program. (1997). Acupuncture. NIH Consensus Development Conference Statement November 3–5, 1997. Retrieved from http://consensus.nih.gov/1997/1997Acupuncture107html.htm
44. Foreman, J. (2005, March 22). Acupuncture has won medical acceptance. *The Boston Globe.* Retrieved from http://www.boston.com/news/globe/health_science/articles/2005/03/22/acupuncture_has_won_medical_acceptance/
45. B. Pomeranz (personal communication, April 8, 2012).
46. The National Institutes of Health Consensus Development Program. (1997). Acupuncture. NIH Consensus Development Conference

Statement November 3–5, 1997. Retrieved from http://consensus.nih.gov/1997/1997Acupuncture107html.htm

47. MedlinePlus. (n.d.). Acupuncture. Retrieved from http://vsearch.nlm.nih.gov/vivisimo/cgi-bin/query-meta?v%3Aproject=medlineplus&query=acupuncture&x=21&y=17

48. Foreman, J. (2005, March 22). Acupuncture has won medical acceptance. *The Boston Globe*. Retrieved from http://www.boston.com/news/globe/health_science/articles/2005/03/22/acupuncture_has_won_medical_acceptance/

49. The National Institutes of Health Consensus Development Program. (1997). Acupuncture. NIH Consensus Development Conference Statement November 3–5, 1997. Retrieved from http://consensus.nih.gov/1997/1997Acupuncture107html.htm

50. Goldman, N., Chen, M., Fujita, T., Xu, Q., Peng, W., Liu, W., et al. (2010). Adenosine A1 receptors mediate local anti-nociceptive effects of acupuncture. *Nature Neuroscience, 13*, 883–888.

51. U.S. National Library of Medicine. (2011). Carpal tunnel syndrome. Retrieved from http://www.ncbi.nlm.nih.gov/pubmedhealth/PMH0001469

52. Napadow, V., Kettner, N., Ryan, A., Kwong, K. K., Audette, J., & Hui, K. K. S. (2006). Somatosensory cortical plasticity in carpal tunnel syndrome—a cross-sectional fMRI evaluation. *NeuroImage, 31*(2), 520–530.

53. Napadow, V., Kettner, N., Liu, J., Li, M., Kwong, K. K., Vangel, M., et al. (2007). Hypothalamus and amygdala response to acupuncture stimuli in carpal tunnel syndrome. *PAIN, 130*(2), 254–266.

54. Napadow, V., Liu, J., Li, M., Kettner, N., Ryan, A., Kwong, K. K., et al. (2007). Somatosensory cortical plasticity in carpal tunnel syndrome treated by acupuncture. *Human Brain Mapping, 28*(3), 159–171.

55. Dhond, R. P., Yeh, C., Park, K., Kettner, N., & Napadow, V. (2008). Acupuncture modulates resting state connectivity in default and sensorimotor brain networks. *PAIN, 136*(3), 407–418.

56. Napadow, V., Lacount, L., Park, K., As-Sanie, S., Clauw, D. J., Harris, R. E., et al. (2010, November). *Intrinsic brain connectivity in fibromyalgia is associated with chronic pain intensity and modulated by acupuncture.* Paper presented at the 40th Annual Meeting of the Society for Neuroscience, San Diego, CA.

57. V. Napadow (personal communication, January 27, 2012).

58. Kong, J., Kaptchuk, T. J., Polich, G., Kirsch, I., Vangel, M., Zyloney, C., et al. (2009). Expectancy and treatment interactions: A dissociation between acupuncture analgesia and expectancy evoked placebo analgesia. *NeuroImage, 45*(3), 940–949.

59. Medical Acupuncture. (2011, May 12). Acupuncture administered by U.S. military physicians growing for a variety of medical conditions [Press release]. Retrieved from http://www.liebertpub.com/global/pressrelease/acupuncture-administered-by-us-military-physicians-growing-for-a-variety-of-medical-conditions/900/

60. Chou, R., & Huffman, L. H. (2007). Nonpharmacologic therapies for acute and chronic low back pain: A review of the evidence for an American Pain

Society/American College of Physicians clinical practice guideline. *Annals of Internal Medicine, 147*(7), 492–504.

61. Berman, B. M., Langevin, H. M., Witt, C. M., & Dubner, R. (2010). Acupuncture for chronic low back pain. *New England Journal of Medicine, 363*(5), 454–461.

62. Ammendolia, C., Furlan, A. D., Imamura, M., Irvin, E., & van Tulder, M. (2008). Evidence-informed management of chronic low back pain with needle acupuncture. *The Spine Journal, 8*(1), 160–172.

63. Berman, B. M., Langevin, H. M., Witt, C. M., & Dubner, R. (2010). Acupuncture for chronic low back pain. *New England Journal of Medicine, 363*(5), 454–461.

64. National Institute for Health and Clinical Excellence. (2009). Low back pain: Early management of persistent non-specific low back pain. NICE clinical guideline 88. Retrieved from http://www.nice.org.uk/nicemedia/live/11887/44343/44343.pdf

65. Trinh, K., Graham, N., Gross, A., Goldsmith, C. H., Wang, E., Cameron, I. D., et al. (2010). Acupuncture for neck disorders [Intervention review]. *Cochrane Database of Systematic Reviews, 2006*(3), CD004870.

66. Furlan, A. D., van Tulder, M. W., Cherkin, D., Tsukayama, H., Lao, L., Koes, B. W., et al. (2008). Acupuncture and dry-needling for low back pain. *Cochrane Database of Systematic Reviews, 2008*(4), CD001351.

67. Vickers, A. J., Cronin, A. M., Maschino, A. C., Lewith, G., MacPherson, H., Foster, N. E., et al. (2012). Acupuncture for chronic pain. *Archives of Internal Medicine, 172*(19), 1444–1453.

68. Berman, B. M., Langevin, H. M., Witt, C. M., & Dubner, R. (2010). Acupuncture for chronic low back pain. *New England Journal of Medicine, 363*(5), 454–461.

69. The National Institutes of Health Consensus Development Program. (1997). Acupuncture. NIH Consensus Development Conference Statement November 3–5, 1997. Retrieved from http://consensus.nih.gov/1997/1997Acupuncture107html.htm

70. Ernst, E., Soo Lee, M., & Choi, T-Y. (2011). Acupuncture: Does it alleviate pain and are there serious risks? A review of reviews. *PAIN, 152*(4), 755–764.

71. Rapaport, M. H., Schettler, P., & Bresee, C. (2010). A preliminary study of the effects of a single session of Swedish massage on hypothalamic-pituitary-adrenal and immune function of normal individuals. *Journal of Alternative and Complementary Medicine, 16*(10), 1–10.

72. Barnes, P. M., Bloom, B., & Nahin, R. L. (2008). Complementary and alternative medicine use among adults and children: United States, 2007 (National Health Statistics Reports No. 12). Retrieved from http://www.cdc.gov/nchs/data/nhsr/nhsr012.pdf

73. Chou, R., & Huffman, L. H. (2007). Nonpharmacologic therapies for acute and chronic low back pain: A review of the evidence for an American Pain Society/American College of Physicians clinical practice guideline. *Annals of Internal Medicine, 147*(7), 492–504.

74. Haldeman, S., & Dagenais, S. (2008). What have we learned about the evidence-informed management of chronic low back pain? *The Spine Journal*, 8, 266–277.

75. Imamura, M., Furlan, A. D., Dryden, T., & Irvin, E. (2008). Evidence-informed management of chronic low back pain with massage. *The Spine Journal*, 8, 121–133.

76. Leavitt, S. B. (2011, October 21). More people turning to clinical massage for pain. Retrieved from http://updates.pain-topics.org/2011/10/more-people-turning-to-clinical-massage.html

77. Chou, R., & Huffman, L. H. (2007). Nonpharmacologic therapies for acute and chronic low back pain: A review of the evidence for an American Pain Society/American College of Physicians clinical practice guideline. *Annals of Internal Medicine*, 147(7), 492–504.

78. Cherkin, D. C., Sherman, K. J., Deyo, R. A., & Shekelle, P. G. (2003). A review of the evidence for the effectiveness, safety, and cost of acupuncture, massage therapy, and spinal manipulation for back pain. *Annals of Internal Medicine*, 138(11), 898–906.

79. Chou, R., & Huffman, L. H. (2007). Nonpharmacologic therapies for acute and chronic low back pain: A review of the evidence for an American Pain Society/American College of Physicians clinical practice guideline. *Annals of Internal Medicine*, 147(7), 492–504.

80. Furlan, A., Imamura, M., Dryden, T., & Irvin, E. (2008). Massage for low back pain. *Cochrane Database of Systematic Reviews*, 2008(4), CD001929.

81. Cherkin, D. C., Sherman, K. J., Kahn, J., Wellman, R., Cook, A. J., Johnson, E., et al. (2011). A comparison of the effects of 2 types of massage and usual care on chronic low back pain. *Annals of Internal Medicine*, 155(1), 1–9.

82. Rapaport, M. H., Schettler, P., & Bresee, C. (2010). A preliminary study of the effects of a single session of Swedish massage on hypothalamic-pituitary-adrenal and immune function in normal individuals. *Journal of Alternative and Complementary Medicine*, 16(10), 1079–1088.

83. Kutner, J. S., Smith, M. C., Corbin, L., Hemphill, L., Benton, K., Mellis, K., et al. (2008). Massage therapy versus simple touch to improve pain and mood in patients with advanced cancer: A randomized trial. *Annals of Internal Medicine*, 149(6), 369–379.

84. Consumer Reports. (n.d.). Alternative treatments. Retrieved from http://www.consumerreports.org/health/natural-health/alternative-treatments/overview/index.htm

85. Leavitt, S. B. (2009). Biofield therapies for pain: Help or hype. Retrieved from http://updates.pain-topics.org/2009/11/biofield-therapies-for-pain-help-or.html

86. Jain, S., & Mills, P. J. (2010). Biofield therapies: Helpful or full of hype? A best evidence synthesis. *International Journal of Behavioral Medicine*, 17(1), 1–16.

87. So, P. S., Jiang, Y., & Qin, Y. (2008). Touch therapies for pain relief in adults. *Cochrane Database of Systematic Reviews*, 2008(4), CD006535.

88. Leavitt, S. B. (2009). Biofield therapies for pain: Help or hype. Retrieved from http://updates.pain-topics.org/2009/11/biofield-therapies-for-pain-help-or.html

89. Singh, S., & Ernst, E. (2008). *Trick or treatment: The undeniable facts about alternative medicine* (p. 327). New York: Norton.

90. Barnes, P. M., Bloom, B., & Nahin, R.L. (2008). Complementary and alternative medicine use among adults and children: United States, 2007. *National Health Statistics Report, 12,* 1-24. Retrieved from http://nccam.nih.gov/sites/nccam.nih.gov/files/news/nhsr12.pdf

91. National Center for Complementary and Alternative Medicine. (n.d.). Health topics A–Z. Retrieved from http://nccam.nih.gov/health/atoz.htm

92. Singh, S., & Ernst, E. (2008). *Trick or treatment: The undeniable facts about alternative medicine* (p. 293). New York: Norton.

93. Stallibrass, C., Sissons, P., & Chalmers, C. (2002). Randomized controlled trial of the Alexander technique for idiopathic Parkinson's disease. *Clinical Rehabilitation, 16*(7), 695–708.

94. Little, P., Lewith, G., Webley, F., Evans, M., Beattie, A., Middleton, K., et al. (2008). Randomised controlled trial of Alexander technique lessons, exercise, and massage (ATEAM) for chronic and recurrent back pain. *British Journal of Sports Medicine, 42,* 965–968.

95. Cacciatore, T. W., Gurfinkel, V. S., Horak, F. B., Cordo, P. J., & Ames, K. E. (2011). Increased dynamic regulation of postural tone through Alexander technique training. *Human Movement Science, 30*(1), 74–89.

96. National Center for Complementary and Alternative Medicine. (n.d.). Get the facts: Headaches and CAM: What the science says about CAM and headaches. Retrieved from http://nccam.nih.gov/health/pain/headache-facts.htm

97. Singh, S., & Ernst, E. (2008). *Trick or treatment: The undeniable facts about alternative medicine* (p. 305). New York: Norton.

98. Barnes, P. M., Bloom, B., & Nahin, R. L. (2008). Complementary and alternative medicine use among adults and children: United States, 2007. *National Health Statistics Report, 12,* 1–24. Retrieved from http://nccam.nih.gov/sites/nccam.nih.gov/files/news/nhsr12.pdf

99. National Center for Complementary and Alternative Medicine. (n.d.). Health topics A–Z. Retrieved from http://nccam.nih.gov/health/atoz.htm

100. Harvard Medical School, Harvard Health Publications. (2005, October). Healing touch therapy: Alternative therapies relax heart patients. Retrieved from http://www.health.harvard.edu/press_releases/healing_touch_therapy

101. National Center for Complementary and Alternative Medicine. (n.d.). Health topics A–Z. Retrieved from http://nccam.nih.gov/health/atoz.htm

102. P.Pettinati (personal communication, December 5, 2011).

103. National Center for Complementary and Alternative Medicine. (n.d.). Health topics A–Z. Retrieved from http://nccam.nih.gov/health/atoz.htm

104. National Center for Complementary and Alternative Medicine. (2006). Reiki: An introduction. Retrieved from http://nccam.nih.gov/health/reiki/introduction.htm

105. Lee, M. S., Pittler, M. H., & Ernst, E. (2008). Effects of Reiki in clinical practice: A systematic review of randomised clinical trials. *International journal of Clinical Practice, 62*(6), 947–954.

106. vanderVaart, S., Gijsen, V. M. G. J., de Wildt, S. N., & Koren, G. (2009). A systematic review of the therapeutic effects of Reiki. *Journal of Alternative and Complementary Medicine, 15*(11), 1157–1169.

107. National Center for Complementary and Alternative Medicine. (n.d.). Health topics A–Z. Retrieved from http://nccam.nih.gov/health/atoz.htm

108. J. Gaffney (personal communication, December 3, 2011).

109. Pettinati, P. M. (2002). The relative efficacy of various complementary modalities in the lives of patients with chronic pain: A pilot study. *United States Association for Body Psychotherapy Journal, 1*(2), 6–15.

110. Rosa, L., Rosa, E., Sarner, L., & Barrett, S. (1998). A close look at therapeutic touch. *Journal of the American Medical Association, 279*(13), 1005–1010.

111. P. Pettinati (personal communication, December 4, 2011).

112. National Center for Complementary and Alternative Medicine. (2008). Spinal manipulation for low-back pain. Retrieved from http://nccam.nih.gov/health/pain/spinemanipulation.htm

113. American Chiropractic Association. (n.d.). What is chiropractic? Retrieved from http://www.acatoday.org/level2_css.cfm?T1ID=13&T2ID=61

114. Chiropractic condemned. (1969). *Journal of the American Medical Association, 208*(2), 352 Retrieved from http://jama.jamanetwork.com/issue.aspx?journalid=67&issueid=8423

115. R. Mills (personal communication, December 9, 2011).

116. National Center for Complementary and Alternative Medicine. (2007). Chiropractic: An introduction. Retrieved from http://nccam.nih.gov/health/chiropractic/introduction.htm

117. Holisticonline.com. (n.d.). Two schools of chiropractors: Straight and mixers. Retrieved from http://www.holistic-online.com/Chiropractic/chiro_straight-and-mixers.htm

118. Consumer Reports. (2009). Relief for aching backs. Retrieved from http://www.consumerreports.org/cro/magazine-archive/may-2009/health/back-pain/overview/back-pain-ov.htm

119. Jensen, M. P., Abresch, R. T., Carter, G. T., & McDonald, C. M. (2005). Chronic pain in persons with neuromuscular disease. *Archives of Physical Medicine and Rehabilitation, 86*(6), 1155–1163.

120. J. Kornfeld (personal communication, December 7, 2011).

121. Liliedahl, R. L., Finch, M. D., Axene, D. V., & Goertz, C. M. (2010). Cost of care for common back pain conditions initiated with chiropractic doctor vs medical doctor/doctor of osteopathy as first physician: Experience of one Tennessee-based general health insurer. *Journal of Manipulative and Physiological Therapeutics, 33*(9), 640–643.

122. Chou, R., Qaseem, A., Snow, V., Casey, D., Cross, J. T., Shekelle, P., et al. (2007). Diagnosis and treatment of low back pain: A joint clinical practice guideline from the American College of Physicians and the American Pain Society. *Annals of Internal Medicine, 147*(7), 478–491.

123. National Center for Complementary and Alternative Medicine. (2008). Spinal manipulation for low-back pain. Retrieved from http://nccam.nih.gov/health/pain/spinemanipulation.htm

124. Chou, R., & Huffman, L. H. (2007). Nonpharmacologic therapies for acute and chronic low back pain: A review of the evidence for an American Pain Society/American College of Physicians clinical practice guideline. *Annals of Internal Medicine, 147*(7), 492–504.

125. Bronfort, G., Haas, M., Evans, R. L., Kawchuk, G., & Dagenais, S. (2008). Evidence-informed management of chronic low back pain with spinal manipulation and mobilization. *The Spine Journal, 8,* 213–225.

126. Bronfort, G., Hass, M., Evans, R. L., & Bouter, L. M. (2004). Efficacy of spinal manipulation and mobilization for low back pain and neck pain: A systematic review and best evidence synthesis. *The Spine Journal, 4*(3), 335–356.

127. Muller, R., & Giles, L. G. F. (2005). Long-term follow-up of a randomized clinical trial assessing the efficacy of medication, acupuncture, and spinal manipulation for chronic mechanical spinal pain syndromes. *Journal of Manipulative and Physiological Therapeutics, 28*(1), 3–11.

128. Senna, M., & Machaly, S. (2011). Does maintained spinal manipulation therapy for chronic nonspecific low back pain result in better long-term outcome? *Spine, 36*(18), 1427–1437.

129. S. Haldeman (personal communication, December 8, 2011).

130. R. Chou (personal communication, December 6, 2011).

131. Hurwitz, E. L., Morgenstern, H., Kominski, G. F., Yu, F., & Chiang, L-M. (2006). A randomized trial of chiropractic and medical care for patients with low back pain: Eighteen-month follow-up outcomes from the UCLA low back pain study. *Spine, 31*(6), 611–621.

132. Cherkin, D. C., Sherman, K. J., Deyo, R. A., & Shekelle, P. G. (2003). A review of the evidence for the effectiveness, safety, and cost of acupuncture, massage therapy, and spinal manipulation for back pain. *Annals of Internal Medicine, 138*(11), 898–906.

133. Russell, I., Underwood, M., Brealey, S., Burton, K., Coulton, S., Farrin, A., et al. (2004). United Kingdom back pain exercise and manipulation (UK BEAM) randomised trial: Effectiveness of physical treatments for back pain in primary care. *British Medical Journal, 329*(7479), 1377.

134. Ferreira, M. L., Ferreira, P. H., Latimer, J., Herbert, R. D., Hodges, P. W., Jennings, M. D., et al. (2007). Comparison of general exercise, motor control exercise and spinal manipulative therapy for chronic low back pain: A randomized trial. *PAIN, 131*(1–2), 31–37.

135. Walker, B. F., French, S. D., Grant, W., & Green, S. (1976). A Cochrane review of combined chiropractic interventions for low-back pain. *Spine, 36*(3), 230–242.

136. Posadzki, P. (2012). Is spinal manipulation effective for pain? An overview of systematic reviews. *Pain Medicine, 13*(6), 754–761.
137. Peterson, C. K., Bolton, J., & Humphreys, B. K. (2012). Predictors of improvement in patients with acute and chronic low back pain undergoing chiropractic treatment. *Journal of Manipulative and Physiological Therapeutics, 35*(7), 525–533.
138. Leavitt, S. B. (2012, August 29). Is chiropractic for low-back pain effective? Retrieved from http://updates.pain-topics.org/2012/08/is-chiropractic-for-low-back-pain.html
139. Rubenstein, S. M., Terwee, C. B., Assendelft, W. J. J., de Boer, M. R., & van Tulder, M. W. (2012). Spinal manipulative therapy for acute low-back pain. *Cochrane Database of Systematic Reviews, 2012*(9), CD008880.
140. Hoving, J. L., Koes, B. W., de Vet, H. C. W., van der Windt, D. A. W. M., Assendelft, W. J. J., van Mameren, H., et al. (2002). Manual therapy, physical therapy, or continued care by a general practitioner for patients with neck pain: A randomized, controlled trial. *Archives of Internal Medicine, 136*(10), 713–722.
141. Vernon, H., Humphreys, K., & Hagino, C. (2007). Chronic mechanical neck pain in adults treated by manual therapy: A systematic review of change scores in randomized clinical trials. *Journal of Manipulative and Physiological Therapeutics, 30*(3), 215–227.
142. Bronfort, G., Evans, R., Anderson, A. V., Svendsen, K. H., Bracha, Y., & Grimm, R. H. (2012). Spinal manipulation, medication, or home exercise with advice for acute and subacute neck pain. *Annals of Internal Medicine, 156*, (1, Part 1) 1–10.
143. Gross, A., Miller, J., D'Sylva, J., Burnie, S. J., Goldsmith, C. H., Graham, N., et al. (2010). Manipulation or mobilisation for neck pain. *Cochrane Database of Systematic Reviews, 2010*(1), CD004249.
144. Ernst, E. (2010). Deaths after chiropractic: A review of published cases. *International Journal of Clinical Practice, 64*(8), 1162–1165.
145. Haldeman, S., Carey, P., Townsend, M., & Papadopoulos, C. (2001). Arterial dissections following cervical manipulation: The chiropractic experience. *Canadian Medical Association Journal, 165*(7), 905–906.
146. Haldeman, S., Kohlbeck, F. J., & McGregor, M. (2002). Stroke, cerebral artery dissection, and cervical spine manipulation therapy. *Journal of Neurology, 249*(8), 1098–1104.
147. Haldeman, S., Carroll, L., Cassidy, J. D., Schubert, J., & Nygren, A. (2008). The bone and joint decade 2000–2010 task force on neck pain and its associated disorders [Executive summary]. *European Spine Journal, 17*(Supplement 1), S5–S7.
148. S. Haldeman (personal communication, December 8, 2011).
149. Cassidy, J. D., Boyle, E., Cote, P., He, Y., Hogg-Johnson, S., Silver, F. L., et al. (2008). Risk of vertebrobasilar stroke and chiropractic care. *Spine, 33*(4S), 176–183.
150. Rubenstein, S. M., Leboeuf-Yde, C., Knol, D. L., de Koekkoek, T. E., Pfeifle, C. E., & van Tulder, M. W. (2007). The benefits outweigh the risks for

patients undergoing chiropractic care for neck pain: A prospective, multi-center, cohort study [Abstract]. *Journal of Manipulative and Physiological Therapeutics, 30*(6), 408–418.

151. Gouveia, L. O., Castanho, P., & Ferreira, J. J. (2009). Safety of chiropractic interventions: A systematic review. *Spine, 34*(11), E405–E413.

152. Wand, B. M., Heine, P. J., & O'Connell, N. E. (2012). Should we abandon cervical spine manipulation for mechanical neck pain? Yes. *British Medical Journal, 344,* e3679.

153. Cassidy, J. D., Bronfort, G., & Hartvigsen, J. (2012). Should we abandon cervical spine manipulation for mechanical neck pain? No. *British Medical Journal, 344,* e3680.

154. Weil, A. (2005). *Healthy Aging* (pp. 141–160). New York: Alfred A. Knopf.

155. Foreman, J. (2004, February 10). Fatty acid imbalance hurts our health. *The Boston Globe.* Retrieved from http://www.boston.com/news/globe/health_science/articles/2004/02/10/fatty_acid_imbalance_hurts_our_health/

156. Maroon, J. C., & Bost, J. W. (2006). Omega-3 fatty acids (fish oil) as an anti-inflammatory: An alternative to non-steroidal anti-inflammatory drugs for discogenic pain. *Surgical Neurology, 65*(4), 326–331.

157. ConsumerLab.com. (n.d.). Product review: Fish oil and omega-3 fatty acid supplements (EPA and DHA from fish, algae and krill). Retrieved from https://www.consumerlab.com/list.asp

158. U.S. National Library of Medicine. (2011). Osteomalacia. Retrieved from http://www.ncbi.nlm.nih.gov/pubmedhealth/PMH0001414/

159. Institute of Medicine. (2010). Dietary reference intakes for calcium and vitamin D. Retrieved from http://www.iom.edu/Reports/2010/Dietary-Reference-Intakes-for-Calcium-and-Vitamin-D.aspx

160. Holick, M. F., Binkley, N. C., Bischoff-Ferrari, H. A., Gordon, C. M., Hanley, D. A., Heaney, R. P., et al. (2011). Evaluation, treatment, and prevention of vitamin D deficiency: An endocrine society clinical practice guideline. *Journal of Clinical Endocrinology & Metabolism, 96*(7), 1911–1930.

161. R. Chou (personal communication, January 3, 2012).

162. McBeth, J., Pye, S. R., O'Neill, T. W., Macfarlane, G. J., Tajar, A., Bartfai, G., Boonen, et al. (2010). Musculoskeletal pain is associated with very low levels of vitamin D in men: Results from the European male aging study. *Annals of Rheumatic Diseases, 69,* 1448–1452.

163. Straube, S., Derry, S., & McQuay, H. J. (2010). Vitamin D for the treatment of chronic painful conditions in adults. *Cochrane Database of Systematic Reviews, 2010*(1), CD007771.

164. Rastelli, A. L, Taylor, M. E., Gao, F., Armamento-Villareal, R., Jamalabadi-Majidi, S., Napoli, N., et al. (2011). Vitamin D and aromatase inhibitor-induced musculoskeletal symptoms (AIMSS): A phase II, double-blind, placebo-controlled, randomized trial. *Breast Cancer Research and Treatment, 129*(1), 107–116.

165. Gopinath, K., & Danda, D. (2011). Supplementation of 1,25 dihydroxy vitamin D3 in patients with treatment naïve early rheumatoid

arthritis: A randomised controlled trial. *International Journal of Rheumatic Diseases, 14*(4), 332–339.

166. Sakalli, H., Arslan, D., & Yucel, A. E. (2011). The effect of oral and parenteral vitamin D supplementation in the elderly: A prospective, double-blinded, randomized, placebo-controlled study. *Rheumatology International, 32*(8), 2279–2283.

167. Song, G. G., Bae, S. C., & Lee, Y. H. (2012). Association between vitamin D intake and the risk of rheumatoid arthritis: A meta-analysis. *Clinical Rheumatology, 1*(12), 1733–1739.

168. Lasco, A., Catalano, A., & Benvenga, S. (2012). Improvement of primary dysmenorrhea caused by a single oral dose of vitamin D: Results of a randomized, double-blind, placebo-controlled trial. *Archives of Internal Medicine, 172*(4), 366–367.

169. Huang, W., Shah, S., Long, Q., Crankshaw, A. K., & Tangpricha, V. (2013). Improvement of pain, sleep, and quality of life in chronic pain patients with vitamin D supplementation. *The Clinical Journal of Pain, 29*(4), 341–347.

170. Mowry, E. M., Waubant, E., McCulloch, C. E., Okuda, D. T., Evangelista, A. A., Lincoln, R. R., et al. (2012). Vitamin D status predicts new brain magnetic resonance imaging activity in multiple sclerosis. *Annals of Neurology, 72*(2), 234–240.

171. Bischoff-Ferrari, H. A., Willett, W. C., Orav, E. J., Lips, P., Meunier, P. J., Lyons, R. A., et al. (2012). A pooled analysis of Vitamin D dose requirements for fracture prevention. *New England Journal of Medicine, 367,* 40–49.

172. L eavitt, S. B. (2012, July 6). Vitamin D—current research roundup. Retrieved from http://updates.pain-topics.org/2012/07/vitamin-d-current-research-roundup.html

173. J. Pereira (personal communication, December 13, 2011).

174. M. F. Holick (personal communication, December 23, 2011).

175. Pietras, S. M., Obayan, B. K., Cai, M. H., & Holick, M. F. (2009). Vitamin D2 treatment for vitamin D deficiency and insufficiency for up to 6 years [Editor's correspondence]. *Archives of Internal Medicine, 169*(19), 1806.

176. Sanders, K. M., Stuart, A. L., Williamson, E. J., Simpson, J. A., Kotowicz, M. A., Young, D., et al. (2010). Annual high-dose oral vitamin D and falls and fractures in older women. *Journal of the American Medical Association, 303*(18), 1815–1822.

177. Dawson-Hughes, B., & Harris, S. S. (2010). High dose vitamin D supplementation: Too much of a good thing? *Journal of the American Medical Association, 303*(18), 1861–1862.

178. Bjelakovic, G., Gluud, L. L., Nikolova, D., Whitfield, K., Wetterslev, J., Simonetti, R. G., et al. (2011). Vitamin D supplementation for prevention of mortality in adults. *Cochrane Database of Systematic Reviews, 2011*(7), CD007470.

179. Holick, M. F., Biancuzzo, R. M., Chen, T. C., Klein, E. K., Young, A., Bibuld, D., et al. (2008). Vitamin D2 is as effective as vitamin D3 in maintaining circulating concentrations of 25-hydroxyvitamin D. *The Journal of Clinical Endocrinology and Metabolism, 93*(3), 677–681.

180. Biancuzzo, R. M., Young, A., Bibuld, D., Cai, M. H., Winter, M. R., Klein, E. K., et al. (2010). Fortification of orange juice with vitamin D2 or vitamin D3 is as effective as an oral supplement in maintaining vitamin D status in adults. *The American Journal of Clinical Nutrition, 91*, 1621–1626.

181. Holmes, E. W., Garbincius, J., & McKenna, K. M. (2012, June). *Analytical performance characteristics of two new automated immunoassays for 25 hydroxy Vitamin D.* Paper presented at the Endocrine Society's 94th Annual Meeting, Houston, TX. Abstract retrieved from http://www.abstracts-2view.com/endo/view.php?nu=ENDO12L_MON-372&terms =

182. Clegg, D. O., Reda, D. J., Harris, C. L., Klein, M. A., O'Dell, J. R., Hooper, M. M., et al. (2006). Glucosamine, Chondroitin Sulfate, and the Two in Combination for Painful Knee Osteoarthritis, *New England Journal of Medicine, 354*, 795–808.

183. Sawitzke, A. D., Shi, H., Finco, M. F., Dunlop, D. D., Bingham, C. O., III, Harris, C. L., et al. (2008). The effect of glucosamine and/or chondroitin sulfate on the progression of knee osteoarthritis: A report from the glucosamine/chondroitin arthritis intervention trial. *Arthritis & Rheumatism, 58*(10), 3183–3191.

184. Sawitzke, A. D., Shi, H., Finco, M. F., Dunlop, D. D., Harris, C. L., Singer, N. G., et al. (2010). Clinical efficacy and safety of glucosamine/chondroitin sulphate, their combination, celecoxib or placebo taken to treat osteoarthritis of the knee: 2-year results from GAIT. *Annals of the Rheumatic Diseases, 69*, 1459–1464.

185. Agency for Healthcare Research and Quality. (2009). Choosing non-opioid analgesics for osteoarthritis (Pub. No. 06(07)-EHC009-3). Retrieved from http://www.effectivehealthcare.ahrq.gov/ehc/products/2/5/Osteoarthritis_Clinician_Guide.pdf

186. Terry, R., Posadzki, P., Watson, L. K., & Ernst, E. (2011). The use of ginger (zingiber officinale) for the treatment of pain: A systematic review of clinical trials. *Pain Medicine, 12*(12), 1808–1818.

187. Sepahvand, R., Esmaeili-Mahani, S., Arzi, A., Rasoulian, B., & Abbasnejad, M. (2010). Ginger (zingiber officinale roscoe) elicits antinociceptive properties and potentiates morphine-induced analgesia in the rat radiant heat tail-flick test. *Journal of Medicinal Food, 13*(6), 1397–401.

188. Black, C., Herring, M. P., Hurley, D. J., & O'Connor, P. J. (2010). Ginger (zingiber officinale) reduces muscle pain caused by eccentric exercise. *The Journal of Pain, 11*(9), 894–903.

189. Zhao, C., Wacnik, P. W., Tall, J. M., Johns, D. C., Wilcox, G. L., Meyer, R. A., et al. (2004). Analgesic effects of a soy-containing diet in three murine bone can pain models. *The Journal of Pain, 5*(2), 104–110.

190. Valsecchi, A. E., Franchi, S., Panerai, A. E., Sacerdote, P., Trovato, A. E., & Colleoni, M. (2008). Genistein, a natural phytoestrogen from soy, relieves neuropathic pain following chronic constriction sciatic nerve injury in mice: Anti-inflammatory and antioxidant activity. *Journal of Neurochemistry, 107*(1), 230–240.

191. Johns Hopkins Medicine. (2002, March 15). Dietary soy reduces pain, inflammation in rats [Press release]. Retrieved from http://www.hopkins-medicine.org/press/2002/MARCH/020315.htm

192. Arjmandi, B. H., Khalil, D. A., Lucas, E. A., Smith, B. J., Sinichi, N., Hodges, S. B., et al. (2004). Soy protein may alleviate osteoarthritis symptoms [Abstract]. *Phytomedicine, 11*(7–8), 567–575.

193. Funk, J. L., Frye, J. B., Oyarzo, J. N., Kuscuoglu, N., Wilson, J., McCaffrey, G., et al. (2006). Efficacy and mechanism of action of turmeric supplements in the treatment of experimental arthritis. *Arthritis & Rheumatism, 54*(11), 3452–3464.

194. The University of Arizona. (n.d.). Tapping the power of turmeric. Retrieved from http://www.arizona.edu/features/tapping-power-turmeric

195. Harrington, A. N., Hughes, P. A., Martin, C. M., Yang, J., Castro, J., Isaacs, N. J., et al. (2011). A novel role for TRPM8 in visceral afferent function. *PAIN, 152*(7), 1459–1468.

196. Gagnier, J. J., van Tulder, M. W., Berman, B. M., & Bombardier, C. (2006). Herbal medicine for low back pain. *Cochrane Database of Systematic Reviews, 2006*(2), CD004504.

197. Haldeman, S., & Dagenais, S. (2008). What have we learned about the evidence-informed management of chronic low back pain? *The Spine Journal, 8,* 266–277.

198. Gagnier, J. J. (2008). Evidence-informed management of chronic low back pain with herbal, vitamin, mineral, and homeopathic supplements. *The Spine Journal, 8,* 70–79.

199. Spigt, M., Weerkamp, N., Troost, J., van Schayck, C. P., & Knottnerus, J. A. (2012). A randomized trial on the effects of regular water intake in patients with recurrent headaches. *Family Practice, 29*(4), 370–375.

200. Westernnaturopathic. (2012, April 25). *Dr Oz PEMF* [Video file]. Retrieved from http://www.youtube.com/watch?v=H8JJiSu1KjY

201. Cepeda, M. S., Carr, D. B., Sarquis, T., Miranda, N., Garcia, R. J., & Zarate, C. (2007). Static magnetic therapy does not decrease pain or opioid require-ments: A randomized double-blind trial. *Anesthesia & Analgesia, 104*(2), 290–294.

202. National Center for Complementary and Alternative Medicine. (2008). Magnets for pain: Introduction. Retrieved from http://nccam.nih.gov/health/magnet/magnetsforpain.htm#hed1

203. Federal Trade Commission. (1999, June 24). "Operation Cure.all" targets internet health fraud [Press release]. Retrieved from http://www.ftc.gov/opa/1999/06/opcureall.shtm

204. Brown, C. S., Ling, F. W., Wan, J. Y., & Pilla, A. A. (2002). Efficacy of static magnetic field therapy in chronic pelvic pain: A double-blind pilot study [Abstract]. *American Journal of Obstetrics and Gynecology, 187*(6), 1581–1587.

205. Weintraub, M. I., Wolfe, G. I., Barohn, R. A., Cole, S. P., Parry, G. J., Hayat, G., et al. (2003). Static magnetic field therapy for symptomatic diabetic

neuropathy: A randomized, double-blind, placebo-controlled trial. *Archives of Physical Medicine and Rehabilitation, 84*(5), 736–746.

206. Winemiller, M. H., Billow, R. G., Laskowski, E. R., & Harmsen, W. S. (2003). Effect of magnetic vs sham-magnetic insoles on plantar heel pain: A randomized controlled trial. (2003). *Journal of the American Medical Association, 290*(11), 1474–1478.

207. Carter, R., Aspy, C. B., & Mold, J. (2002). The effectiveness of magnet therapy for treatment of wrist pain attributed to carpal tunnel syndrome. *The Journal of Family Practice, 51*(1), 38–40.

208. Alfano, A. P., Taylor, A. G., Foresman, P. A., Dunkl, P. R., McConnell, G. G., Conaway, M. R., et al. (2001). Static magnetic fields for treatment of fibromyalgia: A randomized controlled trial [Abstract]. *The Journal of Alternative and Complementary Medicine, 7*(1), 53–64.

209. Harlow, T., Greaves, C., White, A., Brown, L., Hart, A., & Ernst, E. (2004). Randomised controlled trial of magnetic bracelets for relieving pain in osteoarthritis of the hip and knee. *British Medical Journal, 329*(7480), 1450–1454.

210. Cepeda, M. S., Carr, D. B., Sarquis, T., Miranda, N., Garcia, R. J., & Zarate, C. (2007). Static magnetic therapy does not decrease pain or opioid requirements: A randomized double-blind trial. *Anesthesia & Analgesia, 104*(2), 290–294.

211. Khoromi, S., Blackman, M. R., Kingman, A., Patsalides, A., Matheny, L. A., Adams, S., et al. (2007). Low intensity permanent magnets in the treatment of chronic lumbar radicular pain. *Journal of Pain and Symptom Management, 34*(4), 434–445.

212. Pittler, M. H., Brown, E. M., & Ernst, E. (2007). Static magnets for reducing pain: Systematic review and meta-analysis of randomized trials. *Canadian Medical Association Journal, 177*(7), 736–742.

213. National Center for Complementary and Alternative Medicine. (2008). Magnets for pain: Introduction. Retrieved from http://nccam.nih.gov/health/magnet/magnetsforpain.htm#hed1

214. A. Pascual-Leone (personal communication, December 29, 2011).

215. Inoue, S., Ohashi, T., Yasuda, I., & Fukada, E. (1977). Electret induced callus formation in the rat. *Clinical Orthopaedics and Related Research, 124*, 57–58.

216. Morone, M. A., & Feuer, H. (2002). The use of electrical stimulation to enhance spinal fusion. *Neurosurgical Focus, 13*(6), 1–7.

217. Bassett, C. A., Mitchell, S. N., Norton, L., & Pilla, A. (1978). Repair of non-unions by pulsing electromagnetic fields. *Acta Orthopaedica Belgica, 44*(5), 706–724.

218. Bassett, C. A., Pawluk, R. J., & Pilla, A. A. (1974). Augmentation of bone repair by inductively coupled electromagnetic fields. *Science, 184*(136), 575–577.

219. Bassett, C. A. (1989). Fundamental and practical aspects of therapeutic uses of pulsed electromagnetic fields (PEMFs) [Abstract]. *Critical Reviews in Biomed Engineering, 17*(5), 451–529.

220. Colson, D. J., Browett, J. P., Fiddian, N. J., & Watson, B. (1988). Treatment of delayed- and non-union of fractures using pulsed electromagnetic fields. *Journal of Biomedical Engineering, 10*(4), 301–304.

221. Satter, S. A., Islam, M. S., Rabbani, K. S., & Talukder, M. S. (1999). Pulsed electromagnetic fields for the treatment of bone fractures. *Bangladesh Medical Research Council Bulletin, 25*(1), 6–10.
222. Mackenzie, D., & Veninga, F. D. (2004). Reversal of delayed union of anterior cervical fusion treated with pulsed electromagnetic field stimulation: Case report. *Southern Medical Journal, 97*(5), 519–524.
223. Bose, B. (2001). Outcome after posterolateral lumbar fusion with instrumentation in patients treated with adjunctive pulsed electromagnetic field stimulation. *Advances in Therapy, 18*(1), 121–20.
224. Foley, K. T., Mroz, T. E., Arnold, P. M., Chandler, H. C., Dixon, R. A., Girasole, G. J., et al. (2008). Randomized, prospective, and controlled clinical trial of pulsed electromagnetic field stimulation for cervical fusion. *The Spine Journal, 8*(3), 436–442.
225. Trock, D. H., Bollet, A. J., Dyer, R. H., Fielding, L. P., Miner, W. K., & Markoll, R. (1993). A double-blind trial of the clinical effects of pulsed electromagnetic fields in osteoarthritis. *The Journal of Rheumatology, 20*(3), 456–460.
226. Trock, D. H., Bollet, A. J., & Markoll, R. (1994). The effect of pulsed electromagnetic fields in the treatment of osteoarthritis of the knee and cervical spine. Report of randomized, double blind, placebo controlled trials. *The Journal of Rheumatology, 21*(10), 1903–1911.
227. Jacobson, J. L., Gorman, R., Yamanashi, W. S., Saxena, B. B., & Clayton, L. (2001). Low-amplitude, extremely low frequency magnetic fields for the treatment of osteoarthritis knees: A double-blind clinical study. *Alternative Therapies in Health and Medicine, 7*(5), 54–64, 66–69.
228. Nicolakis, P., Kollmitzer, J., Crevenna, R., Bittner, C., Erdogmus, C. B., & Nicolakis, J. (2002). Pulsed magnetic field therapy for osteoarthritis of the knee—a double-blind sham-controlled trial. *Wiener Klinische Wochenschrift, 114*(15–16), 678–684.
229. Henry Ford Health Systems. (2010, March 6). Electromagnetic pulses provide pain relief [Press release]. Retrieved from http://www.henryford.com/body.cfm?id=46335&action=detail&ref=1065
230. Thomas, A. W., Graham, K., Prato, F. S., McKay J., Forster, P. M., Moulin, D. E., et al. (2007). A randomized, double-blind, placebo-controlled clinical trial using a low-frequency magnetic field in the treatment of musculoskeletal chronic pain. *Pain Research and Management, 12*(4), 249–258.
231. McCarthy, C. J., Callaghan, M. J., & Oldham, J. A. (2006). Pulsed electromagnetic energy treatment offers no clinical benefit in reducing the pain of knee osteoarthritis: A systematic review. *BMC Musculoskeletal Disorders, 7*, 51.

CHAPTER 13

1. Rainville, J., Sobel, J., Hartigan, C., Monlux, G., & Bean, J. (1997). Decreasing disability in chronic back pain through aggressive spine rehabilitation. *Journal of Rehabilitation Research and Development, 34*(4), 383–393.
2. Hartigan, C., Rainville, J., Sobel, J. B., & Hipona, M. (2000). Long-term exercise adherence after intensive rehabilitation for chronic low back pain. *Medicine & Science in Sports and Exercise, 32*(3), 551–557.

3. Kernan, T., & Rainville, J. (2007). Observed outcomes associated with a quota-based exercise approach on measures of kinesiophobia in patients with chronic low back pain. *The Journal of Orthopaedic and Sports Physical Therapy, 37*(11), 679–687.

4. Rainville, J., Hartigan, C., Jouve, C., & Martinez, E. (2004). The influence of intense exercise-based physical therapy program on back pain anticipated before and induced by physical activities. *The Spine Journal, 4*(2), 176–183.

5. Mailloux, J., Finno, M., & Rainville, J. (2006). Long-term exercise adherence in the elderly with chronic low back pain. *American Journal of Physical Medicine & Rehabilitation, 85*(2), 120–126.

6. Moffett, J. K., Torgerson, D., Bell-Syer, S., Jackson, D., Llewlyn-Phillips, H., Farrin, A., et al. (1999). Randomised controlled trial of exercise for low back pain: Clinical outcomes, costs, and preferences. *British Medical Journal, 319*(7205), 279–283.

7. Chou, R., & Huffman, L. H. (2007) Nonpharmacologic therapies for acute and chronic low back pain: A review of the evidence for an American Pain Society/American College of Physicians clinical practice guideline. *Annals of Internal Medicine, 147*(7), 492–504.

8. Cohen, I., & Rainville, J. (2002). Aggressive exercise as treatment for chronic low back pain. *Sports Medicine, 32*(1), 75–82.

9. Rainville, J., Hartigan, C., Martinez, E., Limke, J., Jouve, C., & Finno, M. (2004). Exercise as a treatment for chronic low back pain. *The Spine Journal, 4*(1), 106–115.

10. Rainville, J. (2003, December). *Exercise for low back pain: What it can and cannot do for your patients.* PowerPoint slides presented at New England College of Occupational and Environmental Medicine Annual Conference, Newton, MA. Retrieved from http://www.necoem.org/documents/0312Rainville.PDF

11. Rainville, J. (2003, December). *Exercise for low back pain: What it can and cannot do for your patients.* PowerPoint slides presented at New England College of Occupational and Environmental Medicine Annual Conference, Newton, MA. Retrieved from http://www.necoem.org/documents/0312Rainville.PDF

12. Wai, E. K., Rodriguez, S., Dagenais, S., & Hall, H. (2008). Evidence-informed management of chronic low back pain with physical activity, smoking cessation, and weight loss. *The Spine Journal, 8*, 195–202.

13. Naugle, K. M., Fillingim, R. B., & Riley, J. L., 3rd. (2012). A meta-analytic review of the hypoalgesic effects of exercise. *The Journal of Pain, 13*(12), 1139–1150.

14. Consumer Reports. (2011, September). Special report: Working out your back pain. *Consumer Reports on Health, 23*(9), 8–9.

15. Maher, C., Latimer, J., & Refshauge, K. (1999). Prescription of activity for low back pain: What works? *Australian Journal of Physiotherapy, 45*, 121–132.

16. Hagen, K. B., Jamtvedt, G., Hilde, G., & Winnem, M. F. (2005). The updated Cochrane review of bed rest for low back pain and sciatica [Abstract]. *Spine, 30*(5), 542–546.

17. J. P. Schneider (personal communication, August 17, 2011).
18. Lin, C-W. C., McAuley, J. H., Macedo, L., Barnett, D. C., Smeets, R. J., & Verbunt, J. A. (2011). Relationship between physical activity and disability in low back pain: A systematic review and meta-analysis [Abstract]. *PAIN*, 152(3), 607–613.
19. Harreby, M., Hesselsøe, G., Kjer, J., & Neergaard, K. (1997). Low back pain and physical exercise in leisure time in 38-year-old men and women: A 25-year prospective cohort study of 640 school children. *European Spine Journal*, 6(3), 181–186.
20. Suni, J. H., Oja, P., Miilunpalo, S. I., Pasanen, M. E., Vuori, I. M., & Bös, K. (1998). Health-related fitness test battery for adults: Associations with perceived health, mobility, and back function and symptoms. *Archives of Physical Medicine and Rehabilitation*, 79(5), 559–569.
21. Croft, P. R., Papageorgiou, A. C., Thomas, E., Macfarlane, G. J., & Silman, A. J. (1999). Short-term physical risk factors for new episodes of low back pain: Prospective evidence from the South Manchester Back Pain Study. *Spine*, 24(15), 1556.
22. Landmark, T., Romundstad, P., Borchgrevink, P. C., Kaasa, S., & Dale, O. (2011). Associations between recreational exercise and chronic pain in the general population: Evidence from the HUNT 3 study. *PAIN*, 152(10), 2241–2247.
23. Bernstein, C. (2008). *The migraine brain*. New York: Free Press.
24. The National Headache Foundation. (2009). Your migraine brain. *NHF Headlines*. Retrieved from http://www.headaches.org/Members_Area/Head_Lines_Archive/NHF_HeadLines_Issue_170
25. Institute of Medicine, Committee on Advancing Pain Research, Care, and Education. (2011). *Relieving pain in America: A blueprint for transforming prevention, care, education and research* (p. 2–32). Prepublication copy. Washington, DC: National Academies Press.
26. Rainville, J., Ahern, D. K., Phalen, L., Childs, L. A., & Sutherland, R. (1992). The association of pain with physical activities in chronic low back pain. *Spine*, 17(9), 1060–1064.
27. Rainville, J., Ahern, D. K., & Phalen, L. (1993). Altering beliefs about pain and impairment in a functionally oriented treatment program for chronic low back pain. *The Clinical Journal of Pain*, 9, 196–201.
28. Roelofs, J., Goubert, L., Peters, M. L., Vlaeyen, J. W. S., & Crombez, G. (2004). The Tampa Scale for Kinesiophobia: Further examination of psychometric properties in patients with chronic low back pain and fibromyalgia [Abstract]. *European Journal of Pain*, 8(5), 495–502.
29. Waddell, G., Newton, M., Henderson, K., Somerville, D., & Main, C. J. (1993). A Fear-Avoidance Beliefs Questionnaire (FABQ) and the role of fear-avoidance beliefs in chronic low back pain and disability [Abstract]. *PAIN*, 52(2), 157–168.
30. Damsgard, E., Thrane, G., Anke, A., Fors, T., & Roe, C. (2010). Activity-related pain in patients with chronic musculoskeletal disorders [Abstract]. *Disability and Rehabilitation*, 32(17), 1428–1437.

31. Vlaeyen, J., & Linton, S. J. (2000). Fear-avoidance and its consequences in chronic musculoskeletal pain [Abstract]. *PAIN*, *85*(3), 317–332.
32. Wilson, A. C., Lewandowski, A. S., & Palermo, T. M. (2011). Fear-avoidance beliefs and parental responses to pain in adolescents with chronic pain [Abstract]. *Pain Research Management*, *16*(3), 178–182.
33. Picavet, H. S. J., Vlaeyen, J. W. S., & Schouten, J. S. A. G. (2002). Pain catastrophizing and kinesiophobia: Predictors of chronic low back pain [Abstract]. *American Journal of Epidemiology*, *156*(11), 1028–1034.
34. Brox, J. I., Storheim, K., Grotle, M., Tveito, T. H., Indahl, A., & Eriksen, H. R. (2008). Evidence-informed management of chronic low back pain with back schools, brief education, and fear-avoidance training. *The Spine Journal*, *8*, 28–39.
35. Buchbinder, R., & Jolley, D. (2005) Effects of a media campaign on back beliefs is sustained 3 years after its cessation [Abstract]. *Spine*, *30*(11), 1323–1330.
36. Lindström, I., Öhlund, C., Eek, C., Wallin, L., Peterson, L. E., Fordyce, W. E., et al. (1992). The effect of graded activity on patients with subacute low back pain: A randomized prospective clinical study with an operant-conditioning behavioral approach [Abstract]. *Physical Therapy*, *72*(4), 279–290.
37. Taimela, S., Diederich, C., Hubsch, M., & Heinricy, M. (2000). The role of physical exercise and inactivity in pain recurrence and absenteeism from work after active outpatient rehabilitation for recurrent or chronic low back pain: A follow-up study. *Spine*, *25*(14), 1809–1816.
38. Kool, J., de Bie, R., Oesch, P., Knusel, O., van den Brandt, P., & Bachman, S. (2004). Exercise reduces sick leave in patients with non-acute non-specific low back pain: A meta-analysis. *Journal of Rehabilitation Medicine*, *36*(2), 49–62.
39. Maul, I., Laubli, T., Oliveri, M., & Krueger, H. (2005). Long-term effects of supervised physical training in secondary prevention of low back pain. *European Spine Journal*, *14*(6), 599–611.
40. Choi, B. K. L., Verbeek, J. H., Tam, W. W-S., & Jiang, J. Y. (2010). Exercises for the prevention of recurrences of low-back pain. *Occupational and Environmental Medicine*, *67*, 795–796.
41. Hayden, J., van Tulder, M. W., Mlmivaara, A., & Koes, B. W. (2005). Exercise therapy for treatment of non-specific low back pain. *Cochrane Database of Systematic Reviews*, *2005*(3), CD000335.
42. Sofi, F., Molino, L. R., Nucida, V., Taviani, A., Benvenuti, F., Stuart, M., et al. (2011). Adaptive physical therapy and back pain: A non-randomised community-based intervention trial. *European Journal of Physical and Rehabilitative Medicine*, *47*(4), 543–549.
43. Liddle, S. D., Baxter, G. D., & Gracey, J. H. (2004). Exercise and chronic low back pain: What works? [Abstract]. *PAIN*, *107*(1), 176–190.
44. Mayer, J., Mooney, V., & Dagenais, S. (2008). Evidence-informed management of chronic low back pain with lumbar extensor strengthening exercises. *The Spine Journal*, *8*, 96–113.
45. Standaert, C. J., Weinstein, S. M., & Rumpeltes, J. (2008). Evidence-informed management of chronic low back pain with lumbar stabilization exercises. *The Spine Journal*, *8*, 114–120.

46. Hayden, J. A., van Tulder, M. W., Malmivaara, A., & Koes, B. W. (2005). Meta-analysis: Exercise therapy for nonspecific low back pain [Abstract]. *Annals of Internal Medicine, 142*(9), 765–775.

47. Hayden, J. A., van Tulder, M. W., & Tomlinson, G. (2005). Systematic review: Strategies for using exercise therapy to improve outcomes in chronic low back pain. *Annals of Internal Medicine, 142*(9), 776–785.

48. Murtezani, A., Hundozi, H., Orovanec, N., Silamniku, S., & Osmani, T. (2011). A comparison of high intensity aerobic exercise and passive modalities for the treatment of workers with chronic low back pain: A randomized, controlled trial. *European Journal of Physical and Rehabilitative Medicine, 47*(3), 359–366.

49. van der Velde, G., & Mierau, D. (2000). The effect of exercise on percentile rank aerobic capacity, pain, and self-rated disability in patients with chronic low back pain: A retrospective chart review. *Archives of Physical Medicine and Rehabilitation, 81*(11), 1457–1463.

50. Chan, C. W., Mok, N. W., & Yeung, E. W. (2011). Aerobic exercise training in addition to conventional physiotherapy for chronic low back pain: A randomized controlled trial. *Archives of Physical Medicine and Rehabilitation, 92*(10), 1681–1685.

51. Bentsen, H., Lindgarde, F., & Manthorpe, R. (1997). The effect of dynamic strength back exercise and/or a home training program in 57-year-old women with chronic low back pain: Results of a prospective randomized study with a 3-year follow-up period. *Spine, 22*(13), 1494–1500.

52. Bronfort, G., Maiera, M. J., Evans, R. L., Schulz, C. A., Bracha, Y., Svendsen, K. H., et al. (2011). Supervised exercise, spinal manipulation, and home exercise for chronic low back pain: A randomized clinical trial [Abstract]. *The Spine Journal, 11*(7), 585–598.

53. Jordan, J. L., Holden, M. A., Mason, E. E., & Foster, N. E. (2010). Interventions to improve adherence to exercise for chronic musculoskeletal pain in adults. *Cochrane Database of Systematic Reviews, 2010*(1), CD005956.

54. Waller, B., Lambeck, J., & Daly, D. (2009). Therapeutic aquatic exercise in the treatment of low back pain: A systematic review. *Clinical Rehabilitation, 23*(1), 3–14.

55. Lim, E. C. W., Poh, R. L. C., Low, A. Y., & Wong, W. P. (2011). Effects of Pilates-based exercises on pain and disability in individuals with persistent nonspecific low back pain: A systematic review with meta-analysis. *Journal of Orthopaedic and Sports Physical Therapy, 41*(2), 70–80.

56. Broad, W. J. (2012, January 8). All bent out of shape. *The New York Times Magazine,* p. 18.

57. National Center for Complementary and Alternative Medicine. (n.d.). Yoga. Retrieved from http://nccam.nih.gov/health/yoga

58. Williams, K. A., Petronis, J., Smith, D., Goodrich, D., Wu, J., Ravi, N., et al. (2005). Effect of Iyengar yoga therapy for chronic low back pain [Abstract]. *PAIN, 115*(1–2), 107–117.

59. Williams, K., Abildso, C., Steinberg, L., Doyle, E., Epstein, B., Smith, D., et al. (2009). Evaluation of the effectiveness and efficacy of Iyengar yoga therapy on chronic low back pain. *Spine, 34*(19), 2066–2076.

60. Chou, R., & Huffman, L. H. (2007) Nonpharmacologic therapies for acute and chronic low back pain: A review of the evidence for an American Pain Society/American College of Physicians clinical practice guideline. *Annals of Internal Medicine, 147*(7), 492–504.

61. Tilbrook, H. E., Cox, H., Hewitt, C. E., Kang'ombe, A. R., Chuang, L-H., Jayakody, S., et al. (2011). Yoga for low back pain. *Annals of Internal Medicine, 115,* 569–573.

62. Sherman, K. J., Cherkin, D. C., Wellman, R. D., Cook, A. J., Hawkes, R. J., Delaney, K., et al. (2011). A randomized trial comparing yoga, stretching, and a self-care book for chronic low back pain [Abstract]. *Archives of Internal Medicine, 171*(22), 2019–2026.

63. Posadzki, P., & Ernst, E. (2011). Yoga for low back pain: A systematic review of randomized clinical trials. *Clinical Rheumatology, 30*(9), 1257–1262.

64. Posadzki, P., Ernst, E., Terry, R., & Lee, M. S. (2011). Is yoga effective for pain? A systematic review of randomized clinical trials [Abstract]. *Complementary Therapies in Medicine, 19*(5), 281–287.

65. Wren, A. A., Wright, M. A., Carson, J. W., & Keefe, F. J. (2011). Yoga for persistent pain: New findings and directions for an ancient practice. *PAIN, 152,* 477–480.

66. Bussing, A., Ostermann, T., Ludtke, R., & Michalsen, A. (2012). Effects of yoga interventions on pain and pain-associated disability: A meta-analysis. *The Journal of Pain, 13*(1), 1–9.

67. National Center for Complementary and Alternative Medicine (Producer). (2012). Scientific results of yoga for health and well-being [Video]. Available from http://nccam.nih.gov/video/yoga

68. Broad, W. J. (2012, January 8). All bent out of shape. *The New York Times Magazine,* p. 18.

69. Broad, W. J. (2012, January 8). All bent out of shape. *The New York Times Magazine,* p. 16.

70. Faas, A., Chavannes, A. W., van Eijk, J. Th. M., & Gubbels, J. W. (1993). A randomized, placebo-controlled trial of exercise therapy in patients with acute low back pain. *Spine, 18,* 1388–1395.

71. Schaafsma, F., Schonstein, E., Whelan, K. M., Ulvestad, E., Kenny, D. T., & Verbeek, J. H. (2010). Physical conditioning programs for improving work outcomes in workers with back pain. *Cochrane Database of Systematic Reviews, 2010*(1), CD001822.

72. Soukup, M. G., Glömsrod, B., Lönn, J. H., Bö, K., & Larsen, S. (1999). The effect of a Mensendieck exercise program as a secondary prophylaxis for recurrent low back pain: A randomized, controlled trial with 12-month follow-up [Abstract]. *Spine, 24*(15), 1585.

73. Hides, J. A., Jull, G. A., & Richardson, C. A. (2001). Long-term effects of specific stabilizing exercises for first-episode low back pain [Abstract]. *Spine, 26*(11), e243–e248.

74. Hurwitz, E. L. (2011). Commentary: Exercise and spinal manipulative therapy for chronic low back pain: Time to call for a moratorium on future randomized trials? *The Spine Journal, 11*(7), 599–600.

75. Centers for Disease Control and Prevention. (n.d.). Arthritis: The nation's most common cause of disability. Retrieved from http://www.cdc.gov/chronicdisease/resources/publications/AAG/arthritis.htm

76. The Arthritis Foundation. (n.d.). Osteoarthritis, rheumatoid arthritis. Retrieved from http://www.arthritis.org

77. Poirot, L. (2012). High-intensity exercise and arthritis. *Arthritis Today*. Retrieved from http://www.arthritistoday.org/conditions/rheumatoid-arthritis/staying-active/high-intensity-exercise.php

78. Munneke, M., de Jong, Z., Zwinderman, A. H., Ronday, H. K., van den Ende, C. H. M., Vliet Vieland, T. P. M., et al. (2004). High intensity exercise or conventional exercise for patients with rheumatoid arthritis? Outcome expectations of patients, rheumatologists, and physiotherapists. *Annals of the Rheumatic Diseases, 63*, 804–804.

79. de Jong, Z., Munneke, M., Jansen, L. M., Ronday, H. K., van Schaardenburg, D. J., Brand, R., et al. (2004). Differences between participants and nonparticipants in an exercise trial for adults with rheumatoid arthritis. *Arthritis Care & Research, 51*(4), 593–600.

80. Munneke, M., de Jong, Z., Zwinderman, A. H., Ronday, K. H., van Schaardenburg, D., Dijkmans, B. A. C., et al. (2005). Effect of a high-intensity weight-bearing exercise program on radiologic damage progression of the large joints in subgroups of patients with rheumatoid arthritis. *Arthritis Care & Research, 53*(3), 410–417.

81. de Jong, Z., Vlieland, V., & Theodora, P. M. (2005). Safety of exercise in patients with rheumatoid arthritis [Abstract]. *Current Opinion in Rheumatology, 17*(2), 177–182.

82. de Jong, Z., Munneke, M., Zwinderman, A. H., Kroon, H. M., Jansen, A., Ronday, K. H., et al. (2003). Is a long-term high-intensity exercise program effective and safe in patients with rheumatoid arthritis? Results of a randomized controlled trial. *Arthritis & Rheumatism, 48*(9), 2415–2424.

83. Munneke, M., de Jong, Z., Zwinderman, A. H., Jansen, A., Ronday, K. H., Peter, W. F. H., et al. (2003). Adherence and satisfaction of rheumatoid arthritis patients with a long-term intensive dynamic exercise program (RAPIT program). *Arthritis Care & Research, 49*(5), 665–672.

84. de Jong, Z., Munneke, M., Kroon, H. M., van Schaardenburg, D., Dijkmans, B. A. C., Hazes, J. M. W., et al. (2009). Long-term follow-up of a high-intensity exercise program in patients with rheumatoid arthritis. *Clinical Rheumatology, 28*, 663–671.

85. de Jong, Z., Munneke, M., Lems, W. F., Zwinderman, A. H., Kroon, H. M., Pauwels, E. K. J., et al. (2004). Slowing of bone loss in patients with rheumatoid arthritis by long-term high-intensity exercise: Results of a randomized, controlled trial. *Arthritis & Rheumatism, 50*(4), 1066–1076.

86. de Jong, Z., Munneke, M., Zwinderman, A. H., Kroon, H. M., Ronday, K. H., Lems, W. F., et al. (2004). Long term high intensity exercise and damage of small joints in rheumatoid arthritis. *Annals of the Rheumatic Diseases, 63*, 1399–1405.

87. Hurkmans, E., van der Giesen F. J., Vliet Vlieland, T. P. M., Schoones, J., & Van den Ende, E. C. H. M. (2009). Dynamic exercise programs (aerobic

capacity and/or muscle strength training) in patients with rheumatoid arthritis. *Cochrane Database of Systematic Reviews, 2009*(4), CD006853.

88. Bailet, A., Zeboulon, N., Gossec, L., Combescure, C., Bodin, L. A., Juvin, R., et al. (2010). Efficacy of cardiorespiratory aerobic exercise in rheumatoid arthritis: Meta-analysis of randomized controlled trials. *Arthritis Care & Research, 62*(7), 984–992.

89. Cooney, J. K., Law, R. J., Matschke, V., Lemmey, A. B., Moore, J. P., Ahmad, Y., et al. (2011). Benefits of exercise in rheumatoid arthritis. *Journal of Aging Research, 2011*(681640), 1–14.

90. Bartels, E. M., Lund, H., Hagen, K. B., Dagfinrud, H., Christensen, R., & Danneskiold-Samsoe, B. (2007). Aquatic exercise for the treatment of knee and hip osteoarthritis [Abstract]. *The Cochrane Database of Systematic Reviews, 2007*(4), CD005523.

91. Cadmus, L., Patrick, M. B., Maciejewski, M. L., Topolski, T., Belza, B., & Patrick, D. L. (2010). Community-based aquatic exercise and quality of life in persons with osteoarthritis [Abstract]. *Medicine and Science in Sports and Exercise, 42*(1), 8–15.

92. Lim, J. Y., Tchai, E., & Jang, S. N. (2010). Effectiveness of aquatic exercise for obese patients with knee osteoarthritis: A randomized controlled trial [Abstract]. *PM&R, 2*(8), 723–731.

93. Ettinger, W. H., Burns, R., Messier, S. P., Applegate, W., Rejeski, W. J., Morgan, T., et al. (1997). A randomized trial comparing aerobic exercise and resistance training exercise with a health education program in older adults with knee osteoarthritis. The Fitness Arthritis and Seniors Trial (FAST). *Journal of the American Medical Association, 277*(1), 25–31.

94. Messier, S. P., Loeser, R. F., Miller, G. D., Morgan, T. M., Rejeski, W. J., Sevick, M. A., et al. (2004). Exercise and dietary weight loss in overweight and obese older adults with knee osteoarthritis: The Arthritis, Diet, and Activity Promotion Trial [Abstract]. *Arthritis Rheumatism, 50*(5), 1501–1510.

95. Pisters, M. F., Veenhof, C., Schellevis, F. G., Twisk, J. W. R., Dekker, J., & De Bakker, D. H. (2010). Exercise adherence improving long-term patient outcome in patients with osteoarthritis of the hip and/or knee. *Arthritis Care & Research, 62*(8), 1087–1094.

96. Sommer, C. (2010). Fibromyalgia: A clinical update. *PAIN: Clinical Updates, 18*(4), 1–4.

97. Wolf, F., Smythe, H. A., Yunus, M. B., Bennett, R. M., Bombardier, C., Goldenberg, D. L., et al. (1990). The American College of Rheumatology 1990 criteria for the classification of fibromyalgia. *Arthritis & Rheumatism, 33*(2), 160–172.

98. Yeh, G. Y., Kaptchuk, T. J., & Shmerling, R. H. (2010). Prescribing tai chi for fibromyalgia—Are we there yet? *New England Journal of Medicine, 363*(8), 783–784.

99. Spaeth, M. (2009). Editorial: Epidemiology, costs, and the economic burden of fibromyalgia. *Arthritis Research & Therapy, 11*(3), 117.

100. Sommer, C. (2010). Fibromyalgia: A clinical update. *PAIN: Clinical Updates, 18*(4), 1–4.

101. Schweinhardt, P., Sauro, K. M., & Bushnell, M. C. (2008). Fibromyalgia: A disorder of the brain? *Neuroscientist, 14*(5), 415–421.

102. Kuchinad, A., Schweinhardt, P., Seminowicz, D. A., Wood, P. B., Chizh, B. A., & Bushnell, M. C. (2007). Accelerated brain gray matter loss in fibromyalgia patients: Premature aging of the brain? *Journal of Neuroscience, 27*(15), 4004–4007.

103. D. L. Goldenberg (personal communication, August 26, 2011).

104. Ortega, E., Garcia, J. J., Bote, M. E., Martin-Cordero, L., Escalante, Y., Saavedra, J. M., et al. (2009). Exercise in fibromyalgia and related inflammatory disorders: Known effects and unknown chances. *Exercise Immunology Review, 15,* 42–65.

105. McBeth, J., Nicholl, B. I., Cordingley, L., Davies, K. A., & Macfarlane, G. J. (2010). Chronic widespread pain predicts physical inactivity: Results from the prospective EPIFUND study [Abstract]. *European Journal of Pain, 14*(9), 972–979.

106. Goldenberg, D. (2011). *Fibromyalgia: The final chapter* [Kindle version]. Retrieved from Amazon.com.

107. Rooks, D. S., Gautam, S., Romeling, M., Cross, M. L., Stratigakis, D., Evans, B., et al. (2007). Group exercise, education, and combination self-management in women with fibromyalgia [Abstract]. *Archives of Internal Medicine, 167*(20), 2192–2200.

108. Kayo, A. H., Peccin, M. S., Sanches, C. M., & Trevisani, V. F. (2012). Effectiveness of physical activity in reducing pain in patients with fibromyalgia: A blinded randomized clinical trial [Abstract]. *Rheumatology International, 32*(8), 2285–2292.

109. Fontaine, K. R., Conn, L., & Clauw, D. J. (2010). Effects of lifestyle physical activity on perceived symptoms and physical function in adults with fibromyalgia: Results of a randomized trial. *Arthritis Research & Therapy, 12*(2), R55.

110. Jones, K. D., Adams, D., Winters-Stone, K., & Burckhardt, C. S. (2006). A comprehensive review of 46 exercise treatment studies in fibromyalgia (1988–2005). *Health and Quality of Life Outcomes, 4,* 67.

111. Busch, A. J., Barber, K. A., Overend, T. J., Peloso, P. M., & Schachter, C. L. (2007). Exercise for treating fibromyalgia syndrome. *Cochrane Database of Systematic Reviews, 2007*(4), CD003786.

112. Busch, A. J., Schachter, C. L., Overend, T. J., Peloso, P. M., & Barber, K. A. R. (2008). Exercise for fibromyalgia: A systematic review. *The Journal of Rheumatology, 35*(6), 1130–1144.

113. Busch, A. J., Barber, K. A. R., Overend, T. J., Peloso, P. M. J., & Schachter, C. L. (2007). Exercise for treating fibromyalgia (Review). *The Cochrane Collaboration, 2007*(4), CD003786.

114. Hauser, W., Klose, P., Langhorst, J., Moradi, B., Steinbach, M., Schiltenwolf, M., et al. (2010). Efficacy of different types of aerobic exercise in fibromyalgia syndrome: A systematic review and meta-analysis of randomised controlled trials. *Arthritis Research & Therapy, 12*(3), R79.

115. Hauser, W., Thieme, K., & Turk, D. C. (2010). Guidelines on the management of fibromyalgia syndrome—a systematic review [Abstract]. *European Journal of Pain, 14*(1), 5–10.

116. Gusi, N., Tomas-Carus, P., Hakkinen, A., Hakkinen, K., & Ortega-Alonso, A. (2006). Exercise in waist-high warm water decreases pain and improves health-related quality of life and strength in the lower extremities in women with fibromyalgia [Abstract]. *Arthritis & Rheumatism, 55*(1), 66–73.

117. Mannerkorpi, K., Nordeman, L., Ericsson, A., & Arndorw, M. (2009). Pool exercise for patients with fibromyalgia or chronic widespread pain: A randomized controlled trial and subgroup analyses [Abstract]. *Journal of Rehabilitation Medicine, 41*(9), 751–760.

118. Langhorst, J., Musial, F., Klose, P., & Hauser, W. (2009). Efficacy of hydrotherapy in fibromyalgia syndrome—a meta-analysis of randomized controlled trials [Abstract]. *Rheumatology, 48*(9), 1155–1159.

119. Wang, C., Schmid, C. H., Rones, R., Kalish, R., Yinh, J., Goldenberg, D. L., et al. (2010). A randomized trial of tai chi for fibromyalgia. *New England Journal of Medicine, 363*(8), 743–754.

120. National Center for Complementary and Alternative Medicine. (2006). Tai chi: An introduction. Retrieved from http://nccam.nih.gov/health/taichi/introduction.htm

121. National Center for Complementary and Alternative Medicine. (2006). Tai chi: An introduction. Retrieved from http://nccam.nih.gov/health/taichi/introduction.htm

122. P. Wayne (personal communication, March 18, 2012).

123. Taggart, H. M., Arslanian, C. L., Bae, S., & Singh, K. (2003). Effects of t'ai chi exercise on fibromyalgia symptoms and health-related quality of life [Abstract]. *Orthopaedic Nursing, 22*(5), 353–360.

124. Wang, C., Schmid, C. H., Rones, R., Kalish, R., Yinh, J., Goldenberg, D. L., et al. (2010). A randomized trial of tai chi for fibromyalgia. *New England Journal of Medicine, 363*(8), 743–754.

125. Yeh, G. Y., Kaptchuk, T. J., & Shmerling, R. H. (2010). Prescribing tai chi for fibromyalgia—are we there yet? *New England Journal of Medicine, 363*(8), 783–784.

126. Growing Bolder. (2011, June 7). Beating cancer one lap at a time [Video file]. Retrieved from http://growingbolder.com/737153.html#content_tabs.

127. Herbst, A. L., Ulfelder, H., & Poskanzer, D. C. (1971). Adenocarcinoma of the vagina—association of maternal stilbestrol therapy with tumor appearance in young women. *New England Journal of Medicine, 284*, 878–881.

128. S. Helmrich (personal communication, May 4, 2011).

CHAPTER 14

1. Institute of Medicine, Committee on Advancing Pain Research, Care, and Education. (2011). *Relieving pain in America: A blueprint for transforming*

prevention, care, education and research (pp. 1–25). Prepublication copy. Washington, DC: National Academies Press.

2. Cousins, M. J., Brennan, F., & Carr, D. B. (2004). Pain relief: A universal human right. *PAIN, 112*(1–2), 1–4.

3. International Pain Summit of the International Association for the Study of Pain. (n.d.). Declaration of Montreal: Declaration that access to pain management is a fundamental human right. Retrieved from http://www.iasp-pain. org/Content/NavigationMenu/Advocacy/DeclarationofMontr233al/ default.htm

4. Brennan, F., Carr, D. B., & Cousins, M. (2007). Pain management: A fundamental human right. *Anesthesia & Analgesia, 105*(1), 205–221.

5. Rich, B. A. (2001). Physicians' legal duty to relieve suffering. *Western Journal of Medicine, 175*(3), 151–152.

6. Tucker, K. L. (2004). The debate on elder abuse for undertreated pain. *Pain Medicine, 5*(2), 214–217.

7. D. Lohman (personal communication, November 21, 2011).

8. Cousins, M. J. (1999). Pain: The past, present and future of anesthesiology? The E. A. Rovenstine memorial lecture [Special article]. *Anesthesiology, 91*(2), 538–551.

9. D. Lohman (personal communication, November 21, 2011).

10. United Nations General Assembly, Human Rights Council. (2013, February 1). *Report of the special rapporteur on torture and other cruel, inhuman or degrading treatment or punishment. Juan E. Mendez* (p. 22). Retrieved from http://www.ohchr.org/Documents/HRBodies/HRCouncil/Regular Session/Session22/A.HRC.22.53_English.pdf

11. Foley, K. (2010, August). *Advancing pain and palliative care globally: Challenges and opportunities.* Paper presented at the International Association for the Study of Pain's 13th World Conference on Pain, Montreal, Canada.

12. Hill, M. (Writer & director). (2011). Short film #7: Torture in heath care? [Documentary series episode]. In S. Collins & M. Hill (Producers), *Life before death.* St Kilda, Victoria, Australia: Moonshine Movies. Retrieved from http://www.lifebeforedeath.com/movie/short-films.shtml

13. K. Foley (personal communication, October 30, 2011).

14. Loeser, J. D. (2012). Relieving pain in America [Editorial]. *Clinical Journal of Pain, 28*(3), 185–186.

15. A. Jordan (personal communication, October 17, 2011).

16. National Institute of Neurological Disorders and Stroke, National Institutes of Health. (2012, February 13). Members of new interagency pain research coordinating committee announced [Press release]. Retrieved from http:// www.nih.gov/news/health/feb2012/ninds-13.htm

17. National Institute of Neurological Disorders and Stroke, National Institutes of Health. (2012, February 13). Members of new interagency pain research coordinating committee announced [Press release]. Retrieved from http:// www.nih.gov/news/health/feb2012/ninds-13.htm

18. National Institutes of Health. (2010, October 25). National Institute of Dental and Craniofacial Research; Interagency pain research

coordinating committee; Call for nominations [Notice]. *Federal Register: The Daily Journal of the United States Government*. Retrieved from http://www.federalregister.gov/articles/2010/10/25/2010-26937/national-institute-of-dental-and-craniofacial-research

19. The Patient Protection and Affordable Care Act, Pub. L. No. 11–148, § 4305, 124 Stat. 119 (2010). Retrieved from http://www.gpo.gov/fdsys/pkg/PLAW-111publ148/html/PLAW-111publ148.htm

20. Garamone, J. (2011, October 25). Military medicine works on managing pain [Press release]. Retrieved from http://www.defense.gov/news/newsarticle.aspx?id=65812

21. M. Emr (personal communication, February 22, 2012).

22. The Patient Protection and Affordable Care Act, Pub. L. No. 11–148, § 4305, 124 Stat. 119 (2010). Retrieved from http://www.gpo.gov/fdsys/pkg/PLAW-111publ148/html/PLAW-111publ148.htm

23. Center for Practical Bioethics. (2012). Pain Action Alliance to Implement a National Strategy (PAINS). Retrieved from http://practicalbioethics.org/initiatives/pain-action-alliance.html

24. S. Fishman (personal communication, October 10, 2011).

25. Institute of Medicine, Committee on Advancing Pain Research, Care, and Education. (2011). *Relieving pain in America: A blueprint for transforming prevention, care, education and research* (pp. 6–5). Prepublication copy. Washington, DC: National Academies Press.

26. L. Robin (personal communication, October 15, 2011).

27. D. Carr (personal communication, October 5, 2011).

28. Liaison Committee on Medical Education. (2011). Overview: Accreditation and the LCME. Retrieved from http://www.lcme.org/overview.htm

29. Accreditation Council for Graduate Medical Education. (n.d.). Home. Retrieved from http://www.acgme.org/acWebsite/home/home.asp

30. Accreditation Council for Continuing Medical Education. (2012). About us. Retrieved from http://www.accme.org/about-us

31. NIH Pain Consortium. (n.d.). NIH Pain Consortium Centers of Excellence in Pain Education (CoEPEs). Retrieved from http://painconsortium.nih.gov/centers-of-excellence-in-pain-education.html

32. A. McKee (personal communication, October 3, 2011).

33. A. McKee (personal communication, October 3, 2011).

34. Institute of Medicine, Committee on Advancing Pain Research, Care, and Education. (2011). *Relieving pain in America: A blueprint for transforming prevention, care, education and research* (p. S–3). Prepublication copy. Washington, DC: National Academies Press.

35. A. Chatzky (personal communication, October 17, 2012).

INDEX

Page numbers followed by t indicate a table

chronic pain. *See also* "flavors" of pain
  acupuncture and, 258
  acute pain transition to, 16, 31–35
  brain tissue losses from, 37–38
  "catastrophizing" response, 38, 92,
    105–107, 111, 284
  from chemotherapy, 5, 16
  Cindy Steinberg example, 15–16
  classification difficulties, 10–11
  coping (non-drug) techniques, 108–124
  defined, 3–4, 31
  depression and, 102–104
  economic costs, 10–12
  genetic susceptibility to, 46, 52–54
  IOM report (2011), 8, 10–11
  Jeffrey Mogil on, 46
  from muscle spasms, 4–5
  from pemphigus vulgaris, 5
  suicide and, 125
  women's susceptibility to, 62
Cisplatin (chemotherapy drug), 243
clonidine, 168, 253
Coalition for Rescheduling Cannabis
    (CRC), 210
Coates, Thomas, 209
coca leaf, 210
Cochrane Collaboration reviews, 86
  acupuncture, 263
  antidepressants, 104
  energy healing, 265–266
  exercise and fibromyalgia, 295
  injection therapy, 235
  low back pain, 285
  placebo medication, 97
  prolotherapy, 237
  TMS, 234
codeine
  -cough syrup, 162
  CSA Schedule inclusion, 162
  mechanism of action, 46, 75
cognitive behavioral therapy (CBT), 106,
    109–111
Cohen, Mark, 177
Cohen, Steven P., 235–236, 238
Cole, James M., 208
Common Osteopathic Medical Licensing
    Examination (COMPLEX), 304
complementary and alternative medicine
    (CAM), 255–281. *See also* acupuncture
  Chinese medicine, 95, 116, 203, 265
  criticisms of, 255–256

diet, vitamins, herbals, 273–278
energy healing, 265–270
magnets/pulsed electromagnetic fields,
    278–281
massage, 94, 256, 263–266, 283
placebo effect and, 256–257
popularity of, 255, 256–257
spinal manipulation, 240, 255,
    269–273
complex regional pain syndrome (CRPS),
    6, 62
COMT gene research, 57, 72
Consortium to Study Opioid Risks and
    Trends (CONSORT) study,
    151–152
controlled substances, federal
    schedules, 163t
Controlled Substances Act (1970), 161, 162,
    204, 208
Controlled Substances by CSA
    Schedule, 162
Cooper, Mark, 5–6
coping (non-drug) techniques, 108–124
  biofeedback, 21, 113–115, 201, 256
  cognitive behavioral therapy, 106,
    109–111
  distraction, 111–114
  empathy, 121–124, 257
  hypnosis, 86, 119–121
  meditation, 96, 115–119, 255, 283
cordotomies, 238
cortisone (steroid) shots, 3, 234–236
Costa, Pam, 47, 49–50, 56
Costigan, Michael, 196–198
Cowan, Penney, 95
Craig, Kenneth, 44
Craker, Lyle, 207–210
craniosacral therapy, 267
CRI Lifetree Clinical Research, 137
CRPS. *See* complex regional pain syndrome
Current Medication Misuse Measure
    (COMM), 146
Cutler, Michael, 204–205
cyclobenzaprine (Flexeril), 249
Cymbalta (duloxetine), 43, 104, 249
cytokines
  astrocytes comparison, 191
  drugs/potential blocking of, 236
  examples of, 32, 34
  "good" vs. "bad," 34–35, 191–192
  healing promoted by, 23

immune system and pain
  cytokines, 191–193
  glial cells, 189–196
  mechanisms of increasing pain, 189–199
  microglial cells, 20, 24, 196–197
  P2X4 receptor, 196
  pemphigus vulgaris (example), 5,
    148–149
  T cells, 197–198
  TLR-4 receptors, 34, 155, 191–192,
    194–196
implantable pumps, 252–253
IMS Health, drug market research firm, 133
inflammatory pain
  chronic inflammatory pain, 75
  description, 23
  drug treatment, 42–43
  dysfunctional pain comparison, 23
  mechanisms of, 32, 107, 238, 241
  neuropathic pain comparison, 24
  opioids/young patient caution, 85
Institute of Medicine (IOM)
  chronic low back pain report, 286–287
  costs of chronic pain report, 8, 10–11, 14
  estimates of chronic pain in US, 17
  gender and pain report, 64
  hospice pain report, 158
  marijuana review, 216
  vitamin D intake recommendations, 274
Institute on Global Drug Policy, 225
Interagency Pain Research Coordinating
    Committee (IPRCC), 13, 302–303
interleukin 1 (IL-1 cytokine), 34, 191–192
interleukin 1B (IL-1B; cytokine), 32
interleukin-6 (IL-6 cytokine), 107, 191–192
International Association for the Study of
    Pain (IASP), 8, 20, 91, 293
International Narcotics Control Board, 139
investigational new drug (IND) approval
    process, 205
IPRCC. See Interagency Pain Research
    Coordinating Committee
irritable bowel syndrome (IBS)
  brain tissue losses in, 37
  as dysfunctional pain example, 23
  estrogen cycle pain variability, 74
  gender pain studies, 67
  placebo vs. no treatment study, 97
  women vs. men data, 62–63
Israel, fibromyalgia studies, 62

Jain, Shamini, 266
Jamison, Robert, 102, 121, 147, 176, 184
Jeffrey Lawson Award for Advocacy in
    Children's Pain Relief, 89
Jensen, Mark, 111–112, 120
Johnson, Keosha, 167
Johnston, Celeste, 84, 86, 87
Joint Commission on Accreditation of
    Healthcare Organizations, 305
Journal of Law, Medicine & Ethics, 177
Journal of the American Medical Association,
    129, 151, 269

Kabat-Zinn, Jon, 116–117
kappa opioids, 75, 77
Kaptchuk, Ted, 96–97, 100
Katz, Michael, 185
Katz, Mitchell, 176–177
Katz, Nathaniel, 180
Kauffman, Jan, 146, 169
Keefe, Francis, 93
Kennedy, Edward, 207
Kerlikowske, Gil, 133
knee injections, 237
knockout/knockdown mice studies, 55
Konowitz, Paul, 5, 167
Krane, Elliot, 86, 193
Kroenke, Kurt, 102–103

Landis, Story, 303
Lawson, Jeffrey, 79–81, 89
Lazar, Sara, 117, 119
Lazarus Project (naloxone program),
    165–166
Leavitt, Stew, 308
Leonhart, Michele, 207–208
LeResche, Linda, 72–73
Levine, Jon, 71
lidocaine (sodium-channel blocker), 51–52
Lifetree Clinical Research (Utah), 172
Living With Chronic Pain (Schneider), 285
Loeser, John, 9, 230–232, 252, 302
loss-of-function genetic mutation, 48–49
low back pain
  acupuncture treatment, 258, 259, 263
  Alexander technique, 266
  bed rest contraindication, 285
  brain function and, 38
  catastrophizing score, 106
  chronic, 106, 229–230, 235, 259

Neizer, Hyrum, 125–126
neonatal abstinence syndrome, 129
nerve blocks, 236
nerve growth factor (NGF), 32
nerve killing, 237–239
nerve transplantation, 253–254
nervous system
    action potentials (of nerves), 27–28,
        48, 113
    acute pain to chronic pain transition,
        31–35
    autonomic nervous system, 25, 118
    male/female, secondary messenger
        differences, 71
    pain transmission role, 24–31, 34
    peripheral nervous system, 25, 114–115
Netherlands, fibromyalgia studies, 62
Neuman, Herbert, 184
neural plasticity, 31
neuromatrix theory of pain (Melzack), 21
Neurontin (gabapentin), 43, 103,
        248–249, 294
neuropathic pain. *See also* complex regional
        pain syndrome
    causes, 23–24, 42
    drug treatment, 103–104
    effects from, 23–24
    IL-10 treatment, 193
    inflammatory comparison, 24
    mechanism of, 33
    mice/neuropathic pain trial, 24, 253
    nociceptive comparison, 24
    subtype classification, 22
    in women, 62
neuropeptide Y, 33
neurotransmitters, 27. *See also* gamma-ami-
        nobutyric acid
New England Journal of Medicine, 138, 235,
        247
Nigeria, facial pain studies, 62
Nixon, Richard, 130
NMDA receptors, 32
nocebo effect, 95–96
nociceptive pain
    in combination, in cancer, 22
    description, 22–23
    neuropathic comparison, 24
nonsteroidal anti-inflammatory drugs
        (NSAIDs)
    deaths data, 129–130
    marijuana comparison, 203

placebo experiment, 1, 99–100
    risk factors, 250–251
    with tanezumab: side-effects, 247
    variety of, 249–250
Norpramin (desipramine), 103, 249
North American Spine Society, 263
nortriptyline, 103, 249
Nubain (nalbuphine hydrochloride), 75, 77
Nucynta ER (by Janssen), 174
numerical scales (for pain assessment), 41

Oaklander, Anne Louise, 68
Obama, Barack, 134–135, 208
O'Connor, Mary I., 69–70
Ogden, David, 208
olanzapine (Zyprexa), 103–104, 249
Opana ER (by Endo), 174
"Operation Pill Nation" (DEA; 2011),
        135
opioid abstinence syndrome, 167
opioid conundrum, 127
opioid drugs, 3. *See also* opioid drugs,
        withdrawal from; individual
        opioids
    abuse-deterrent opioids, 172–174
    acupuncture comparison, 261
    addiction/dependence risks, 127,
        139–150
    death risk from, 151
    difficulties getting, ix
    effectiveness, long term, 158–162
    falling risks in older people, 155
    gender and effectiveness, 74–78
    guidelines for use, 184–187
    hormonal changes from, 154–155
    immune system suppression from,
        149, 155
    increased pain from, 155
    kappa opioids, 75, 77
    limited effects in depression, 102
    mechanisms of action, 169
    overdose and death risks, 150–154, 165
    pain patients vs. street abusers,
        127–137
    Physicians for Responsible Opioid
        Prescribing, 128
    risk reduction efforts, 166–167
    suicide risk factor, 147–150
    undertreatment of pain and, 137–139
    use in children, 81, 85, 86
    U.S. usage data, 136–137

opioid drugs, withdrawal from
in children, 85
drugs for treatment of, 152–153, 165,
168–171
limited doctor education for, 149
medication contracts and tests, 175–179
opioid rotation strategy, 171–172
pain control and, 167
prescription monitoring programs,
179–182
risk evaluation and mitigation strategy,
182–184
symptoms, 147–148, 150, 167–168
opioid-induced hyperalgesia (OIH), 155
opioid-receptor controlling gene research, 58
Opioids911-Safety (educational group), 185
Osher Center for Integrative Medicine,
259, 295
osteoarthritis, 22, 38, 46, 53, 62, 105, 151,
237, 276–277
The Other Brain (Fields), 198
over-the-counter pain relievers
NSAIDs, 129–130, 203, 247, 249–251
topical treatments, 251–252
oxycodone, 156, 159
in combinations, 174, 183
CSA classification, 162, 163t
extended-release, 172, 182–183
Florida problems with, 135
prescription data, 133
withdrawal from, 167–168, 172
OxyContin, 126, 127, 132–135, 154,
173–174

P2X4 receptor, 196
Paclitaxel (chemotherapy drug), 243
pain. *See also* "flavors" of pain
assessment of, 39–44
caring for, 299–306
gender and, 61–78
genetics of, 45–59
hormones and, 70–74
immune system and, 189–199
marijuana and, 214–216
mind-body in, 91–124
nervous system transmission of, 24–31
phantom limb pain, 30–31, 37, 238
Pain Action Alliance to Implement a
National Strategy (PAAINS), 303
Pain Catastrophizing Scale, 106

The Pain Chronicles (Thernstrom), 21
Pain Consortium (NIH), 13, 303
pain education of doctors. *See* medical
school, lack of pain education at
Pain Genes Database, 56
Pain Medicine journal, 165–166
pain relievers. *See also* complementary and
alternative medicine; Western medicine
drugs originally for other purposes,
248–249
over-the-counter, 249–251
topical treatments, 251–252
pain tracking programs, 42
Palliative Medicine journal, 139
Pamelor (nortriptyline), 103, 249
PAP gene research, 58
parasympathetic nervous system, 25
Parazin, Stephen, 230, 240
paroxysmal nocturnal hemoglobinuria, 5
Pascual-Leone, Alvaro, 233
Patterson, David, 111–112
Paul, Ron, 131, 225
pelvic inflammatory disease, 67
pemphigus vulgaris, 5
pentazocine (Talwin), 75, 77
Pentostatin (deoxycoformycin), 245
peppermint, 277
Percocet, 131, 142, 148, 162, 183, 250
Pereira, John, 275
peripheral nerve field stimulation
(PNFS), 231
Pertofrane (desipramine), 249
Pettinati, Pamela, 267
phantom limb pain, 30–31, 37, 238
phenotypes, of pain, 22
phenotypes of pain, 22
physical therapy, 3, 15, 94, 240,
270–271, 283
Physicians for Responsible Opioid
Prescribing (PROP), 128, 141, 160,
185–187
Pizzo, Philip, 14
"placebo by proxy" effect, 96
placebos (medication/placebo effect),
95–100
body part effectiveness variability, 99
buprenorphine vs., 170
in circumcision, 94
in distraction study, 113
endocannabinoid system role, 99–100

selective serotonin reuptake inhibitors
(SSRIs), 103, 104, 249
self-hypnosis, 86, 119–120
sensitization (of nerve cells), 31–34, 155
Serhan, Charles, 244
serotonin norepinephrine reuptake
inhibitors (SNRIs), 103, 249
shingles pain, 4
Shir, Yoram, 11–12
short-term pain. *See* acute (short-term) pain
Shultz, George P., 130
Singer, Tania, 123
Singh, Simon, 258, 266, 267
Single Convention on Narcotic Drugs
(UN), 130, 206, 207
sleep medications, 162. *See also* Ambien
SNRIs. *See* serotonin norepinephrine
reuptake inhibitors
sodium-channel blocking drugs, 51–52.
See also carbamazepine; lidocaine;
mexiletine
sodium channels, 27–28
message transmission role of, 48
SCN9A gene mutation and, 48, 49, 51
voltage-gated, 48, 52
soldiers, wound management, 92
Soma (carisoprodol), 249
somatic nervous system, 25
somatization theory, 101
soy, 273, 277
spasmodic torticollis, 5–6
spinal cord stimulation (SCS), 231, 232
spinal fusion surgery, 240–242
spinal manipulation, 240, 255, 269–273
The Spine Journal, 291
spondylolisthesis, 2
Sprenger, Christian, 113
SSRIs. *See* selective serotonin reuptake
inhibitors
Stadol (butorphanol tartrate), 75, 77
Standardized Evaluation of Pain (StEP), 42
Stanford Systems Neuroscience and Pain
Lab, 114
Starrels, Joanna, 176
Staud, Roland, 49
Steinberg, Cindy, 15–16, 182
steroid injections, 3, 234–236
Substance Abuse and Mental Health Services
Administration (SAMHSA), 134
sucrose, for children's pain management,
86–87

suicide
chronic pain risk factor, 4, 47
migraine pain and, 125–127
opioid dependence and, 147–150
surface electromyography (sEMG), 113
surgery, 239–242
Sweden
facial pain studies, 62
fibromyalgia studies, 62
gender and pain study, 70
placebo-PET scan study, 98–99
swimming (inspirational example), 296–298
sympathetic nervous system, 25, 118

tai chi, 116, 295–296
Talwin (pentazocine), 75, 77
tanezumab, 246–247
Tarlov cysts, 68
Tawfik, Vivianna, 212, 222
Taylor, Jill Bolte, 91
temporomandibular joint disorder(TMD)
biofeedback treatment, 113
CBT for, 110
estrogen cycle pain variability, 74
pre-/postpuberty data, 71
in women, 62
women, HRT and, 73
testosterone, role in pain, 72
tetrahydrocannabinol (THC)
absence of lethal dose, 203
biology of marijuana and, 211–213
concentration-benefit connection, 215
pharmaceuticals made from, 209
vapor inhalation effectiveness, 223
Therapeutic Touch, 269
Thernstrom, Melanie, 21
TLR-4 receptors (toll-like receptor number
4), 34, 155, 191–192, 194–196
TMD. *See* temporomandibular joint disorder
TNF (tumor necrosis factor), 34
TNF-a, 32
topical treatments, 251–252
torticollis, 6, 283
Toxicology Investigators Consortium
(ToxIC), 130
Tracey, Irene, 37, 38
traditional Chinese medicine (TCM), 203
transcranial magnetic stimulation (TMS),
233–234
transcutaneous electric nerve stimulation
(TENS), 231